CHILDHOOD OBESITY

Edited by **Sevil Ari Yuca**

Childhood Obesity
Edited by Sevil Ari Yuca

Published by InTech
Janeza Trdine 9, 51000 Rijeka, Croatia

Publishing Process Manager Martina Blecic

Technical Editor Teodora Smiljanic

Cover Designer InTech Design Team

Additional hard copies can be obtained from orders@intechopen.com

Childhood Obesity, Edited by Sevil Ari Yuca
p. cm.
ISBN 978-953-51-0374-5

For EU product safety concerns:
IN TECH d.o.o., Prolaz Marije Krucifikse Kozulić 3, 51000 Rijeka, Croatia,
info@intechopen.com or visit our website at intechopen.com.

Meet the editor

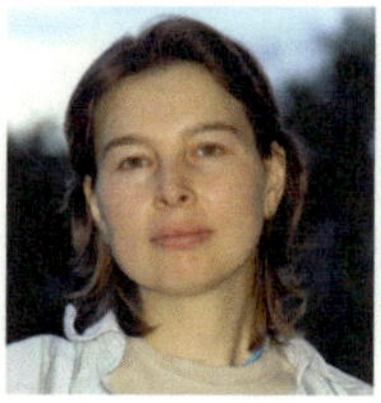

Sevil Ari Yuca is an Assistant Professor at the Department of Pediatric Endocrinology of the Selcuk University, Meram Medical Faculty, Turkey. Since 2005 she has been working on subjects from the field of pediatric endocrinology, childhood obesity, diabetes and thyroid disease.

Contents

Preface

Childhood obesity has been one of the major problems for children in the last century and it still is a widespread condition all over the world. The metabolic effect of early-onset obesity is more severe in children than in adults. This process may start in early infancy or even in the uterus. Obesity in children is a very complex and difficult issue for endocrinologists. This book aims to draw attention to the various aspects of this disease.

The following chapters are presented:

- "Behavioral and Psychosocial Factors in Childhood Obesity " by Fernando L. Vazquez and Angela Torres; a review of the relevant literature concerning both behavioral and psychosocial factors involved in childhood obesity, and the impact of childhood obesity on mental health.

- "Childhood Immigration and Obesity - An Emerging Problem " by I. Díez López and M. Carranza Ferrer; a review on immigration and its role in the etiology of childhood obesity.

- "Childhood Obesity: The Need for Practice Based Solutions – A South African Perspective" by A.E. Pienaar and G.L. Strydom; a review with the focus on childhood obesity in South Africa which discusses the extent of this problem within the complex context of the South African demographics.

- "Comorbidities Of Childhood Obesity " by Ambar Banerjee and Dara P. Schuster; a review on the complications of childhood obesity in childhood and adulthood.

- "Critical Periods for the Development of Obesity" by C. Campoy, T. Anjos and E. Martín-Bautista; a review on etiology and mechanisms of obesity.

- "Can Breastfeeding Reduce the Risk of Childhood Obesity?" by Laurie Twells et. al.; a review on the protective role of breastfeeding in the development of obesity later in life.

- "Epidemiological and Clinical Aspects in a Developing Country" by Ana Mayra Andrade de Oliveira; a review on the impact of obesity on cardiometabolic risk factors in youth, Metabolic syndrome.

- ''Early Infant Feeding Influences and Weight of Children'' by Elizabeth Reifsnider and Elnora Mendias; a review on the effects of early feeding on the development of obesity in infancy.

- ''Jugando a Ganar Salud" ("Playing to Gain Health"): A Summer-Vacation Physical Activity and Correct Eating Workshop for School-Aged Children – A Pilot Study'' by Karime Haua-Navarro et. al.; a review on the results of regular physical activity and nutrition in school aged children.

- ''Obesity and Quality of Life in Communities of Diverse Ethnicity and Low Socioeconomics'' by Joan Griffith; a review on quality of life, socioeconomic status or position, prevailing obesity prevalence disparity and the role of behavioral and social factors.

- ''Waist Circumference in Children and Adolescents from Different Ethnicities'' by Peter Schwandt and Gerda-Maria Haas; a comparison of waist circumference of adolescents in Germany, Iran and Brazil.

Sevil Ari Yuca, MD,
Selcuk University, Meram Medical Faculty, Department of Pediatric Endocrinology
Turkey

Part 1

Childhood Obesity – Epidemiology and Risk Factors

1

Epidemiological and Clinical Aspects in a Developing Country

Ana Mayra Andrade de Oliveira
Department of Health, State University of Feira de Santana, Feira de Santana, Bahia, Brazil

1. Introduction

There is growing prevalence of cardiovascular diseases (CVD) and diabetes mellitus type 2 (DM2) in the child and youth population, and particularly in young adults, secondary to an increase in their risk factors, which present themselves at very early stages of life. Among these, the most prevalent is obesity, which may increase rates of dyslipidemia, arterial hypertension (AH) and carbohydrate metabolism disorders, which are also recognized risk factors for cardiometabolic diseases (CMD).

High prevalence of obesity has also been found in the pediatric population worldwide. An epidemiological study conducted in Feira de Santana, a city in the northeast of Brazil, including children from 5 to 9 years old showed rates of 9.1% and 4.4% for overweight and obesity respectively, confirming the finding of obesity at early stages of life.

The literature has pointed out to the relationship between obesity in youth and premature death due to endogenous causes of cardiac/metabolic origin. It is therefore fundamental to know how and when the risk factors for CMD begin to affect vascular function and structure, and particularly, how to detect them early in order to enable the development of truly primary preventive strategies. This would make it possible to change the epidemiology of these chronic diseases, with consequent reduction in psychosocial and economic cost to the population and Health System, which is especially important in factor in developing countries.

2. Impact of obesity on cardiometabolic risk factors in youth

Obesity (defined as body mass Index [BMI] > 95th percentile, or BMI score z > 2.0) is a well defined and very complex disease of which overweight is merely one of the signs. Increasing obesity prevalence in youth over the last three decades has led to growing evidence of its implications for human health. Based on longitudinal studies, overweight has been shown to be an important risk factor for the development of atherosclerotic CVD, carbohydrate metabolism disorders, obstructive sleep apnea, cancers, intellectual deterioration, among others, therefore presenting elevated cumulative morbid-mortality.

A follow-up study of American indigenous children over a mean period of 23.9 years, demonstrated that factors such as obesity, particularly the abdominal type (defined as waist circumference [WC] > 75th percentile), diminished glucose tolerance, and childhood AH are involved in the development of premature death and DM. In addition to obesity being the earliest event in this chain of morbidity, the deregulation of glycemic homeostasis is probably the most important mediator between overweight and death.

Nevertheless, a significant proportion of obese individuals may attain longevity without the previously mentioned comorbidities. This is due to the fact that the determinant of individual metabolic risk associated with accumulation of adipose tissue (AT) is not represented by its excess only, but above all, by its distribution, which can be determined by means of simple and available techniques such as WC measurement, as previously mentioned.

AT is recognized as the largest energy store of free fatty acids (FFA) and triglycerides (TG), and more recently as an endocrine organ that regulates the secretion of adipokines, which coordinate energy metabolism, insulin sensitivity and feeding behavior, not only in adults but also in pediatric populations. Imbalance between visceral and subcutaneous AT is capable of altering its physiology. In obese individuals, especially those with abdominal obesity, there is an increase of cytokines, such as interleukins (IL), tumor necrosis factor-alpha (TNF-α), c-reactive protein (CRP), plasminogen activator inhibitor (PAI-1) and fibrinogen among others, known for their proinflammatory, prothrombotic and proatherogenic actions, and a decrease in a cytokine with opposite characteristics, called adiponectin. In addition, the adipocytes that constitute visceral AT present intense lipolytic activity and when in excess, promote an increase of FFA circulanting levels that contribute to the presence of ectopic fat deposition.

These two basic mechanisms (imbalance in cytokine production and increase in FFA) favor both fat deposition in non habitual sites essential to the maintenance of glucose homeostasis, such as pancreas, liver and muscle, among others. This may lead to the development of insulin resistance (IR) and states of chronic inflammation with significant impact on carbohydrate metabolism and vascular system, promoting endothelial dysfunction. The inflammatory state is recognized by the increase in some cytokines (CRP, IL-6, TNF-α, etc) and is a great predictor of CVD. Therefore, it is rational to include CRP, especially high-sensitivity CRP (hs-CRP), in screening for the risk of CVD, also in the pediatric population at risk of these diseases.

Fatty liver deposition or hepatic steatosis (HS) is considered a hepatic component of the metabolic syndrome (MS) by the International Diabetes Federation (IDF), and in adult population it is an established predictor of dysglycemia and DM2. In youth, an association between obesity, particularly abdominal obesity and HS has been confirmed. Furthermore, the degree of steatosis in the liver has a decisive influence on the development of alterations in glycidic metabolism, with an important increase in hepatic glucose production, due to increase in gluconeogenesis.

It is thus imperative to conduct studies on ectopic fat deposits in youths with excessive weight in order to diagnose individuals with this alteration and calculate a risk score for CVD and DM. This screening may be done by means of simple techniques such as hepatic enzyme measurements (aspartate aminotransferase [AST], alanine aminotransferase [ALT] and hepatic ultrasound and/or sophisticated techniques (not always available in developing countries) such as nuclear magnetic resonance (NMR) with spectroscopy or hepatic biopsy, which is an invasive method, especially for children. Research in intramyocellular fat using NMR is also fundamental for determining peripheral muscle insulin sensitivity however the technique is not available for clinical use.

2.1 Cardiovascular system

Cardiovascular screening is normally recommended for adults, especially those with a family history positive for CVD. Nevertheless the combination of atherogenic diet, sedentary lifestyle and genetic have resulted in overweight and atherogenic dyslipidemia (decrease in high-density-lipoprotein cholesterol [HDL-C], increase in low-density-lipoprotein cholesterol [LDL-C] and TG at very early stages of life, thus anticipating the need for screening the cardiovascular system.

Although the vascular pathology in children with obesity and DM has been described, the course of development of these abnormalities has not yet been fully explained. In adults, abnormalities in vascular function precede the development of the anatomic or structural pathology. Vascular dysfunction, including reduction in endothelial function and vascular complacency and increase in inflammatory markers are therefore the initial findings in subjects with obesity, dyslipidemia, AH and carbohydrate metabolism disorders. Inflammation and maintenance of these risk factors subsequently lead to the development of atherosclerosis with alteration in vascular structure and increase in its rigidity.

2.2 Mechanism of atherogenesis

When elevated, LDL-C infiltrates the arterial endothelium, producing fat striae, even at very early ages in life (1st and 2nd decades) and if dyslipidemia persists, various subtypes of white globules, similar in shape, infiltrate the vascular wall and secrete inflammatory cytokines and oxidative molecules, with development of an inflammatory state and oxidative stress (OS).

OS, defined as imbalance between the concentrations of reactive oxygen species (ROS), such as superoxide and antioxidants (superoxide dismutase and catalase, among others), are essential for the development of endothelial damage, representing the initial and fundamental stage that is interposed between the formation of atherosclerotic plaque and the thrombus. Signaling pathways that regulate cytokine expression, such as the nuclear factor kappa B transcriptional pathway (NF-kB), is also activated by OS, resulting in the induction of adhesion molecule expression and inflammation on the vascular wall, contributing to the atherogenic process. In association, the clotting cascade and platelet aggregation are activated in an effort to repair the atheromatous lesion. This process can induce occlusive thrombi, infarctions and generalized micro and macro-vascular disease. Some systemic markers that represent OS have been identified in youngsters, confirming early onset of the atherosclerotic process.

In various studies, including our study in adolescents, inflammation markers, such as the simple overall leukocyte count and high-sensitivity CRP (hs-CRP) have been shown to be elevated in this group with clear demonstration of the relationship between inflammation and obesity, MS and a number of its components. The clinical usefulness of monitoring these markers in the pediatric population has not been well studied, nevertheless, some authors recommend that it should be measured, based on the hypothesis that the subclinical inflammation present in MS results from a silent and progressive atherosclerotic process that started in the first decade of life that could be stopped or at least delayed if identified.

In addition, thrombosis markers, such as fibrinogen, IL (6,8, 1 B), TNF-α, monocyte chemotactic protein-1 (MCP-1) and PAI-1 have elevated levels in obese youngsters with MS.

Up until very recently, only necropsy studies warned about the beginning of atherogenesis early in life, and non invasive techniques have attested to this sequence of events.

Ultrasound of the neonatal and fetal aorta have indicated that retardation of fetal growth, *in utero* exposure to hypercholesterolemia and maternal smoking habits, in addition to diabetic macrossomia may also contribute as risk factors for CVD.

Endothelial function may be investigated invasively or non-invasively by means of various techniques, in several vascular sites and by diverse pharmacological or mechanical stimuli. The non invasive technique most frequently used clinically, involves capturing images by high resolution ultrasound after stimulation determined by ischemia induced by brachial artery occlusion (reactive hyperemia test). A similar non invasive ultrasound technique is used to evaluate the vascular structure by measuring the thickness of the intima media layer of the common carotid (IMCC). Larger IMCC thickness has been observed in youngsters with traditional risk factors for CMD, such as obesity, dyslipidemia and hypertension.

Another study of our group was conducted in 128 adolescents (age 14.6 ± 2.7 years, BMI z score 1.9 ± 0.8). The IMCC thickness was measured and the reactive hyperemia test performed. We found a statistically significant positive correlation between BMI and reactive hyperemia test. Levels of soluble intercellular adhesion molecule (sICAM-1), soluble vascular cell adhesion molecule (sVCAM-1) and PAI-1 was also measured and the it was found positive association between abdominal obesity and sVCAM-1 and also with adiposopathy (defined as the presence of three or more adipocitokines such as IL-6, FNT-α, CRP, leptin and high molecular weight adiponectin) and sICAM-1 confirming the hypotheses of early onset of the atherosclerotic process.

Although atherosclerosis is clinically manifested in adult life, it is clear that a long and asymptomatic phase precedes its development. Apparently it begins in childhood and there are evidences in populations of developed and developing countries that the proinflammatory state and OS are triggers for atherogenesis. Therefore, in order to be effective, primary prevention of CVD must occur in this age group, especially in those with excessive weight. Even more important is the fact that the major determinant of both inflammation and OS is abdominal obesity, which constitutes a risk factor believed to be modifiable, therefore, intervention is recommended, and with adequate control its consequences are reversible.

2.3 Insulin resistance and carbohydrate metabolism disorders

Insulin plays a vital role in glucose metabolism and energy homeostasis. Its action depends on two basic factors: pancreatic secretion and tissue sensitivity. Peripheral insulin sensitivity is responsible for glucose uptake (by the muscle) and for suppression of glucose production (by the liver).

IR occurs when a defined quantity of insulin produces a subnormal biologic response, more specifically, it is characterized by reduction in the ability of insulin to stimulate the use and uptake of glucose by peripheral tissues and suppress hepatic glyconeogenesis. As an anabolic and mitogenic hormone, insulin acts on stimulating the synthesis of glycogen, FFA, TG and proteins and also in reducing proteolysis and lipolysis.

One of the major consequences of obesity is IR, and is almost a consensus that it represents the link between some cardiovascular and metabolic risk factors in both, adults and youngsters. There is also association between this state and the polycystic ovary syndrome, nonalcoholic fatty liver disease, obstructive sleep apnea and some specific types of cancer.

Fasting insulinemia is not a good marker for IR diagnosis, due to the lack of standardization among the tests and non definition of normal values, particularly for youngsters. The gold standard method for the diagnosis of insulin sensitivity in adults as well as children and youngsters is the hyperinsulinemic-euglycemic clamp, however it is difficult to use clinically. One simple and validated index is the homeostasis model f insulin resistance (HOMA-IR) ([fasting insulin (U/mL)] x [fasting glycemia (mg/dL)]/405). Nevertheless, there is no consensus about the cut-off point for the pediatric population. Keskin and collaborators, after a study with adolescents proposed the value > 3.16.

Glycemia per *se* is an important risk factor for adverse cardiovascular events, and its control leads to cardioprotection, particularly when early intervention is provided. Several studies with strict glycemic control, such as The Diabetes Control and Complications Trial (DCCT) , The Epidemiology of Diabetes Interventions and Complications Study (EDIC) among others confirmed this hypothesis. Various mechanisms have been proposed to explain this relationship: 1. Protein glycation: this process leads to the production of advanced glycation end products (AGE) which, after activation of their receptor (RAGE) in endothelial cells, smooth muscle cells and macrophages, determine both increase in the activation of transcription factors in the vessel that favor atheroma plaque formation, increase in adhesion molecule expression and cytokine secretion; 2. Circulating lipoprotein glycation: potentiates the atherogenicity of LDL-C, thus contributing to atherogenesis; and 3. Direct effect glucose on the vascular wall: contributes to endothelial dysfunction by increasing adhesion molecule expression, reducing plasminogen activator production and increasing PAI-1 production, generating a hypofibrinolytic and inflammatory state

3. Metabolic syndrome

3.1 Epidemiology

Since 1970, in the United States, the prevalence of overweight among children from 2 to 5 years of age has doubled, and among children and adolescents from 6 to 19 years of age, tripled. At present 17% of the pediatric population is overweight. In Brazil the panorama is no different, with growing rates ranging between 4.4% and 33.6%, depending on the methodology used for defining obesity and the characteristic of the sample studied. It is always important to remember that biological, social, cultural and economical factors are involved in the development of obesity and Brazil is a country with heterogeneous characteristics in terms of these factors. The Brazilian Institute of Geography and Statistic in 2012 showed rate of 10% of overweight and 7.3% of obesity among children and adolescents. An epidemiologic study conducted with 699 children in Feira de Santana, BA, has confirmed this fact by finding prevalence of 8.6%, 9.1% and 4.4% of underweight, overweight and obese children, respectively as already mentioned.

In this same population blood pressure levels were analyzed and even at a mean age of 7.1 years, 3.6% of the sample presented elevated arterial pressure, with an odds ratio of 4.4 and 13.0 higher for those who were overweight and obese respectively.

Data obtained from the four largest regions in the world (United States of America, Latin America, Europe and Asia) reinforce the importance of MS in the pediatric population because it affects individuals of both sexes, in the major ethnic groups, but above all, those who are overweight.

The estimated prevalence of MS among individuals aged 2 to 19 years is ~10% (1,2% to 22,6%), from ~2% among children and adolescents with normal weight and ~32% among the obese, but with prevalence of up to 60% in this special group. Thus the odds of presenting MS is 15 times higher among overweight youngsters when compared with individuals of normal weight. The information with regard to sex is conflicting, but there is a trend towards higher prevalence among men, because they have greater predisposition for abdominal obesity. Age is another factor that must be taken into consideration, and adolescents are affected to a larger extent than children.

The National Health and Nutrition Examination Survey (NHANES) was the population study that analyzed ethnic differences, and it pointed out a higher rate of MS among Caucasians, and a lower rate among Afro-Americans. This fact is surprising, since the outcomes of MS (acute myocardial infarction and DM2) are more frequent among Afro-Americans, probably due to greater IR found among the youngsters in this ethnic group.

Nevertheless, this IR is initially compensated by increased insulin secretion and clearance, consequently with less risk of MS. As the increased insulin secretion probably precedes the state of IR, this high level of insulin, plays a fundamental role in the physiopathology of the syndrome. Hyperinsulinemia and IR are linked to endothelial dysfunction (ED) in adults, a relationship between HOMA-IR and IMCC thickness.

In Brazil the prevalence of MS among youngsters is very similar to that in developed countries, particularly among the obese. A study conducted with 548 school children in Feira de Santana, BA, with a mean age of 11.1 years, showed a prevalence of 31.3% among those who were overweight (BMI z score > 1.5). Abdominal obesity was the most frequent traditional component of MS found in the total sample (68.3%) confirming the fundamental role of visceral AT accumulation in development of the syndrome. This was followed by hypertriglyceridemia (29.3%), reduction in HDL-C (28.4%) and elevation of arterial blood pressure (17.4%). Interestingly, no alteration in carbohydrate metabolism was detected, in spite of the oral glucose tolerance test having been performed for diagnosis of carbohydrate metabolism disorders. Another study, also conducted in the Brazilian northwest confirmed the association between overweight and diagnosis of the syndrome, with rates of 22.6% and 59.3% in the total sample and in the obese subgroup, respectively. An analysis of 99 adolescents in the southeast of Brazil demonstrated a lower prevalence of the syndrome (6%) and also no cases of it were observed among those with normal weight and overweight (BMI z score > 1.5 and < 2.0). Nevertheless, among the obese (BMI z score > 2.0), the rate increases to 26.1% and once again, no cases of carbohydrate metabolism disorders were detected. Thus, the Brazilian data with regard to the component "glucose metabolism disturbance" of MS, diverge from those in the literature, particularly the North American data, which point towards and increase in the rates of pre-diabetes and DM2 in the obese pediatric population. The possible causes of this divergence, apart from the non uniformity of diagnostic criteria for the syndrome, would be the lower severity of obesity in the Brazilian population, which is a recognized factor for the development of alteration in glycid metabolism, in addition to the probable presence of protective genetic and environmental factors.

This epidemiologic profile indicates that obese youngsters must be considered at risk for cardiometabolic diseases and therefore considered targets for preventive and therapeutic strategies. However, in developing countries it has been suggested that screening for MS should also be done in normal weight individuals if the objective is prevention of CVD and DM2, because, in the same way as with obese individuals, this population may present disorders linked to metabolism and the cardiovascular system.

3.2 Definition, diagnosis and clinical importance

MS is defined as a constellation of specific anthropometric, physiological and biochemical abnormalities that predispose affected individuals to the development of CVD and DM2, described in adults in 1988 by Reavan and collaborators.

In youngsters the non existence of a universally accepted definition for the diagnosis of the syndrome is recognized, probably because of the dynamic aspects related to growth and development, and it is a real barrier. For example, individuals develop IR during puberty, and the normal levels of lipids and arterial blood pressure vary according to age and sex.
Another complicating factor is the absence of standardization of the measurement of abdominal obesity, as well as its cut-off points. Thus, the criteria used for defining MS in the pediatric population are adaptations of criteria used for adults, and none of them are widely accepted. Nevertheless, the majority of them include the following elements: 1. Elevation of TG; 2. Reduction in HDL-C; 3. Increase in arterial blood pressure; 4. Alteration in plasma glucose; and, 5. Increase in abdominal obesity.
Based on data from NHANES III (1988 - 1994), Cook and collaborators have suggested a definition adapted from the criteria defined by the National Cholesterol Education Program - Adult Treatment Panel III, NCEP/ATP-III), since Ferranti and collaborators, in spite of proposing definition also based on the NCEP/ATP-III criteria, used different cut-off points for each criteria. A study conducted at the School of Medicine of Yale University by Weiss and collaborators, used another criterion, replacing WC used in the previously described definitions, by the BMI, because they proved this index to be less subject to variations resulting from age and ethnic group (Table 1).

Epidemiological and clinical aspects in developing country			
Criteria / components	**Cook et al.**	**de Ferranti et al.**	**Weiss et al.**
Abdominal obesity	$WC^1 > 90^{th}$ percentile	$WC^1 > 70^{th}$ percentile	$z\,(BMI)^6 > 2$
Glycid metabolism	$FG^2 > 110$ mg/dL	$FG^2 > 110$ mg/dL	Glycemia ($OGTT^7$) of 140 to 200 mg/dL
Dyslipidemia	$TG^3 > 110$ mg/dL or $HDL^4 > 40$ mg/dL	$TG^3 > 110$ mg/dL or $HDL^4 > 45$ mg/dL (men) and < 50mg/dL (women)	$TG^3 > 95^{th}$ percentile or $HDL^4 < 5^{th}$ percentile
Arterial hypertension	$BP^5 > 90^{th}$ percentile	$BP^5 > 90^{th}$ percentile	$BP^5 > 95^{th}$ percentile

*WC = waist circumference; 2FG = fasting glycemia; 3TG = triglycerides; 4HDL-C = high density cholesterol; 6z BMI = z score of body mass index; 7 OGTT = oral glucose tolerance test; 8 BP = blood pressure.
Source: Adapted from Pergher et al (2010).

Table 1. Criteria for classification of the metabolic syndrome in children and adolescents, proposed by Cook et al., de Ferranti et al. and Weiss et al. in the presence of at least three of the five criteria

The organizations, NCEP/ATP, World Health Organization and IDF have suggested criteria for the child and young population based on the criteria proposed for the adult population (Table 2). The new IDF definition is interesting as it divides the groups according to age: from 10 to 16 years and over 16 years, children under the age of 10 years being excluded due to the non existence of data related to this age range. The authors also suggested that in children under the age 6 - 10 years the syndrome should not be diagnosed, but that the need for weight reduction must be emphasized in those with abdominal obesity. For children over the age of 10 years, the syndrome is diagnosed by the presence of abdominal obesity, defined by the WC measurement, associated with two or more clinical criteria (hypertriglyceridemia, low levels of

HDL-C, AH and hyperglycemia). For the other factors, cut-off points were established by means of a fixed value, which in truth, is contrary to the other proposals for child and young populations. Nevertheless, the use of percentiles is also criticized, particularly in the transition to the adult stage, since the cut-off points for the criteria for this population are fixed and not based on percentiles. Thus, when an individual aged 18 years is analyzed using the fixed cut-off points and those based on the percentile tables, there may be a difference in the diagnosis.

As there is increasing prevalence of childhood obesity, as well as other risk factors for CVD and DM2, it has become necessary to conduct studies for standardizing criteria that are simple to apply for the diagnosis of MS in the child and young populations. Early diagnosis followed by treatment, which up to now has been directed towards individual components of the syndrome, particularly intervention in lifestyle, is fundamental for reducing the progression of MS rates in children and adolescents.

Over the last decade questions have arisen about the real existence of the syndrome, especially in the child and young populations, in terms of whether the syndrome represents a distinct clinical entity, or only a constellation of factors linked to obesity, occurring in the same individual, since its diagnosis does not aggregate greater risk of cardiometabolic disease than its components evaluated individually (visceral obesity, dyslipidemia, AH, alteration in carbohydrate metabolism and IR). In a concrete manner, however, there are: 1. Alarming data on the prevalence of the syndrome and the relationship between its components and cardiometabolic complications at a very early age, with thickening of the IMCC layer and atherosclerotic lesions in the arterial network; 2. Information that confirms that the diagnosis of overweight and MS in childhood are predictors of MS and its consequences in the adult population; 3. Relationship between MS and DM2 in adult life and similar association in children and adolescents; 4. Association between this syndrome in childhood and other disorders, including hyperuricemia, HE, polycystic ovary syndrome and obstructive sleep apnea; and 5. That it has been accepted as a simple clinical instrument for the early detection of DM2 and ACVD and individuals at risk for these conditions.

In addition to all these affirmations, the recognition of a probable physiopathological basis linked to visceral obesity/IR as a link between the components of MS, enables the clinician to have a broader vision of the risks of excess AT, even in very young individuals, thus changing his/her practical conduct, by systematic investigation of the factors that constitute the syndrome and its consequences. Thus, preventive and therapeutic measures are adopted earlier, thereby reducing the chance of development of cardiovascular outcomes.

Nevertheless, it is worth emphasizing that there is no consensus about the benefits of diagnosing MS in the pediatric population, and future studies will probably be developed with the aim of establishing which individual component of MS creates the greatest future risk and should be the target for therapy.

1. National Cholesterol Education Program - Adult Treatment Panel III: modified criteria for children and adolescents

Definition of MS: presence of three or more of these conditions (A-B-C-D-E):

A	FG1	> 110 mg/ dL (6.1 mmol/L) or >100 mg/ dL (5.6 mmol/L)
B	WC2	> 90th percentile of sample distribution
C	TG3	> 110 mg/ dL (1.13 mmol/L)
D	HDL-C4	< 40 mg/ dL (1.04 mmol/L)
E	BP5	> 90th percentile of sample distribution

2. International Diabetes Federation (IDF) criteria for children and adolescents

Definition of MS: presence of central obesity (A) in addition two or more of the conditions (B-C-D-E)

Criteria according to age

		6 to <10 years of age	10 to 16 6 to <10 years of age	16 years of age
A	WC2	MS cannot be diagnosed, but future evaluation must be made if there is presence of family history of MS, DM2, dyslipidemia, cardiovascular disease, hypertension and / or obesity.	> 90th percentile	Use existing IDF criteria for the adult population
B	TG3		> 150mg/ dL (1.7mmol/L)	
C	HDL-C4		< 40 mg/dL (1.03 mmol/L)	
D	BP5		Systolic BP5 >130 mmHg or Diastolic BP5 > 85 mmHg	
E	FG1 or previous diagnosis of diabetes mellitus type 2 (DM2)		>100 mg/dL (5.6 mmol/L)	

3. World Health Organization (WHO) criteria modified for children and adolescents

Definition of the MS: presence of three of more of these conditions (A-B-C-D-E):

A	BMI6	> 95th percentile
B	Abnormal Glucose Homeostasis	Hyperinsulinaemia or IFG7 or IGF8
C	BP5	> 952th percentile
D	TG3	> 105/136 mg/dL (1.2/1.5 mmol/L) for children aged <10 years and > 10 years respectively
E	HDL-C4	< 35 mg/ dL (0.9 mmol/L)

[1]FG = fasting glycemia [2]WC = waist circumference; [3]TG = triglycerides; [4]HDL-C = high-density cholesterol; [5]BP = blood pressure, [6]z BMI = z score of body mass index. Source: Adapted from Tailor et al. (2009).

Table 2. Summary of the Metabolic Syndrome (MS) definitions used in the studies.

4. Conclusions

The prevalence of obesity among youngsters presents epidemic proportions with significant implications for cardiovascular and metabolic health at a very early age in life. There are increasing rates of MS in children and adolescents, which points towards the premature development of CVD and DM2 in the next generation of adults. IR, determined by abdominal obesity appears to represent the link between the components of MS in this age range, and functions as a predictor for CVD and disturbances in carbohydrate metabolism. Therefore, the WC measurement should be considered a screening instrument for the identification of youngsters with a cardiometabolic disease phenotype.

As a consequence of this abdominal obesity-IR binomial, a systemic inflammatory state is produced, which functions as a trigger for the atherogenic process. The earlier the onset of overweight, the more prematurely this will manifest clinically. Therefore, in order to implement primary prevention of CMD, investigation/prevention/treatment of risk factors, such as obesity, dyslipidemia, AH and disturbances in carbohydrate metabolism and its consequences must begin in the initial stages of life.

5. Acknowledgements

Special thanks to Bridget Pierpont of Yale University and undergraduates in Medicine Atila Oliveira, Ana Luisa Oliveira, Marcele Almeida, Yanna Alves, Maria Rosa Dantas and Lorena Veneza.

6. References

[1] Alberti KG, Eckel RH, Grundy SM, Zimmet PZ, Cleeman JI, Donato KA, et al. Harmonizing the metabolic syndrome: a joint interim statement of the International Diabetes Federation Task Force on Epidemiology and Prevention; National Heart, Lung, and Blood Institute; American Heart Association; World Heart Federation; International Atherosclerosis Society; and International Association for the Study of Obesity. Circulation 2009 Oct: 120(16):1640-5.

[2] Baker JL, Olsen LW, S0rensen TI. Childhood body-mass index and the risk of coronary heart disease in adulthood. N Engl J Med 2007 Dec: 357(23):2329-37.

[3] Bibbins-Domingo K, Coxson P, Pletcher MJ, Lightwood J, Goldman L. Adolescent overweight and future adult coronary heart disease. N Engl J Med 2007 Dec:357(23):2371-9.

[4] Bitsori M, Linardakis M, Tabakaki M, Kafatos A. Waist circumference as a screening tool for the identification of adolescents with the metabolic syndrome phenotype. Int J Pediatr Obes 2009; 4(4):325-31.

[5] Cali AM, Oliveira AM, Kim H, Chen S, Reyes-Mugica M, Escalera S, et al. Glucose dysregulation and hepatic steatosis in obese adolescents: is there a link? Hepatology 2009 Jun: 49(6):1896-903.

[6] Cali AM, Caprio S. Obesity in children and adolescents. J Clin Endocrinol Metab 2008 Nov: 93(11 Suppl 1):S31-6.

[7] Cole TJ, Bellizzi MC, Flegal KM, Dietz WH. Establishing a standard definition for child overweight and obesity worldwide: international survey. BMJ 2000 May:320(7244):1240-3.

[8] Cook S, Weitzman M, Auinger P, Nguyen M, Dietz WH. Prevalence of a metabolic syndrome phenotype in adolescents: findings from the third National Health and Nutrition Examination Survey, 1988-1994. Arch Pediatr Adolesc Med 2003 Aug:157(8):821-7.

[9] Definition, Diagnosis and Classification of Diabetes Mellitus and its Complications. Part 1: Diagnosis and Classification of Diabetes Mellitus. Geneva. Geneva: WHO Department of Noncommunicable Disease Surveillance; 1999.

[10] Duvnjak L, Duvnjak M. The metabolic syndrome - an ongoing story. J Physiol Pharmacol 2009 Dec: 60 Suppl 7:19-24.

[11] Expert Panel on Detection, Evaluation, and Treatment of High Blood Cholesterol in Adults. Executive Summary of The Third Report of The National Cholesterol

Education Program (NCEP) Expert Panel on Detection, Evaluation, And Treatment of High Blood Cholesterol In Adults (Adult Treatment Panel III). JAMA 2001 May:285(19):2486-97.
[12] Fernandez JR, Redden DT, Pitrobelli A, Allison DB. Waist circumference percentiles in nationally representative samples of African-American, European-American, and Mexican-American children and adolescents. J Pediatr 2004; 145:439-44.
[13] Ferranti SD de, Gauvreau K, Ludwig DS, Neufeld EJ, Newburger JW, Rifai N. Prevalence of the metabolic syndrome in American adolescents: findings from the Third National Health and Nutrition Examination Survey. Circulation 2004 0ct:110(16):2494-7.
[14] Ford ES, Li C, Zhao G, Pearson WS, Mokdad AH. Prevalence of the metabolic syndrome among U.S. adolescents using the definition from the International Diabetes Federation. Diabetes Care 2008 Mar: 31(3):587-9.
[15] Guimaraes IC, Moura de Almeida A, Guimaraes AC. Metabolic syndrome in Brazilian adolescents: the effect of body weight. Diabetes Care 2008 Feb: 31(2):4.
[16] Hoffman RP. Metabolic syndrome racial differences in adolescents. Curr Diabetes Rev Nov: 5(4):259-65.
[17] Hong YM. Atherosclerotic Cardiovascular Disease Beginning in Childhood. Korean Circ J 2010 Jan: 40(1):1-9.
[18] Hossain P, Kawar B, El Nahas M. Obesity and diabetes in the developing world-a growing challenge. N Engl J Med. 2007 Jan: 356(3):213-5.
[19] International Diabetes Federation. The IDF consensus worldwide definition of the metabolic syndrome. 2005. Dispornvel em < http:// www.idf.org.> [2010 abr20]
[20] Juonala M, Magnussen CG, Berenson GS, Venn A, Burns TL, Sabin MA, et al. Childhood Adiposity, Adult Adiposity, and Cardiovascular Risk Factors. N Engl J Med 2011 Nov; 365(20):1876-85.
[21] Keskin M, Kurtoglu S, Kendirci M, Atabek ME, Yazici C.Homeostasis model assessment is more reliable than the fasting glucose/insulin ratio and quantitative insulin sensitivity check index for assessing insulin resistance among obese children and adolescents. Pediatrics 2010; 115:500- 3.
[22] Kimani-Murage EW, Kahn K, Pettifor JM, Tollman SM, Dunger DB, Gomez-Olive XF, et al, Norris SA. The prevalence of stunting, overweight and obesity, and metabolic disease risk in rural South African children. BMC Public Health 2010 Mar: 10:158.
[23] Mauras N, Delgiorno C, Kollman C, Bird K, Morgan M, Sweeten S, et al. Obesity without established comorbidities of the metabolic syndrome is associated with a proinflammatory and prothrombotic state, even before the onset of puberty in children. J Clin Endocrinol Metab 2010 Mar: 95(3):1060-8.
[24] McGill HC Jr, Geer JC, Strong JP. Natural history of human atherosclerotic lesions. In: Sandler M, Bourne GH, editors. Atherosclerosis and Its Origin. New York: Academic Press, 1963. p. 39-65.
[25] Nelson RA, Bremer AA. Insulin resistance and metabolic syndrome in the pediatric population. Metab Syndr Relat Disord. 2010 Feb: 8(1):1-14.
[26] Oliver SR, Rosa JS, Milne GL, Pontello AM, Borntrager HL, Heydari S, et al. Increased oxidative stress and altered substrate metabolism in obese children. Int J Pediatr Obes 2010 Mar doi: 10.3109/17477160903545163.
[27] Oliveira AC, Oliveira AM, Almeida MS, Silva AM, Adan L, Ladeia AM. Alanine aminotransferase and high sensitivity C-reactive protein: correlates of cardiovascular risk factors in youth. J Pediatr 2008 Mar: 152(3):337-42.

[28] Oliveira AM, Cerqueira EM, Oliveira AC. Prevalencia de sobrepeso e obesidade infantil na cidade de Feira de Santana-BA: detecgao na famflia x diagnostico cllnico. J Pediatr 2003;79(4): 325-8.
[29] Oliveira AM, Oliveira AC, Almeida MS, Almeida FS, Ferreira JB, Silva CE, et al. Fatores ambientais e antropometricos associados a hipertensao arterial infantil. Arq Bras Endocrinol Metab 2004;48(6), 849-54.
[30] Oliveira AM, Oliveira AC, Almeida MS, Oliveira N, Adan L. Influence of the family nucleus on obesity in children from northeastern Brazil: a cross-sectional study. BMC Public Health 2007 Sep: 7:235.
[31] Oliveira AM, Oliveira N, Reis JC, Santos MV, Silva AM, Adan L. Triglycerides and alanine aminotransferase as screening markers for suspected fatty liver disease in obese children and adolescents. Horm Res 2009;71(2):83-8.
[32] Oliveira AM, Pinto A, Almeida MS, Oliveira N, Silva AM, Dantes MR, et al. Echocardiographic Abnormalities in Childhood: The Effect of Obesity. Diabetes 2009;58:A453.
[33] Olshansky SJ, Passaro DJ, Hershow RC, Layden J, Carnes BA, Brody J, et al. A potential decline in life expectancy in the United States in the 21st century. N Engl J Med 2005 Mar: 352(11):1138-45.
[34] Pergher RN, de Melo ME, Halpern A, Mancini MC; Liga de Obesidade Infantil. Is a diagnosis of metabolic syndrome applicable to children? J Pediatr 2010 Mar-Apr:86(2):101-8.
[35] Reaven GM. Banting lecture 1988: role of insulin resistance in human disease. Diabetes. 1988;37:1595-607.
[36] Rein P, Saely CH, Beer S, Vonbank A, Drexel H. Roles of the metabolic syndrome, HDL cholesterol, and coronary atherosclerosis in subclinical inflammation. Diabetes Care May doi: 10.2337/dc09-2376.
[37] Short KR, Blackett PR, Gardner AW, Copeland KC. Vascular health in children and adolescents: effects of obesity and diabetes. Vasc Health Risk Manag 2009; 5:973-90.
[38] Silva RC da, Miranda WL, Chacra AR, Dib SA. Metabolic syndrome and insulin resistance in normal glucose tolerant Brazilian adolescents with family history of type 2 diabetes. Diabetes Care 2005 Mar: 28(3):716-8.
[39] Tailor AM, Peeters PH, Norat T, Vineis P, Romaguera D. An update on the prevalence of the metabolic syndrome in children and adolescents. Int J Pediatr Obes 2010 May 3;5(3):202-13.
[40] Weiss R. Fat distribution and storage: how much, where, and how? Eur J Endocrinol 2007 Aug: 157 Suppl 1:S39-45.
[41] Weiss R, Dziura J, Burgert TS, Tamborlane WV, Taksali SE, Yeckel CW, et al. Obesity and the metabolic syndrome in children and adolescents. N Engl J Med 2004 Jun:350(23):2362-74.
[42] Weiss R, Shaw M, Savoye M, Caprio S. Obesity dynamics and cardiovascular risk factor stability in obese adolescents. Pediatr Diabetes 2009 Sep;10(6):360-7.
[43] Zimmet P, Alberti KG, Kaufman F, Tajima N, Silink M, Arslanian S, et al. The metabolic syndrome in children and adolescents - an IDF consensus report. Pediatr Diabetes 2007 Oct: 8(5):299-306.

2

Early Infant Feeding Influences and Weight of Children

Elizabeth Reifsnider[1] and Elnora Mendias[2]
[1]*College of Nursing and Health Innovation, Arizona State University*
[2]*School of Nursing, University of Texas Medical Branch, Galveston*
USA

1. Introduction

Childhood obesity has become a major health concern in nearly every country in the world. In the United States, the number of overweight children aged 2 to 5 years has more than doubled in the past 30 years. Overweight and obesity, already epidemic among the world's adults and children in both developed and developing countries, is escalating. While 61% of U.S. adults and almost 12% of U.S. children were overweight in 2001, a decade later, over two thirds of U.S. adults and almost one-third of U.S. children and adolescents were overweight or obese (Satcher, 2011). A 2010 estimate by the World Health Organization (WHO, n.d.[a]) indicated 42 million overweight children under five years of age worldwide, with 35 million living in developing countries. However, 2010 estimates provided by the International Association for the Study of Obesity International Obesity Taskforce (IASO/IOTF, n.d.) indicated one billion overweight (and another nearly half billion obese) adults internationally, with even higher estimates if adjusted for Asian-specific obesity measures. Moreover, the IASO International Obesity Taskforce's 2010 estimated 200 million obese or overweight school-aged children (IASO/IOTF, n.d.[b]).

Global trends toward childhood overweight or obesity have been attributed to two major factors: 1) increasing intake of energy-dense foods, high in sugars and fats and nutrient-poor (low in beneficial nutrients, such as minerals, vitamins, and healthy micronutrients); and 2) increasingly sedentary lifestyles, with low physical activity (Corvalan et al., 2009; Satcher, 2011; WHO, n.d.[b],). However, though primarily associated with unhealthy nutrition and limited physical activity, WHO (n.d.[b]) suggests that increased childhood obesity rates are related to child behaviors and numerous economic or social changes, as well as environmental, educational, urban planning, agricultural, transportation, and food policies.

Polhamus et al. (2009) reported that data from 1998–2008 Pediatric Nutrition Surveillance System indicate prevalence of overweight/obese preschool children as 14.7%, and this prevalence is higher among Hispanic preschoolers (18.5%). Infant and toddler stages are a time of transition from dependent feeding to independent feeding. During early life, weight trajectories and food preferences predict trends and preferences throughout life (Allen & Myers, 2008). Early childhood is a crucial stage for monitoring growth and BMI and the most opportune time to prevent obesity in children by promoting healthy dietary and physical activity behaviors (Hawkins & Law, 2006a; He, 2008; Story et al., 2002). Many factors contribute to the alarming rates of childhood obesity. Childhood obesity has a strong hereditary tendency (American Academy of Pediatrics [AAP], 2003; Barsh et al., 2000); however, there is evidence that a child's size (height, weight, and BMI) is influenced by factors in the family's environment. Many researchers have examined the relationship between childhood obesity and individual and family risk factors (Hawkins & Law, 2006b), such as parental BMI (Burke et al., 2001; Wardle et al., 2001), childhood television use (Adachi-Mejia et al., 2007; Dennison et al., 2002; Faith et al., 2001), and diet (Dennison et al., 1997; Welsh et al., 2005).

Sturm (2002) is among the many researchers who have noted that obesity has the same association with chronic health conditions as does 20 years of aging, and the cost of obesity exceeds the costs of smoking and drinking for national health care use. According to a study of costs attributed to adult overweight (BMI 25–29.9) and obesity (BMI > 30), these expenses accounted for 9.1% of the total U.S. medical expenditures in 1998 and reached $92.6 billion in 2002 dollars. In 2008 dollars, these costs totaled about $147 billion (Finkelstein et al., 2003, 2009). Some investigators predict that adolescent obesity may result in up to 1.5 million life-years lost, with total costs of $294 billion if lost productivity is counted along with medical costs (Inge & Xanthakos, 2010; Lightwood et al., 2009). Being overweight or obese carries considerable consequences. Substantial research has linked child obesity/overweight to increased risks for serious health outcomes, which include adverse physical, psychological/behavioral, or social consequences (AAP, 2005; Levi et al., 2011; Monasta, Batty, Cattaneo, et al., 2010; Monasta, Batty, Macaluso et al., 2010). Overweight or obese children tend to remain overweight or obese as they become adults, and these children also tend to develop illnesses, such as cardiovascular diseases, hypertension, or diabetes, at younger ages (Horta et al., 2007; WHO, n.d.[a],). Barker (1990) has been credited with first relating infant birth weight with adult illness such as hypertension, cardiovascular disease, and diabetes. Since then a number of studies, some of which are reviewed below, have examined relationships between obesity and these or other illnesses.

Recent studies have indicated that obesity has negative outcomes on very young children and contributes to health problems as obese children age. Investigators found that 3-year-old children who were very obese at < 2 years had multiple markers of inflammation associated with numerous chronic diseases (Skinner et al., 2010). Rising BMIs in childhood are also associated with increased risk for coronary heart disease in adulthood. Obese children have higher rates of asthma (Al-Shawwa et al., 2007; Rodriguez-Artalejo et al., 2002), hepatic steatosis (fatty degeneration of the liver; Dietz, 1998), sleep apnea (Kaditis et al., 2008), and type 2 diabetes (Must & Anderson , 2003). Risks of developing diabetes by the late teens can be predicted as early as age six based on blood pressure, BMI, fasting glucose, insulin and lipid values (Morrison et al., 2008, 2010). Most researchers now realize that by the time a child is 5, the prime years for prevention of obesity have passed. By this age, many children and families are set in patterns of eating and activity that are difficult to modify. Infancy and early childhood are now viewed as the prime ages for preventing obesity (Birch & Ventura, 2009; McCormick et al., 2010; Taveras et al., 2010).

Several systematic reviews have examined the relative contributions of a host of factors that contribute to childhood obesity. Hawkins and Law (2006b) reported on 59 studies (out of 1,923 originally identified) that met the inclusion criteria of accurate body-size measures and including children between the ages of six months and five years. Their review was organized as an ecological model with concentric circles expanding outwards to represent the spheres of influence on the development of child obesity. They identified the levels of child characteristics (infant feeding, weaning, bottle use, diet, snack foods, physical activity and sedentary behavior, amount of screen time and use); family characteristics (parental factors, maternal pre-pregnancy weight, maternal smoking during pregnancy, maternal employment, social disadvantage); community-level factors (neighborhood, day care); and policy implications (dietary intake, opportunities for physical activity). These factors were largely reiterated in a systematic review by Monasta, Batty, Macaluso et al. (2010), who conducted a systematic review of 22 systematic reviews but in a different arrangement of factors. Monasta's et al. systematic review reported strong evidence from the constellation of reviews for the following factors as contributors to child obesity: genetics, maternal factors (including gestational diabetes and smoking), infant birth weight; size; and rate of growth; infant feeding, sleep duration, abuse/neglect and other negative social experiences, physical activity and sedentary behavior, and society and the built environment. A recent systematic review of interventions to prevent obesity in children birth to age five examined 18 studies and reported that few showed any evidence of effectiveness regardless of the location or components of the study. The authors concluded by stating that prevention of obesity and early intervention at its earliest sign is the most effective means to combat child obesity, as interventions later in childhood are not very effective (Hesketh & Campbell, 2010).

Whincup et al. (2008) conducted a systematic review examining the relationship between birth weight and type II diabetes in adults. The authors reported an inverse relationship between birth weight and risk for Type II diabetes (pooled OR, adjusted for age and gender: 0.75; 95% Confidence interval (CI): 0.70-0.81). Harder et al. (2009) conducted a systematic review and meta-analysis of studies examining relationships between diabetes and birth weight or weight gain during an infant's first year of life. The authors reported a significant association between higher birth weight (e.g., >4,000 grams) and increased risks for subsequent later development of Type I diabetes (OR: 1.17; 95% (CI): 1.09- 1.26). Harder et al. (2009) also noted studies supported a relationship between rapid weight gain in early life and later Type II diabetes development, though a meta-analysis was not possible due to differences in studies' time measurements and parameters for weight gain.

Recently, Monasta, Batty, Cattaneo, et al. (2010) conducted a systematic review of 22 published systematic reviews examining determinants of overweight/obesity in children in early life (e.g., conception to 5 years). Monasta, Batty, Cattaneo, et al. (2010) concluded that breastfeeding may be protective against later overweight/obesity and identified multiple factors that may affect risks for obesity. The researchers noted difficulty extricating "the complex web of associations and of reciprocal influences of all these factors" (Monasta, Batty, Cattaneo, et al., 2010, p. 703) and called for early-life intervention studies to substantiate protective and risk factors.

Hurley et al. (2011) conducted a systematic review of child obesity and responsive feeding (caregiver recognition and response to a child's hunger or satiety cues) in high-income countries. The majority of studies reviewed (24/31) reported significance between child BMI z-scores and nonresponsive feeding (e.g., caregiver lack of recognition of or response to child hunger/satiety cues; Hurley at al., 2011). This could be an interesting area to explore in breastfed children, where babies are much more "in charge" of their breast milk intake.

Along with birth weight and parental body size, infant feeding is recognized as one of the most influential biological and environmental factors that affect weight gain during infancy (Griffiths et al., 2009). Parental feeding practices have a strong impact on children's food availability (Keller et al., 2006), eating behaviors, and weight (Birch & Fisher, 1998, 2000). Parental involvement in feeding is essential for children to grow, and parental knowledge, parenting style, modeling of food choices, and eating environment all have a strong impact on an infant's and child's weight (Campbell et al., 2008). Johnson and Birch (1994), for example, reported that parental over-control of child eating was associated with poorer eating regulation by the child and increased BMI. Helping parents acquire health-promoting parenting techniques is thus a key component in addressing the growing epidemic of childhood obesity in infants and toddlers (Anderson & Whitaker, 2010; Olstad & McCargar, 2009), yet systematic reviews have recognized that opportunities for prevention of obesity are plentiful but poorly recognized (Monasta, Batty, Macaluso et al., 2010) by health care providers and parents.

This chapter will review the current research on gestational programming of growth, maternal factors, and early infant feeding and the subsequent impact on the development of overweight, obesity, or both. As the earliest infant feeding is milk based, the review will discuss the research on breastfeeding as to whether the evidence shows a clear link between breastfeeding and obesity and present issues concerning maternal obesity and breastfeeding. The problems of early and rapid weight gain will be discussed. We will also discuss the factors associated with the development of overweight/obesity among a specific population, namely low-income Hispanic children in the southwest United States, as that is the first author's field of expertise. Recommendations for health care providers, researchers, and parents on ways to prevent the development of overweight/obesity among infants and young children will be presented for clinicians.

2. Programming of growth

Although the focus of this chapter is not on fetal growth and development, it is necessary to briefly review the contributions of fetal nutrition on infant growth and development. The fetal environment can set in motion developmental changes in metabolism to promote the survival of a fetus and neonate, so that his/her postnatal life will be enhanced. The developmental origins of disease, or developmental programming as it is also known, were popularized by the work of Barker and colleagues two decades ago (Barker et al., 1989, 1990; Hales et al., 1991). They proposed that developmental changes in key tissues and organ systems at critical periods of fetal growth can influence the long-term risk of metabolic and cardiovascular diseases (Warner & Ozanne, 2010). Fetal malnutrition from poor maternal diet or impaired placental blood flow can "program" the fetus to spare the development of the nervous system to the detriment of the endocrine system, for example. The poorly fed fetus results in a small for gestational age (SGA) or low birth weight (LBW) infant. If these infants are born into a poor nutritional environment, they are equipped through fetal development to grow appropriately for the available food and to survive through abdominal storage of fat. If however, the SGA or LBW infants have been born into an abundant nutritional environment, they rapidly gain weight (experience catch-up growth) and have been shown in numerous epidemiological studies to be at higher risk for hypertension, cardiovascular disease, insulin resistance and type 2 diabetes, renal disease, skeletal muscle alterations, and increased fat storage (Warner & Ozanne). A recent systematic review of 22 studies examining 40,000 deaths among 400,000 people reported that for deaths from all causes, there was a 6% lower risk per kg higher birth weight for men and women (adjusted HR = 0.94; 95% CI: 0.92-0.97, Risnes et al., 2009). The association was stronger for deaths from cardiovascular diseases (HR =0.88; 95% CI: 0.85-0.91).

The hazard ratio was increased for men and cancer mortality but not significant for women. These results from a strong systematic review show that birth weight is an indicator of in utero developmental processes that influence long-term health. However, the available data do not allow us to determine whether sociocultural factors, genetic factors, the intrauterine environment or life course exposures are more influential in explaining the observed associations. The type of nutritional support for appropriate catch-up growth that will allow a SGA or LBW infant to thrive without becoming at risk for later metabolic disease is still unknown.

While maternal undernutrition has received the most attention for its contribution to metabolic programming for infants and children, maternal overnutrition is now recognized for its role in creating detrimental health outcomes. Infants who are born large for gestational age (LGA) are also at risk for developing metabolic and cardiovascular diseases similar to infants born SGA and exposed to plentiful postnatal nutrition (Warner & Ozanne, 2010). Infants born to mothers who have gestational diabetes often are LGA and at risk for adult disease, due to the higher glucose maternal blood levels they are exposed to during gestation. In fact, researchers now believe that a U-shaped curve of risk exists for both ends of the birthweight spectrum, as SGA and LGA infants are both at risk for developing metabolic disorders later in life (Curhan, Chertow et al. 1996; Curhan, Willett, et al. 1996). Overfeeding and accelerated postnatal (catch up) growth appears to be the trigger that establishes the trajectory for at-risk status for SGA infants (Eriksson et al., 1999; Cheung et al., 2000) while the link between accelerated postnatal growth and metabolic disease for the LGA infants has not been as clearly identified (Cottrell & Ozanne, 2008).

Maternal smoking is a factor other than maternal diet that can influence a fetus's growth and impact the infant's risk of becoming overweight or obese. Maternal smoking during the first trimester and through the entire pregnancy has been associated with childhood obesity at age 5 (Toschke et al., 2003a), with more than twice the odds (OR 2.22; 95% CI: 1.33-3.69) for obesity at 5 years of age for maternal smoking in the first trimester and nearly twice (OR 1.70; 95% CI: 0.1.02-2.87) for smoking throughout pregnancy. Mizutani et al. (2007) reported that maternal smoking habits were associated with overweight in the 5-year-old children (OR 2.15; 95% CI: 1.12-4.11) among children of Japanese mothers who smoked during pregnancy. Mangrio et al. (2010) found that smoking worked synergistically with maternal obesity in that the odds for obesity were greater when the mothers were obese and smoked (OR 3.12; 95% CI: 1.13-8.63), while smoking did not appear to increase child obesity if the mother was not obese.

The reasons for the association of smoking and obesity are not well understood. Smoking can reduce blood flow to the placenta, which in turn can promote development of SGA or LBW. Magee et al. (2004) found that LBW was 58% more common among smokers than among non-smokers, and LBW can lead to accelerated postnatal growth, which itself can lead to obesity (Institute of Medicine [IOM], 2011). It has been demonstrated in animal models that maternal under-nutrition leads to LBW offspring who have altered leptin levels, hyperphagia, and increased weight gain (Plagemann & Harder, 2009). Smoking in pregnancy is implicated in appetite control and impulse control among offspring (Montgomery et al., 2005). Toschke et al. (2003b) described self-reported appetite among adults who were 42 years old and had been followed from birth. The proportion with poor appetite increased with levels of maternal smoking during pregnancy: from 4.5% with maternal non-smoking to 7.7% with maternal heavy smoking. BMI or levels of obesity among the adults were not reported. Montgomery et al. (2005) reported that compared with non-smoking mothers, the adjusted odds ratios (95% confidence intervals) for bulimia in offspring were 0.74 (0.25-2.21) for those who gave up before pregnancy, 3.04 (1.16-7.95) for giving up smoking during pregnancy and 2.64 (1.47-4.74) for smoking throughout pregnancy. Smoking during pregnancy was not associated with anorexia nervosa in offspring. Neither BMI nor variation between childhood and adult BMI explain the association. If the association of smoking during pregnancy with bulimia in offspring is causal, then it may operate through compromised central nervous system development and its influence on impulse or appetite control. The increased risk associated with mothers who gave up smoking during pregnancy emphasizes the importance of smoking cessation prior to conception.

The Millennium Cohort Study (a longitudinal study of 11,653 preschool children) Child Health Group reported significant factors that impacted rapid weight gain at age three included parental weight status (maternal and paternal), pre-pregnancy maternal obesity, and maternal smoking; they were highly significant in predicting high BMI at age three (Griffiths et al., 2010) The BMI at age three was also a risk factor for subsequent excessive weight gain. However, how smoking may also affect the activity levels, appetite, or metabolism of the infants is currently unknown but may be through neurobehavioral changes in the developing neural system of the fetus.

Moran and Phillip (2003) reviewed studies of leptin, a hormone involved in human food intake and energy expenditure and nutritional balance, which is produced primarily by fat cells and elevated in obesity. They concluded a growing body of evidence linked leptin and diabetic pathophysiology. Some researchers have suggested that increased obesity rates are related to earlier puberty onset (precocious puberty), as both trends occurred over a similar time period. A review by Kaplowitz (2008) reported linkages between higher BMIs and earlier onset of puberty, especially in girls, identifying leptin as the key connection between body fat and early puberty.

Maternal prenatal behaviors such as diet and rest also contribute to infant obesity. The odds of obesity among children whose mothers did not eat breakfast was 1.78 (95% CI: 1.14-2.77), but if the mothers had a long sleep duration during pregnancy, the odds of obesity were 0.37 (95% CI: 0.15-0.88), showing a protective effect of maternal rest (Mizutani et al., 2007). Poor maternal diet among women who are normal or underweight at conception contributes to LGA and LBW infants (Fall, 2009; Scholl, 2008), and the link between maternal intake, LBW infants, and later development of metabolic disease in adults was the basis for the theory of metabolic programming, discussed earlier. Maternal rest and sleep has not been as well established as a contributor to LBW, but was linked to LBW by Abeysena et al. (2010) who studied paid employment, sleep, and levels of psychosocial stress, and found that standing more than 2.5 hours per day and sleeping less than 8 hours at night were significantly associated with LBW, while levels of psychosocial stress were not.

3. Early infant feeding

Although the link between infant feeding and overweight/obesity is established for preschoolers and younger school-aged children, not all studies have established a link between infant feeding and overweight/obesity at later age. Michels et al. (2007) examined the relation between infant feeding and the development of overweight/obesity throughout the life course. They utilized the Nurses' Health Study II, a prospective cohort of 116,678 female nurses. The mothers of the nurses in the study were contacted and queried about the type of feeding given to the nurse subject when she was an infant. The mothers reported if they had breast-fed and if so, for how long, and if the subject was bottle-fed, the type of milk used in the bottle. Breastfeeding, regardless of its duration, did not influence the adult BMI of the nurse subjects, and there was also a lack of relationship between breastfeeding and the recalled weight of the nurse subjects at age 18. Although the feeding was reported as exclusively breast-fed or not, the type of associated food (liquid or solid) that was provided if the infant was not exclusively breast-fed was not addressed.

The type of formula fed to infants is also studied for its relation to later obesity risk. Breast milk has lower protein content than does formula that is based on cow's milk (Alexy et al., 1999) and formula fed infants have been found to have higher postprandial insulin than breast-fed infants, which enhances growth and stimulates adipocyte activity (Lucas et al., 1981) and results in earlier adiposity rebound and higher childhood BMI (Scaglioni et al., 2000). This is known as the early protein hypothesis (Koletzko et al., 2009) and was tested in the European Childhood Obesity Trial. Infants whose mothers chose to formula feed were randomly assigned to infant formula with higher protein content or lower protein content (Grote et al., 2010). Infants whose mothers chose to breast-fed were also followed as the standard growth group to which the growth of the formula fed infants was compared. All three groups of infants were followed for 2 years for growth. Significant differences in weight and weight-for-length emerged by 6 months in the 2 groups of formula fed infants and remained stable, with the higher protein-fed infants having a .20 higher z-score for growth than the lower protein-fed infants (Grote et al.). There was no difference in length at 2 years of age. Compared to the breast-fed group, the lower protein formula-fed infants had similar growth, while the higher protein infants had significantly higher weight and weight-for-length z-scores at 2 years of age. The researchers note that the lower-protein-formula group still had a higher intake of protein than did the breast-fed infants, and that the difference in protein content between the higher-protein-formula infants and the breast-fed infants would produce a 13% higher risk for later obesity.

3.1 Rapid growth

The growth rate of infants in the first six months of life has been suggested as an early indicator of risk status for becoming overweight/obese or as a cause of later obesity. A population-based study in the Netherlands (Generation R Study) examined the development and health of 1,232 infants. Their mothers consented during pregnancy, and the growth of the infants was examined from fetal life until six months of age. Body composition was ascertained through skinfold thickness. The investigators found that infants who had the greatest increase in weight from birth to six months of age had the highest percentage of body fat, regardless of their BMI, and concluded that rapid postnatal weight gain represents the early onset of adiposity (Holzhauer et al., 2009). Rapid weight gain during infancy of Chilean SGA children was associated with insulin resistance which preceded the weight gain, although the overall body weight was similar to children who had been born at normal weight (Mericq et al., 2005).

Several systematic reviews have been conducted on the issue of rapid weight gain, rapid growth, or both in infancy and the later development of overweight/obesity. Monteiro and Victora (2005) conducted a systematic review of 15 articles on rapid early growth and its association with obesity in later life. They reported that 13 of the studies found strong associations between rapid early growth and the occurrence of overweight, obesity, and increased adiposity in spite of the ages at which the children were measured for follow-up of early growth. In their systematic review, Baird et al. (2005) reported on 24 studies out of 27,949 references originally identified. All studies were observational in design. The studies were remarkably consistent, in that they found that infants who were defined as obese in infancy were more likely to be obese in childhood, adolescence, or adulthood. Rapid growth was especially predictive, with odds ratios of 1.06 to 5.70 for rapid early growth and later obesity. They did not find an association between the timing of the rapid growth; any periods of rapid growth in the first or second year led to later obesity. Ong and Loos (2006) conducted a systematic review of 21 articles reporting on weight gain during infancy and risk for obesity in later life. They defined rapid infant weight gain as >0.67 SD in weight, as this SD represents the change from one centile line on the standard infant growth charts (e.g., 2nd, 10th, 25th, 50th, 75th, 90th, 98th centiles). All examined studies showed evidence of a positive association of infant weight gain that crosses percentiles upwards and a subsequent risk of obesity. They found that weight gain very early in life is a critical time for later obesity risk and that increasing weight gain from 1 to 2 years of age presents a 60% increased risk of obesity. They also reported that the effects of rapid early weight gain are similar in normal birth weight infants and LBW infants, demonstrating that rapid weight gain and catch-up growth are both important contributors to obesity development.

Owen et al. (2005) conducted a systematic review of published studies examining influences of types of initial infant feeding (breast vs. formula) on later development of obesity. Breastfeeding was associated with lower obesity risk, compared with formula feeding (OR: 0.87; 95% CI: 0.85, 0.89); this effect was stronger in smaller studies (<500 participants) but also apparent in larger studies (Owen et al., 2005). In another study, Owen et al. (2006) conducted a systematic review of published research examining relationships between initial infant feeding (breast vs. formula) and type 2 diabetes and glucose and insulin concentrations. Breastfeeding was associated with lower risks for type 2 diabetes in later life, compared to formula (OR: 0.61; 95% CI: 0.44, 0.85: p = 0.003, Owen et al., 2006).

3.2 Breastfeeding

There are many conflicting research studies about the effects of breastfeeding on later childhood obesity. Many studies acknowledge that breastfeeding is beneficial in reducing morbidity and mortality from gastrointestinal and respiratory infections, necrotizing enterocolitis in preterm infants, sudden infant death syndrome, and results in reduced atopic eczema, and higher IQ and academic performance (Kramer, 2010). However, the studies that also examine the risk for obesity have had conflicting results. This is partially due to the high level of confounding inherent in examination of the effects of breastfeeding on infant outcomes, as it is not possible to randomly assign infant feeding methods to mothers and infants. The choice to breast-feed is highly associated with education, income level, culture, influence of family and friends, and these variables are also associated with risk for adult obesity. This brief review of the conflicting studies will present the research that supports the effect of breastfeeding on lower risk for obesity initially and then present the studies that indicate that breastfeeding is not protective against later obesity risk.

3.2.1 Breastfeeding trends

Numerous international and national health organizations and professional groups have supported and continue to support breastfeeding as the optimal infant nutrition, for a variety of psychological, development, nutrition, immunological, environmental, and economic reasons ([AAP], 2005). WHO for many years has endorsed exclusive breastfeeding (e.g., the infant receiving only breast milk, though vitamins, medicine, and minerals may also be received) from birth to six months of age in both developed and developing countries (Kramer & Kakuma, 2002) or longer. UNICEF (n.d.) also has promoted exclusive breastfeeding for the first six months of life, with continued breastfeeding for two or more years, as well as responsive, appropriate complementary food added at six months of age.

Despite this support and endorsement, global breastfeeding rates, especially for exclusive breastfeeding, are still less than optimal. U.S. breastfeeding rates have increased recently, with infants reported as ever breastfed rising from 60% to 77% of infants born (1993-94 vs. 2005-2006; McDowell et al., 2008). Moreover, U.S. breastfeeding rates remained significantly affected by race/ethnicity (80% for Mexican American, 79% for non-Hispanic white, and 65% for non-Hispanic black infants), family income (74% for higher income v 57% lower income infants), and maternal age (43% for women less than 20 years old v 65% of mothers 20-29 and 75% of mothers 30 or older; McDowell et al.). While recent data indicated that about three-fourths of U.S. infants were ever breastfed (Centers for Disease Control and Prevention [CDC], 2010), rates for exclusive breastfeeding for six months (e.g., only breast milk, with no other liquids or foods) were much lower at 13.3% (Levi et al., 2011). Moreover, only 35% of infants in the 94 countries monitored by WHO or 65% of global infant population) are exclusively breastfed for the first 4 months of life (WHO, 2006).

3.2.2 Breastfeeding and child health

Although multiple factors have been examined for their relationship to overweight/obesity (Lamb et al., 2010), a large body of evidence has established linkages between breastfeeding and breastfeeding mothers' and children's health outcomes (Metzger & McDade, 2010). Breastfeeding benefits for the infant are thought to be both short term, such as protection from infection and morbidity (Horta et al., 2007; UNICEF, n.d.), and longer term (Horta et al.). A stunning amount of research has examined breastfeeding and child health outcomes. A comprehensive summary of breastfeeding is beyond the scope of this chapter.

Breast milk has long been viewed as the ideal infant food (AAP, 2005; Kramer, 2010; McDowell et al., 2008). Nevertheless, past debate focused on weighing exclusive breastfeeding benefits and concerns that exclusive breastfeeding might be insufficient to meet infants' energy and micronutrient needs after four months of age (Kramer & Kakuma, 2002). Kramer and Kakuma conducted a systematic review of studies that compared maternal or child health outcomes for exclusive breastfeeding > six months of age vs. exclusive breastfeeding between three to four months as well as complementary liquids or foods through six months of age or longer. The authors concluded that evidence failed to support increased risks in infants exclusively breastfed for six months in developed or developing countries.

Druet and Ong (2008) examined the early childhood predictors of adult body composition, and support the view that breastfeeding has a protective effect against later obesity. They believe that the effect may be due to the slower weight gain that breastfed infants maintain compared to formula fed infants and reduced protein intake. The WHO has identified breastfeeding as the normal feeding for infants and the growth of breastfed infants as the norm to which the growth of formula fed infants should be compared. The WHO 2006

Growth Standards are based on the growth of breastfed infants worldwide whose mothers were provided with lactation support for exclusive or predominant breastfeeding (de Onis et al., 2004).

3.2.3 Breastfeeding reduces childhood obesity

Breast milk contains many biologically active substances, some of whom have functions as yet unknown. The composition of milk varies throughout the feeding, throughout the day, and from day to day. Leptin, a hormone released by adipocytes to regulate energy balance by decreasing food intake and increasing energy expenditure, is present in breast milk (Palou & Picó, 2009). It allows for the body to maintain fat stores within a certain range but appears to lose its effect with weight gain, in that most obese individuals are resistant to leptin (Ahima & Flier, 2000). The effect of leptin on breastfed infants may regulate their feeding, although this remains unknown. Palou and Picó examined the effects of leptin provided to suckling rats and found that these rats as adults were more resistant to age-related weight increases and less likely to gain weight when provided with a high-fat diet. They conclude that leptin plays a critical role in assisting with the development of brain regions that regulate body weight.

Since so many of the confounding variables that accompany infant feeding choices cannot be controlled through random assignment, researchers have attempted to control these variables through intra-family studies of feeding choices and through large scale, nationally representative cohort studies. An interesting study, conducted by Metzger and McDade (2010), examined breastfeeding effects on obesity prevention, using a sibling difference model. The children of women who chose different feeding methods for their infants (formula feeding or breastfeeding) were studied as part of the Panel Study of Income Dynamics (PSID), a longitudinal examination of representative families in the United States on child development. Children who were not breastfed had lower birth weights and were more likely to be preterm; their mothers were more likely to be teens at the time of birth and their income lower. There were 118 children who differed by feeding method within families and they were much more similar to each other than the overall comparisons of formula fed or breastfed children. The breastfed children, when compared to their formula fed siblings, were 0.4 SD thinner, which amounts to 14 pounds for a 14 year old boy, and the breastfed children were less likely to be at the upper end of the BMI distribution (Metzer & McDade).

The growth velocities of 2 cohorts of infants in Germany were examined (Rzehak et al., 2009) as part of the GINI and LISA birth cohort studies. Infant feeding method was noted, along with many socioeconomic variables and was studied in 7,643 infants. The investigators found that the velocity of weight gain was lower for exclusively breastfed infants than formula fed infants, and the larger difference between velocities was between 3 and 6 months. The velocity of length gain did not differ between infants with different feeding methods. For each time period, exclusively breastfed infants had lower velocity of monthly weight-for-length (BMI) gain than did formula fed or mixed (formula- and breast milk–fed) infants.

The growth of 10,533 children from birth to age 3 was examined as part of the Millennium Cohort Study in the United Kingdom in which parental confounding factors were adjusted in the analyses (Griffiths et al., 2009). The researchers noted that infants who received no breast milk gained weight most rapidly and infants who were breastfed for fewer than 4 months gained weight more quickly than those who were breastfed longer than 4 months. These differences in weight gain were significantly associated with BMI z-score at age 3, although there was no significant difference in height z-score. The researchers also reported that early introduction of solid foods was not associated with greater BMI at age 3 in contrast to earlier research. The researchers from both the U.S. cohort study (PSID), the U.K. cohort study, and the German cohort studies conclude that their finding are consistent with the early programming hypothesis that breast milk and breastfeeding have biological and physiological effects on brain development that impact on the risk for later weight gain and development of obesity. The mechanisms that foster the effects remain to be determined but may also be due to infant self-regulation of hunger and satiety.

Kramer was credited with first proposing that breastfeeding provides a protective effect against childhood obesity (Arenz et al., 2004; Horta et al., 2007). In 1981, Kramer conducted an epidemiological case-control study including 639 children 12-18 years of age attending a clinic at which obesity was a frequent reason for care and 533 high school students of similar age, where lower rates of obesity were deemed likely. In the study, participants were first classified as non-obese, overweight, and obese based on anthropomorphic measurements (height, weight, and subscapular and triceps skinfold thickness), then demographic, family history, and feeding history were obtained by phone interviews with participants' mothers. The school participants' obesity prevalence rate was lower than that of clinic participants (11.3% vs. 20.3%), and school participants' breastfeeding rates were higher (36.2% vs. 21.6%). Kramer (1981) concluded that breastfeeding significantly reduced subsequent obesity through adolescence, with a slight increase with duration greater than two months. There was little additional benefit from delaying solid food introduction, and findings remained significantly protective after controlling for several confounders, including race, socioeconomic status, and birth order

Harder et al. (2005) completed a meta-analysis of studies examining breastfeeding duration and risk for later overweight. Breastfeeding duration was significantly negatively associated with risk for overweight in later life (regression coefficient: 0.94, 95% CI 0.89, 0.98). Categorical analysis of five breastfeeding duration categories (<1 month, 1-3 months, 4-6 months, 7-9 months, and >9 months) confirmed a dose-response association between duration and risk of later overweight, beginning at one month and plateauing at nine months. Each month of breastfeeding was associated with a 4% decrease in risk for later overweight (OR=0.86, 95%CI: 0.50, 0.91).

3.2.4 Breastfeeding has no impact on childhood obesity

In contrast to mechanistic and cohort studies that conclude that breastfeeding is protective against childhood obesity, some researchers have found no effect of type of infant feeding on obesity using samples from different cohort studies than described above. Kramer et al. (2009) recently published the effects of their large randomized intervention trial of a breast-feeding promotion intervention in Belarus. The PROBIT (Promotion of Breastfeeding Intervention Trial) design randomized lactation support interventions by hospital and was conducted in Belarus from June 1996 to December 1997 with a sample size of 16,491 infants. The exclusive breastfeeding rate at 3 months of age among infants born at the intervention hospitals was 43% compared to 6.4% among infants born at control hospitals. The mothers in the study were not significantly different by group. At age 6 there were no significant differences between the children in the intervention group and the children in the control group for height, BMI, waist circumference or skinfold thickness. The children in the intervention group had significantly improved cognitive ability (higher IQ and academic performance) at age 6 and reduced atopic eczema in infancy (Kramer et al., 2009, 2010). Though the intervention was effective in producing exclusive breastfeeding at 3 months of age (43.3 % v. 6.4%, P <0.001) and higher rates of breastfeeding throughout infancy, they observed no significant intervention effects of their breast-feeding promotion intervention on measures of height, blood pressure, BMI, or adiposity. However, one critique of this study is that it appeared not to have originally been designed to examine overweight/obesity outcomes (Monasta, Batty, Macaluso, et al., 2010).The children who were breastfed were not compared to the children who were bottle-fed regardless of their group membership and so this was not a true comparison of the effect of breastfeeding on obesity; rather it was a test of the effectiveness of hospital-based lactation support on increasing rates of breastfeeding. The PROBIT study provides information for policy changes on lactation support as it demonstrated that lactation support can increase breastfeeding rates among postpartum hospitalized mothers.

A sample of 2,291 Kuwaiti 3 to 6 year old children were examined for height and weight and were taken from the larger Kuwait Nutrition Surveillance System (Al-Qaoud & Prakash, 2009). The children's early feeding histories were obtained by questionnaire and were categorized by breastfed or never breastfed, and duration of breastfeeding. The investigators found no significant differences between the children who were breastfed regardless of duration and children who were not breastfed after adjusting for confounding variables such as time of introduction of solid foods, mother's socio-economic status, and child's birth weight and gestational age. The majority of the infants were breastfed for fewer than 4 months. The investigators note that Kuwait has undergone a nutrition transition that has resulted in increased high-fat food consumption and a more sedentary lifestyle and that these environmental impacts may also affect infants' and young children's size and growth.

The Copenhagen Perinatal Cohort, consisting of 9,125 individuals, was begun in 1959. Information on the infants' feeding history was collected when they were 1 year old and rates of breastfeeding were high, with only 9% of infants not receiving breast milk during 1st week of life. Data on the timing of solid food introduction and the type of solid foods were also measured at age 1. The participants' BMIs were measured longitudinally throughout their lives, and the relationship between early infant feeding and BMI was examined at age 42 (Schack-Nielsen et al., 2010). A longer duration of breastfeeding was associated with a lower BMI at age 1, but no effect was seen at older childhood or in adulthood. A later introduction of solid food was associated with a lower BMI at age 42 but no effect was seen at earlier ages. The authors conclude that early introduction of solid food is related to adult obesity, and adult obesity is not related to breastfeeding in infancy. It is possible that a longer duration of breastfeeding is related to a later introduction of solid foods. Mothers who determine that their breastfed infants are satisfied with breast milk and are growing adequately may not introduce solid foods as soon as mothers who perceive that their infants are not getting full with breast milk and want more to eat.

A similar cohort study examined the relationship of early infant feeding and adult BMI among the participants of the Nurses Health Study II, a prospective cohort of 116,678 female registered nurses ages 25-42 in 1989 and residing in the US. In 2001, the mothers of the study participants were asked about the infant feeding their daughters received. The data collected from the mothers included type of feeding (breast or bottle), duration of breastfeeding and bottle feeding, and use of formula or evaporated milk. The ages of introduction of solid food and cow's milk was also obtained. There were 41% of nurse participants who were breastfed for longer than 1 week and no effect type of infant feeding was found in adulthood for overweight or obesity (Michels et al., 2007). The duration of breastfeeding was also not associated with adult BMI as women who were breastfed for 9 months had the same risk of obesity as did women who were exclusively bottle-fed, although the women who were breastfed had a lower risk of being overweight during early childhood.

Though a number of reviews in this paper have agreed that breastfeeding has a protective effect again later obesity, others have been less conclusive (Monasta, Batty, Cattaneo, et al., 2011). Neutzling et al. (2009) studied relationships between breastfeeding duration, introduction of complementary solid/semi-solid foods before age four months, and overweight/obesity at eleven years of age in adolescents born in Pelotas, Brazil. They reported that the lowest prevalence of overweight or obesity was observed in participants breastfed one-three months, noting that their findings did not indicate consistent relationships between breastfeeding and introduction of complementary food or risks for later obesity. However, they recommended caution in interpreting their findings, due to several limitations, including a very short duration of breastfeeding in their participants.

3.2.5 Impact of maternal obesity on breastfeeding

An association between maternal obesity and reduced breastfeeding incidence and duration has been known since 1992 (Rutishauser & Carlin, 1992); subsequently, other researchers have found lower rates of breastfeeding among women who are overweight or obese (Donath & Amir, 2008). The reasons suggested for the association are cultural, physiological, and physical (results of pregnancies and deliveries complicated by obesity). The Third National Health and Nutrition Survey (Li et al., 2002) and the Pediatric Nutrition Surveillance System and the Pregnancy Nutrition Surveillance System (Li et al., 2003), established that obese women were less likely to have ever breast-fed. Two factors, both independently associated with reduced breastfeeding incidence, are higher maternal BMI before pregnancy and higher gestational weight gain. A dose-response was evident from the Longitudinal Study of Australian Children (Donath & Amir), with increasing rates of obesity among women associated with reduced incidence of breastfeeding. The women least likely to breastfeed are obese women with a BMI > 40. Danish women also demonstrated this dose response relationship between increased obesity and a lower incidence of breastfeeding (Baker et al., 2007). Finding this association in societies that are very supportive of breastfeeding (Denmark and Australia) suggests that the association may be due to physiological factors, in addition to psychological or cultural factors.

3.2.6 Physiological factors impacting breastfeeding

Lactogenesis II, the postpartum onset of copious lactation, is also known colloquially as when the milk "comes in" and usually occurs between 48 and 72 hours postpartum. Delayed lactogenesis II occurs when copious milk is not available more than 72 hours after delivery. Delayed lactogenesis II is associated with a high maternal pre-pregnancy BMI, and a delay in copious milk production may predict shorter breastfeeding duration. The negative effects of greater maternal BMI can, however, be overcome if in-depth breastfeeding support is present (Chapman & Perez-Escamilla, 2000).

The discrepancy between normal weight and obese postpartum women in lactogenesis II may be due to several factors. First, lower levels of prolactin in the first 48 hours after delivery are found in obese new mothers (Rasmussen & Kjolhede, 2004). Release of prolactin is reduced in obese women more than in lean women, and it is connected to the numerous hormonal changes that occur postpartum (Rasmussen, 2007). Obese women have reduced prolactin response to an infant's sucking at 2 and 7 days postpartum, and this may reduce the mother's confidence that her milk is sufficient for her child and lead to early cessation of breastfeeding. In addition, obese women have a less steep decline in insulin concentrations from the end of pregnancy to the initiation of lactation, perhaps leading to less glucose available for milk synthesis (Lovelady, 2005). Higher leptin levels, which have been found in obese women postpartum, can inhibit oxytocin's effect on muscle contractions in vitro, leading to an increased incidence of dysfunctional labor and higher cesarean section rates among obese women (Moynihan et al., 2006). Oxytocin is also necessary for the milk ejection reflex, which allows milk to be available to the sucking infant.

An interesting hypothesis related to the interaction of early feeding and life course development may also partially explain why obese women have lower rates of breastfeeding initiation and duration (Rasmussen 2007). Studies in domesticated animals (such as cows, pigs, sheep, and laboratory animals) have shown that a high-energy intake during early development and gestation can lead to reduced growth of the mammary glands and reduced milk yield. This has been extensively studied in dairy cows and has the name of "fat cow syndrome" (Morrow, 1976). However, the ways in which early feeding contributes to development of connective, adipose, and epithelial tissue, all of which constitute human breasts, remains unclear. It is not yet known if breast development in obese women mimics the reduced mammary development that occurs in overfed animals.

3.2.7 Medical/physical factors impacting breastfeeding

Obese women are more likely to have comorbid conditions and to develop certain pregnancy-related diseases such as preeclampsia, gestational hypertension, and gestational diabetes, leading to higher rates of complicated labor, higher rates of cesarean delivery, and more postpartum complications such as hemorrhage (Hadar & Yogev, 2011; Rasmussen & Kjolhede, 2008). Recovery is longer after difficult labors, cesarean deliveries, or both than after spontaneous labors and vaginal deliveries. Women with difficult labors and deliveries experience more infections, pain from incisions, and greater delay in putting the infant to breast (Sebire et al., 2001). Delays in putting the infant to breast can result from the need to attend to the health of the mother after the complicated delivery, pain from incisions, or from separation of the newborn from the mother for observation in the newborn nursery. It is also more difficult to hold an infant in the traditional "Madonna" position (a common breastfeeding position) after a cesarean section because of pain from an abdominal incision. In addition, the mechanical difficulties of latching an infant onto a large breast may require specialized lactation expertise unavailable to the new mother (Jevitt et al., 2007). Kitsantas and Pawloski (2010) found that obesity impacts the initiation and duration of breastfeeding only among mothers who experienced medical complications during pregnancy or labor and delivery complications. They reported that obese women who had no pregnancy, labor, and delivery complications initiated breastfeeding at the same rate as women who were not overweight/obese. Lactation education and assistance can make a difference in breastfeeding initiation and duration among obese women.

3.2.8 Sociocultural factors impacting breastfeeding

Sociocultural factors may exert an indirect effect on lactation, while physiological or medical factors among obese women can have direct effects on lactation. The National Immunization Survey conducted by the Centers for Disease Control and Prevention (CDC, 2007) revealed that rates of exclusive breastfeeding were lowest among infants of mothers who were under 20 years of age, with a high school education or less, unmarried, living in rural areas, and at the federal poverty level or below. In population-based studies, obese women have been found to be more likely to be lower income, with less education, and with higher rates of smoking than women of normal weight (Donath & Emir, 2008; Eriksson et al., 2003). Even as obesity has been found to be an independent risk factor for low rates of breastfeeding (Oddy et al., 2006), the constellation of obesity, low levels of education, rural residence, poverty, smoking, and being unmarried combine to predict a high risk of not breastfeeding. Women with these risk factors will need special lactation education, counseling, and support to overcome the risk of failing to breastfeed.

3.2.9 The impact of breastfeeding on maternal obesity

Breastfeeding can have short- and long-term effects on the weight of postpartum women (Walker et al., 2004). It is important to include these effects in this review because retained weight from each pregnancy is a risk factor for maternal obesity, which perpetuates the cycle of LGA infants. Breast milk contains varying amounts of calories based on the child's age, the mother's diet, and the amount of milk produced by the mother. Calories in milk can range from 53 to 75 kcal/100 ml, also depending on the mother's dietary intake and the timing of the feeding as milk produced later in the feeding is higher in fat (hindmilk). Mothers in developed countries produce breast milk with higher calories than mothers in developing countries (Lauber & Reinhardt, 1979), probably because women in developed countries are better nourished. The mother whose infant consumes a liter of breast milk a day may use 600 kilocalories a day in milk production and in the content of the milk. If the breastfeeding woman does not increase her dietary intake by a corresponding number of calories, postpartum weight loss can result. Araujo et al. (2006) found that in Brazil, postpartum weight retention was lowest in women who breast-fed for 4 to 12 months and highest for mothers who breast-fed for less than 1 month or more than 12 months. In a related study, Gigante et al. (2001) reported that 5 years after the birth of their children, BMI did not significantly differ between women who had breast-fed and those who had not. Brazilian researchers also found that breastfeeding did not have a significant effect on postpartum weight retention in obese women, although it did on women with a normal pre-pregnancy BMI (Kac et al., 2004). It may be necessary to include the maternal pre-pregnancy weight status when examining the effect of breastfeeding on postpartum weight loss.

Studies from the Danish National Birth Cohort have shown that if obese women breastfeed as recommended (exclusively to 6 months, and continuing in addition to solid food to 12 months) postpartum weight retention could be eliminated and BMI could be reduced by 18 months postpartum (Baker et al., 2008). The Stockholm Pregnancy and Weight Development Study provided 15 years of follow-up of women who delivered in 1984-1985. Women with a higher BMI at the 15-year follow-up had a higher pre-pregnancy BMI and more gestational weight gain (Linne et al., 2003); women who remained normal weight had breast-fed longer and more exclusively than women who became overweight across the 15 years of follow-up. In a related study, the long-term impact of lactation on women's health was examined in the

Women's Health Initiative (WHI). Thirty-five years after childbearing, women who had breast-fed for cumulative lifetime duration of 12 months or longer were less likely to have hypertension, diabetes, hyperlipidemia, or cardiovascular disease (Schwarz et al., 2009). In summary, breastfeeding can promote postpartum weight loss depending on breastfeeding intensity (exclusive or supplemental), duration in months, the woman's pre-pregnancy BMI, and the woman's dietary intake. Breastfeeding can thus be beneficial not only for the infant but also for the breastfeeding mother.

3.2.10 Recommendations for promoting breastfeeding among obese women

Given the findings that breastfeeding is beneficial to women's and infants' health, that obese women are at more risk to deliver LGA infants who are at risk to develop cardiovascular disease as adults, and that obese women are less likely to breastfeed, it is important for obstetric care providers to assist obese postpartum women to breastfeed (Reifsnider, 2011). Many clinicians are unaware of the research showing that obese women have lower rates of breastfeeding or of the reasons for the lower rates (Rasmussen et al., 2006). Thus, clinicians need to be aware of the risks of lactation failure in obese women and target these women for additional education and support during pregnancy and after delivery. It may be more difficult for an infant to latch onto the breast of an obese mother, and obese women will benefit from specific counseling on latching on and from breast support with a towel placed under the breast (Jevitt et al., 2006; Rasmussen et al.). Pumping from both breasts using a double-pump system between infant feedings can increase milk production and promote the woman's sense of accomplishment in feeding her infant (Jevitt et al.).

Encourage skin-to-skin contact and put newborn to breast as soon after birth as possible
Limit maternal-newborn separation, encourage mother-baby in same room
Carefully observe latch-on and correct any incorrect placement of infant's jaw and assist with latch-on until mother is competent
Encourage frequent sucking and ad lib newborn feeding at breast
Demonstrate variety of nursing positions to relieve pressure on nipples
Assist mothers with flat or inverted nipples to use shields to allow for nipple protrusion
Support large breasts with towel placed under breast
Teach mothers how to use breast pump and encourage pumping between feedings to increase milk supply
Teach mothers how to wake a "sleepy baby" and encourage the neonate to nurse
Teach mothers how to recognize neonate swallowing of breast milk
Teach mothers to recognize signs of adequate infant intake (to 5-6 stools per day and first appearance of yellow stool by Day 6) to reassure her that her milk is sufficient for her infant. This can promote breastfeeding duration and exclusivity (Shrago et al., 2006).
Refer to lactation specialist if needed

Table 1. Clinical Lactation Support for Obese Breastfeeding Mothers

4. Timing of weaning/introduction of solid foods

The age at which an infant is introduced to foods other than breast milk or formula has been examined as one factor influencing the risk for obesity. The American Heart Association (AHA) has released dietary recommendations for children and adolescents, and the recommendations have been endorsed by the American Academy of Pediatrics (AHA, 2006). The recommendations recognize that the period from weaning (introduction of solid foods) to consumption of a mature diet, occurring from 4 to 6 months to 2 years of age, represents a major developmental time point for children, but there has been very little research on the best methods to achieve optimal nutrition during this transition. Transition to solid foods and sources of nutrients other than breast milk or formula should begin at 4 to 6 months of age to ensure sufficient nutrition in the diet, but the best methods for accomplishing this task are essentially unknown. A recent examination of the timing of solid food introduction and obesity at three years of age was reported by Huh et al. (2011). The children were in a prospective cohort study from birth and the primary outcome was obesity at age three. The exposure to solid foods at < 4 months, 4-5 months, or ≥ 6 months was examined along with the type of feeding (breast-fed or formula fed). Infants who were breast-fed for less than four months were categorized in the formula-fed group. Among breast-fed infants, 9% were obese at three years of age, and the timing of solid food introduction was not associated with obesity. Among formula-fed children, introduction of solid foods before four months was associated with a six times higher increase in the odds ratio for obesity (OR 6.3; 95% CI: 2.30-6.90). Only 8% of breast-fed infants were introduced to solid foods before four months, compared with 33% of formula fed infants. Introduction of solid foods between four and six months did not increase the odds for obesity at age 3.
These finding are similar to those reported almost two decades ago by researchers with the DARLING study, who found that solid foods displaced milk intake in breast-fed infants but not in formula fed infants, who consumed the same amount of formula while adding solid foods as well (Heinig et al., 1993). A prospective cohort followed from birth in the United Kingdom found that energy intake at four months was higher in formula fed or mixed feeing (formula and breast milk) infants who were fed solid foods earlier (some starting at 1-2 months). The higher energy intake at four months predicted greater weight gain from birth to age 1, age 2, and age 3, and resulted in larger BMI at age 3. No effect of early feeding on BMI at age 3 was found in breast-fed infants. In the formula and mixed-feeding group, each 100 kcal increase in energy intake at age four months was associated with increased risk of obesity at age three (OR 1.46; 95% CI:1.20-1.78) and at five years of age as well (OR 1.25; 95% CI: 1.00-1.55). The authors noted that the larger energy intake and the increased weight gain from year to year contributed to the risk of obesity at age three (Ong et al., 2006). A prospective cohort study from Australia enrolled 620 pregnant women and followed their children until they were 10 years old, when their BMI was assessed (Seach et al., 2010). The duration of breastfeeding (whether exclusive or mixed) was not associated with BMI, but the age of solid food introduction and parental smoking were both significantly associated with higher BMIs. Healthy-weight children started solid foods on average at 20.5 weeks of age, while the obese children started solid foods at 18.7 weeks of age. The prevalence of obesity in the group that started solids before 20 weeds was 34.7%, while it was 19.4% among the children who started solid foods at 24 weeks or later. The researchers did not find any interaction effects with duration of breastfeeding and introduction of solid foods, as opposed to the findings of Huh et al., discussed earlier.

However, they recommend that solid foods not be introduced until the infant is six months of age to provide the strongest protection against obesity, both as an infant and as a child. Adiposity rebound is the time when the fatness of children accelerates and usually occurs between the ages of 4 to 6. Children's growth rate slows after age 1 and the children become thinner, but with the advent of the adiposity rebound, the fatness and the weight increase. Children who become obese have an earlier rebound (approximately age 3) than those who do not (ages 4 to 6). The Raine prospective cohort study followed 1,330 children from birth to adolescence and collected detailed infant feeding data during their first year. The investigators conducted repeated anthropometric measurements (Chivers et al., 2010) and found that at 14 years of age, BMI was consistently higher for the group breast-fed less than four months. Adiposity rebound occurred on average at age 5.3 years for the normal weight group, age 3.8 for the overweight group, and age 2.6 for the obese group. Adiposity rebound was earlier and the BMI at the nadir was earlier for the group that was breast-fed less than four months. The impact of other feeding (besides formula) on the adiposity rebound or later obesity was not reported in this study, while the authors concluded that the early introduction of formula is associated with accelerated growth and later obesity.

In a retrospective study in Brazil of 566 children, investigators collected data on infant feeding from their parents along with types of feeding and dates of weaning (Simon et al., 2008). The children were between the ages of two and six, with the older children being significantly heavier than the younger children. The duration of exclusive breastfeeding was found to be protective of being obese as a preschooler as infants who were exclusively breast-fed for six months having nearly half the odds of being obese (OR .57; 95% CI: 0.38-0.86). In addition, the duration of breastfeeding also contributed to the reduction of obesity, as being breast-fed until 24 months results in OR of 0.13; 95% CI: 0.05-0.37) for obesity. There were no significant differences between rates of obesity and the timing or the type of solid foods given to the infants. The foods the infants were given included tea, fruit, non-maternal milk, cold cuts, sugar, meat, and eggs.

An interesting examination of how infants consume their food revealed that infants who were breast-fed less than 20% of milk feedings (included pumped breast milk and formula) were two times more likely to have excess weight between 6 to 12 months, and infants who often emptied their bottles were 70% more likely to have excess weight (Li et al., 2010). Maternal encouragement to finish the bottle was not significantly associated with excess weight; only the infants' own initiated bottle-emptying behavior predicted later obesity. Nursing from the breast was not associated with excess weight. The authors recommend that mothers be taught to recognize satiety in infants and provide less formula in bottles to reduce the amount of intake at each bottle feeding. Parenting education is also needed to recognize signs of infant temperament and use other soothing techniques besides providing a bottle of formula or juice. Wasser et al. (2011) found that among mothers and infants in the Special Supplemental Nutrition Program for Women, Infants, and Children (WIC program), infants were introduced to solids and juice by the first and second months. The most common sources of nutrition other than formula were juice and cereal in formula bottles. Mothers who perceived that their children were "fussy" were twice as likely to be fed solid food before six months. The formula fed infants who received solid or juice consumed approximately 100 kcal more than infants who consumed only formula. This amount mirrors the amount of extra kcal reported by Ong et al. in the U.K. (see above). Clearly, parenting education is needed to promote delaying introduction of solids and juice until six months, to provide appropriate amounts of formula, and to use techniques other than bottle feeding when a child is fussing or crying.

5. First author's research with obesity and low-income Hispanic families in the southwest United States

The toddler stage is a time of transition from dependent feeding to independent feeding. During this early time in life, food preferences develop, and often they predict preferences throughout life (Allen & Myers, 2006). Not only is this a crucial stage for monitoring growth and BMI, it is the most opportune time to prevent obesity in children by promoting healthy nutrition and increased physical activity behaviors (He, 2006; Story et al., 2002). The majority of intervention studies on pediatric obesity have been conducted with white, middle-class samples (Ward-Begnoche et al., 2009), thus providing scant knowledge for intervening with low-income, Hispanic populations. Hispanics of Mexican American origin are at an increased risk for obesity, particularly among those in the lower socioeconomic level (Fisher-Hoch et al., 2010). Treviño et al. (2008) found rates of obesity of 33% among low-income, school-aged Hispanic children in rural south Texas. McCormick et al. (2010) have documented that 16% of infants in their practice in Galveston, Texas are obese, as measured by weight for length calculations. More Hispanic infants were obese than were children of other ethnicities with no significant differences in sex or financial status. Only 14% of the obese infants and 23% of the obese 24 month olds were diagnosed as obese by their primary care provider, demonstrating that obesity may not be acknowledged by parents or health care providers. The first author's work has focused on the causes and elimination of these health disparities in growth.

The ecological model of growth (EMG; Reifsnider & Ritsema, 2008) has been used as the framework for all the first author's studies and directs the choice of conceptual and operational variables to measure. The EMG is a heuristic model that explains the levels of a child's environment that contribute to a child's growth (Reifsnider, 1995; Reifsnider et al., 2005). The EMG is a combination of Human Ecology (Bronfenbrenner, 1979) and epidemiology and illustrates influences at the host (child) and agent (food) levels as they interact in the environment (microsystem and mesosystem). The host variables are those that are characteristics of the child, such as a child's anthropometric measurements, a child's diet, and level of activity or inactivity. The agent is viewed as the proximate cause of the problem, in this case, nutrition that is not balanced with the child's needs. The ecological environment is conceived as a set of connected structures, each influencing the other structures within the set. The microsystem is the immediate setting containing the parent and child. In the studies reviewed below, the family, the family's home situation, other children in the family, and the interaction between parent and child are all considered characteristics of the microsystem.

Since first noticing the rising rates of obesity among the WIC population, the first author has worked extensively with low-income, predominately Hispanic families on issues of maternal child nutrition and growth. The samples have been drawn from the population of women and children who qualified for food subsidies from WIC, a program funded by the U.S. Department of Agriculture for families who are at 185% of the federal poverty level or below. The WIC program provides to pregnant and breastfeeding women and children up to the age of five with nutritional needs, specified foods to be purchased using vouchers that include (for pregnant women) milk, cheese, fresh fruits and vegetables, whole wheat breads (including brown rice and corn tortillas), eggs, peanut butter, breakfast cereals that are low in sugar and high in vitamins and minerals, fruit juice, and for breastfeeding women, tuna and salmon. Infants are provided vouchers for baby fruits and vegetables, cereal, and infant formula. If infants are breast-fed, they can also receive vouchers for infant canned meat. Multiple studies have found that the rates of breastfeeding are lower and the early introduction of cow's milk is higher if pregnant women receive WIC. These differences persist after the women receiving WIC are compared with women in similar socioeconomic situations (Ziol-Guest & Hernandez, 2010). Overall, breastfeeding rates of initiation and duration are lower in low-income women than are the rates in middle- and higher-income women, although the reasons for the lower rates have not been clearly elucidated.

The first author conducted studies on breastfeeding promotion using qualitative methods with Hispanic families who were WIC clients, consisting of pregnant and postpartum women, the mothers of the women receiving WIC, and male partners of the women receiving WIC. The findings revealed that all participants viewed breastfeeding as the healthier choice for the infant, and some perceived it also as a cheaper choice than formula feeding. The women chose breastfeeding without input from their partners. All the respondents felt that breastfeeding in public, with its attendant risk of an exposure of a breast, to be unacceptable. The women believed it was appropriate to breastfeed around their intimate partners and perhaps other female relatives. Other barriers to breastfeeding concerned nipple pain and inconvenience, in that no one could feed an infant other than the mother (Gill et al., 2004). A similar study was conducted with staff at WIC clinics (clerks, educators, nutritionists) who were WIC providers (92% Hispanic) of the subjects described in the previous study. They were asked similar questions and encouraged to share what they had heard about breastfeeding from their WIC clients. The WIC staff reported that their WIC clients did not breastfeed because of work, lack of family support, or misinformation about diet during lactation. They believed that they would encourage a WIC client to breastfeed, and that after delivery, she would be exposed to bottle-feeding in the hospital, and would choose not to breastfeed. They felt that the hospitals could make a better effort with teaching and supporting a new mother to breastfeed (Reifsnider et al., 2003).

These qualitative studies laid the groundwork for intervention studies on supporting breastfeeding among the WIC population, and a study was conducted with 200 low-income pregnant women who were followed for six months after delivery. The intervention group received telephone support and, if indicated by concerns elicited during the phone calls, home visits from lactation educators and lactation consultants. The home visits consisted of observation of breastfeeding, weighing of the infant, and discussion of any other problems the new mothers were having. Often, receiving reassurance that the infant was gaining weight and growing was enough to encourage the women to continue to breastfeed. The control group received regular WIC support, which included WIC peer counseling for breastfeeding if requested by the new mother. The results showed that the intervention group had twice (OR 2.31) the odds of starting breastfeeding, twice (OR 1.84-3.15) the odds of continuing to breastfeed for 6 months, and only half (.50-.54) the tendency to quit at any one time than did the control group (Gill et al., 2007).

The first author and research team also conducted qualitative studies on Hispanic mothers' perceptions of their children's growth, health, and body size (Reifsnider et al., 2000a, 2000b, 2006). These studies revealed that mothers perceived their children's growth as determined by heredity, over which they had little influence. Growth charts that demonstrated their children's BMI, or pictures of children of differing sizes, were not useful to mothers when considering their children's own sizes. Hispanic mothers relied more heavily on comparing their children's sizes with other children of their acquaintance to determine if they were underweight, normal weight, overweight, or obese. Another method used by mothers to monitor size and growth was the size labels on the children's clothing. Both of these methods have flaws, as individuals tend to have affiliations with others of their similar size (Valente et al., 2009), and clothing sizes vary depending on the type of garment and its maker. The mothers' views of health did not consider a child's size but rather focused on a child's mood, activity level, and appearance. The first author found that Hispanic mothers defined a healthy child as one who has chubby legs and arms with round cheeks, and an unhealthy child as one who is thin. If a child is chubby, happy, active, and appears well-cared for, the child is considered healthy. An unhealthy child is described as thin, unhappy, lacking in energy, and unkempt. When asked directly if an overweight child is a healthy child, the mothers denied this but used descriptions such as "plump, dimples, rolls, round" to describe health in children. A thin child was evidence that the mother was not "doing a good job caring for her child." This theme was corroborated by Sussner et al. (2009), who documented that Hispanic mothers described how providing a lot of food to children is consistent with good parenting. Hispanic mothers and grandmothers traditionally are the primary health caretakers for their families, and altering their views of appropriate child weight may have long-term benefits for the child as well as other siblings and family members.

The first author also conducted descriptive and quantitative studies of low-income Hispanic children who received food assistance through the WIC program. The sample size was 100 children ages 12 to 24 months in each of three conditions (stunted, normal sized, and obese) and their mothers (N = 600), and a cross-sectional design was used. The WIC program in this health district had an average monthly enrollment of 50,000 women and children, and the clinic where the data collection occurred was its largest site. By virtue of qualifying for WIC, all the families were at 185% of federal poverty level or lower. All children had documented residence in the city. To be included in the study, the children had to fit anthropometric criteria for being stunted, normal-sized, or obese. In addition, they had to live with a parent or guardian (no foster children), not have any metabolic or major illnesses or any neurological or developmental delays, and not have an organic cause for stunted growth or obesity. No inclusion or exclusion criteria existed for the children's mothers.

Data were collected from children and their mothers on weight and height (weight for height for children and BMI for mothers), 24-hour diet recall of child's diet from mothers, social and demographic variables from mothers (income, educational level of parents, parental employment, number and relation of people in the household, receipt of food stamps and monthly amount, receipt of free or reduced lunches for any siblings in the family, length of residence in current house, generation of residence in United States, ethnicity, and language spoken at home). Acculturation was measured by the Acculturation Rating Scale for Mexican Americans-II (ARSMA-II; Cuéllar et al., 1995). The variable of parent–child interaction was measured by the Nursing Child Assessment Teaching Scale (NCATS; Barnard et al., 1989). The mother's activity level was measured by the Baecke Questionnaire, which is designed to measure three aspects of an adult's daily activities: work, leisure, and sports (Baecke & Frijters, 1982).

The child-focused agent variables that showed significant differences between the groups were dietary intake, as well as length of time breast-fed and daily ingestion of fluoride. The normal-weight group was breast-fed the longest and the obese group the shortest length of time. The stunted group received fluoride more often than did either of the other two groups. The obese group had significantly higher daily intakes of Mexican rice and Kool-Aid and showed a trend to significance for higher intakes of water and bread, while the normal-weight group had the highest daily intake of American cheese, raw apple with peel, and pancakes and showed a trend to significance for Vitamin C. The stunted group showed a trend to significance for the highest daily intake of vegetables.

Analysis of the food intake indicates that diets featuring dairy protein (American cheese) and fruit (apple with peel and Vitamin C) are a characteristic of the normal-sized group, while diets featuring starches (Mexican rice, breads) and sweetened beverages (Kool-Aid®) are characteristic of the obese group. Dairy consumption has been inversely associated with components of the metabolic syndrome in adults in several studies (Pfeuffer & Schrezenmeir, 2007). Zemel (2005), in a review on the role of dairy foods in weight management, postulated that high-calcium diets reduce fat accumulation and play an important role in maintenance of normal weight and management of overweight. Ariza et al. (2004) found that overweight Hispanic children (ages 5-6 years) were more likely to consume sweetened beverages (including Kool-Aid®) daily. Vegetables are generally low in calories, and the finding that the stunted group ate the most vegetables could indicate their lower caloric intake. The diet differences are only suggestive at this time but do lend support to advising mothers to provide dairy protein and fresh fruit to encourage normal growth and discouraging intake of many servings of starches and sweetened beverages to prevent overweight. In one of the largest studies (N=428, children aged 4-5 years) to investigate appetite and activity preferences in children at risk of becoming obese, Wardle et al. (2001) found that children of obese or overweight families had a higher preference for fatty foods in a taste test, lower preference for vegetables, and a more "overeating-type" eating style. In addition, children of overweight or obese families had a stronger affinity for sedentary activities. Similarly, in a longitudinal study of older children, Burke et al. (2001) found that obese or overweight parents had children with higher BMIs.

The differences in the parent variables, regarding size of parents, are consistent with previous findings. The BMI of the parents of the obese children was significantly larger than the BMI of the parents of the normal-sized children. Of note is the finding that the mean BMI for parents in both groups, both mothers and fathers, was in the range considered overweight (BMI >25), and the BMI of the mothers of the obese children was in the obese range (BMI > 30). The finding that the mother's participation in activity during leisure time decreased as the children's BMI increased has not been previously reported. The finding that more leisure-time physical activity is associated with a lower BMI was expected because Mouton et al. (2000) have shown that leisure-time physical activity was inversely associated with obesity among repeated samples of Mexican American adults from family practice clinics in South Texas. Increasing a mother's leisure-time physical activity could be one way to promote normal child size and decrease risk of overweight in children (Fogelholm et al., 1999).

Our finding that as more parents and grandparents are born in the United States the children's BMI increases mirrors the finding of Duerksen et al. (2007), who noted that parental overweight is associated with eating at American restaurants, while child and parental BMI were lowest in families that ate predominately at Mexican restaurants. However, Ariza et al. (2004) found no association between children's overweight and the mother's score on the acculturation scale in their study of 250 kindergarten children who were primarily Mexican American. The effect of acculturation and generation in the United States on health and weight gain is complex, and it calls for models that examine the patterns of health and disease outcomes for distinct ethnic and cultural subgroups, according to Castro (2007).

The children in the original cross-sectional study were followed for six months while they remained clients of the WIC Program. The differences between the normal-weight and obese groups on dietary intake were grouped into fluids, fat, protein, carbohydrates, and total calories. The differences occurred between the normal-weight and obese groups, across time from time 1 to time 2 (six months apart), and in some cases, resulted in significant group by time interaction effects. There were significant differences between the groups at Time 1 in their water intake and within the normal-weight group across time as they significantly increased their intake of water. These differences also resulted in a significant group-by-time interaction effect. The obese group significantly increased their juice intake across time but did not differ from the normal-weight group in total intake. Both groups significantly decreased their intake of soda across time. Both groups also significantly increased their intake of fat, meat, and protein across time, but the intake did not differ between groups. Both groups significantly increased their intake of bread across time, with the obese group eating significantly more bread and other carbohydrates at Time 1 and Time 2. The obese group consumed more calories than the normal-weight group at Time 2 and also had higher rate of calorie increase than did the normal-weight group. This resulted in a trend to significance for an interaction effect.

The dietary intake of the groups revealed areas of significant differences between the groups in fluid, fat, bread and carbohydrate intake, and total calories, with the obese group consuming more servings. These differences, however, resulted in an alarming increase in calories, with the overweight group consuming a mean of 300 more calories per day by Time 2. Across time, the overweight group increased significantly in water, juice, meat, and protein. Both groups significantly decreased their soda intake across time. Adjustments to dietary intake such as a reduction in fruit juice intake may alter weight at an early age. These dietary changes may reflect the emphasis on the food pyramid when it included breads and carbohydrates as its bottom tier, encouraging consumption of 6-11 servings a day. The increase in fruit juices and the decrease in soda may reflect the impact of nutrition education since all the children were in WIC and their mothers were receiving nutrition education every six months.

The first author found both clinically and statistically significant differences in various aspects of the microsystem such as (home), agent (food), but not in the mesosytem (neighborhood) of normal and obese preschoolers. A variety of factors influence the development of obesity in young children. The greater BMI measures of the obese group at time 1 and time 2 were expected and support the view that the microsystem influences body size. The mothers of the overweight participants had significantly higher BMIs at time 1 and remained higher across the six months of measurement. If children reflect or imitate parental behavior in diet, activity, or both, then it appears that obese children in this study could be destined to follow their mothers. It would thus be important to follow these mothers and children to see whether the trend continues or whether reversals in both occur.

For example, a child may be encouraged to consume more when accompanied by a parent than when eating alone. Those who sit with children tend to influence their intake at meal time. At both time 1 and time 2, more of the overweight children did not eat alone. One feature of the home environment was that mothers of both groups at Time 1 were twice more likely to sit with their children at mealtime than were fathers (p=.00); however, this difference was not significant at Time 2. The obese children more often ate with someone at mealtime (100%) while 93% of the time the normal-weight children (p=.02) had someone sitting with them at mealtime. This suggests that both groups received attention at meals (by mothers most often), even though the obese group received attention more often.

The parent-child interaction scores overall indicated that mothers of the obese group had more positive interactions with their children in all areas except for response to distress. Mothers of normal-weight children responded more to their children's distress than did mothers of obese children. The mothers of both groups significantly increased in their responsiveness to their children. However, in all the subscales except clarity of cues, the mothers of obese children had a greater increase in being responsive to their children than did the mothers of the normal-weight children. We hypothesize that in this sample, the mothers of the obese children viewed feeding their children as an important way to interact with their children and show them affection. Findings from the earlier qualitative studies suggest that Hispanic mothers may view a thin child as an unloved or uncared for child, and the mothers took pride in caring for their children. The mothers of the obese children were more likely to be overweight themselves, and perhaps they associated food with positive emotion and were repeating that pattern with their children. It is important to educate mothers of overweight children to interact with their children in more active ways that do not involve food, such as reading stories, going on walks, and paying attention to their children at other times than mealtimes. This will also help the children learn that there are other positive ways to receive attention and affection than through meals and food.

The studies by the first author, reported above were limited to Mexican American, low-income children participating in a WIC program in a large city. Generalization to other Hispanic populations may be possible, but similarities in acculturation and economic situations must be taken into consideration.

6. Conclusions and recommendations

It is important to recognize that childhood obesity is a complex systems problem that has resulted from environmental changes and biological dispositions. For millennia, parents had to struggle to obtain sufficient food for their children, and a 'plump' child was evidence that the parents were good providers. In times of food scarcity, the children at either end of the growth spectrum would be more likely to survive; those born LBW/SGA as they were prenatally programmed to use nutrients efficiently, and those who were large with extra adipose tissue. Society has now changed from times of food scarcity to the easy provision of calorie-dense food and elimination/reduction of daily activities that could consume calories. Biology and culture have not adapted as rapidly as humans are still programmed to gain weight for survival and large children are a sign of successful parenting in many cultures. We need to create and encourage interventions that integrate multiple levels of influence, and note the intervention effects on social and environmental change as well as behavioral and clinical changes at the individual and family level (Huang & Story, 2010).

Though a number of studies have studied prevention of child obesity, great gaps exist in identifying effective interventions. Three issues related in general to child obesity prevention are worth mentioning as appropriate considerations when conducting studies of obesity prevention. First, a Cochrane Review examined evidence related to intervention effectiveness of obesity prevention in children and found insufficient evidence to prove that any single program could prevent child obesity (Summerbell et al., 2005). On a positive note, Summerbell et al. reported a trend for more recent interventions to include communities. Second, Saunders's (2007) literature review of studies examining prevention of obesity in children less than 5 years of age pointed to overall poor study quality, inconsistencies in research themes and findings, and absence of comprehensive evidence related to intervention effectiveness. Finally, a systematic review of randomized control trials of overweight or obesity prevention interventions for preschool children (<5 years of age) reported that none of the reviewed interventions demonstrated effectiveness (Monasta, Batty, Macaluso, et al., 2010). Reviewers recommended more rigorous examination of interventions and of social/environmental factors affecting lifestyle (Monasta, Batty, Macaluso, et al.).

Although many studies have been conducted on prevention and treatment of pediatric obesity, the prevalence remains high, especially among populations affected by health disparities. Family-based treatment is effective yet time-consuming and requires adherence by parents, while population-based efforts require political will that can be easily diverted to other pressing problems. Epstein and Wrotniak (2010) propose a multi-pronged approach from numerous fields of science to address the epidemic of childhood obesity. They recommend contributions from the fields of molecular genetics, basic behavioral science, educational science, developmental science, decision science, and sociology (social networks). Findings from each of these fields can be integrated into culturally-competent, community-specific interventions. Each culture and community must be considered and the persons affected by the issue of childhood obesity must be included when interventions are created with the community.

The IOM's recent report (2011) recommended 5 areas of focus to reduce childhood obesity. They recommend that all children be screened, monitored, and have their growth tracked from birth to age 5 to detect and treat obesity as soon as the child's growth begins to accelerate. They recommend that children increase physical activity and reduce sedentary behavior, and that parents be helped to find ways to accomplish this. All children should consume a variety of nutritious food and breastfeeding should be supported during infancy. Access to affordable healthy foods is a priority. Parents need to be taught how to recognize children's cues of hunger and satiety. Children's screen time should be monitored and limited to 2 hours a day or fewer, depending on the age of the child. Age appropriate sleep durations are important for healthy growth, and parents can be assisted with creating restful environments for their children. These recommendations are family and community focused and have been supported through clinical trials.

Based on findings briefly reviewed, several recommendations appear relevant for future studies. Among these are:

1. Increase study quality and rigor, with improved design and data analysis;
2. Consider prenatal, infancy, and early childhood periods when examining development and prevention of obesity and obesity consequences (Taveras et al., 2010);

3. Emphasize intervention studies focused on obesity determinants (Monasta, Batty, Macaluso, et al., 2010);
4. Approach child obesity as a social problem, using population-based, multisectoral, culturally appropriate, and multi-disciplary approaches (WHO, n.d.[b]);
5. Use community-based participatory research and other models that view community as active participants in research; and
6. Emphasize bench-to-bedside/community research that links study of complex bio-physiological factors, such as leptin and other adipocyte-produced compounds, to clinical outcomes.

7. References

Abeysena, C., Jayawardana, P., & Seneviratne Rde, A. (2010). Effect of psychosocial stress and physical activity on low birthweight: A cohort study. *Journal of Obstetrics and Gynaecology Research,* Vol. 36, No. 2, pp. 296-303.

Adachi-Mejia, A.M., Longacre, M.R., Gibson, J.J., Beach, M.L., Titus-Ernstoff, L.T., & Dalton, M.A. (2007). Children with a TV in their bedroom at higher risk for being overweight. *International Journal of Obesity,* Vol. 31, No.4, pp. 644-651.

Ahima, R.S., & Flier, J.S. (2000) Leptin. *Annual Review of Physiology,* Vol.62, pp. 413-437.

Alexy, U., Kersting, M., Sichert-Hellert, W., Manz, F., &. Schoch G. (1999). Macronutrient intake of 3- to 36-month-old German infants and children: Results of the DONALD Study. Dortmund Nutritional and Anthropometric Longitudinally Designed Study. *Annals of Nutrition & Metabolism,* Vol. 43, No. 1, pp. 14-22.

Allen, R.E., & Myers, A.L. (2006). Nutrition in toddlers. *American Family Physician,* Vol. 74, No. 9, pp.1527-1532.

Al-Qaoud, N., & Prakash, P. (2009). Can breastfeeding and its duration determine the overweight status of Kuwaiti children at the age of 3-6 years? *European Journal of Clinical Nutrition,* Vol. 63, No. 8, pp. 1041-1043.

Al-Shawwa, B.A., Al-Huniti, N.H., DeMattia, L., & Gershan, W. (2007). Asthma and insulin resistance in morbidly obese children and adolescents. *Journal of Asthma: Official Journal of the Association for the Care of Asthma,* Vol. 44, No. 6, pp. 469-473.

American Academy of Pediatrics (APA), Committee on Nutrition. (2003). Policy statement: Prevention of pediatric overweight and obesity. *Pediatrics,* Vol. 112, No. 2, pp. 424-430.

American Academy of Pediatrics (APA). (2005). Policy statement: Breastfeeding and the use of human milk. Accessed August 21, 2011, available from: http://aappolicy.aappublications.org/cgi/reprint/pediatrics;115/2/496.pdf

American Heart Association. (2006). Dietary recommendations for children and adolescents: A guide for practitioners. *Pediatrics,* Vol. 117, No. 2, pp. 544-559; doi:10.1542/peds.2005-2374

Anderson, S.E., & Whitaker, R.C. (2010). Household routines and obesity in US preschool-aged children. *Pediatrics,* Vol. 125, No. 3, pp. 420-428.

Araujo, C.L., Victora, C.G., Hallal, P.C. & Gigante, D.P. (2006). Breastfeeding and overweight in childhood: Evidence from the Pelotas 1993 birth cohort study. *International Journal of Obesity,* Vol. 30, No. 3, pp. 500-506.

Arenz, S., Ruckert, R., Koletzko, B., & von Kries, R. (2004).Breast-feeding and childhood obesity—A systematic review. *International Journal of Obesity,* Vol. 28, pp. 1247-1256. DOI:10.1038/sj.ijo.0802758

Ariza, A. J., Chen, E. H., Binns, H. J., & Christoffel, K. K. (2004). Risk factors for overweight in five- to six-year old Hispanic American children: a pilot study. *Journal of Urban Health,* Vol. 81, No. 1, pp. 150-161.

Baecke, J., & Frijters, J. (1982). A short questionnaire for the measurement of habitual physical activity in epidemiological studies. *American Journal of Clinical Nutrition,* Vol. 36, pp. 936-942.

Baird, J., Fisher, D., Lucas, P., Kleijnen, J., Roberts, H., & Law, C. (2005). Being big or growing fast: Systematic review of size and growth in infancy and later obesity. *BMJ.* doi:10.1136/bmj.38586.411273.EO (published 14 October 2005)

Baker, J.L., Gamborg, M., Heitmann, B.L., Lissner, L., Sorensen, T.I., & Rasmussen, K.M. (2008). Breastfeeding reduces postpartum weight retention. *American Journal of Clinical Nutrition,* Vol. 88, pp. 1543-1551.

Baker J.L., Michaelsen, K.F., Sorensen, T.I., & Rasmussen, K.M. (2007). High prepregnant body mass index is associated with early termination of full and any breastfeeding in Danish women. *American Journal of Clinical Nutrition,* Vol. 86, No. 2, pp. 404-411.

Barker, D.J. (1990). The fetal and infant origins of adult disease. *BMJ,* Vol. 301, No. 6761, p. 1111.

Barker, D.J., Winter, P.D., Osmond, C., Margetts, B. & Simmonds, S.J. (1989). Weight in infancy and death from ischaemic heart disease. *Lancet,* Vol. 2, No. 8663, pp. 577-580.

Barnard, K., Hammond, M., Booth, C., Bee, H., Mitchell, S., & Spieker, S. (1989). Measurement and meaning of parent–child interaction. In: F. Morrison, C. Lord, D. Keating (Eds.), *Applied Developmental Psychology,* Vol. III (pp. 39–80). Academic Press, ISBN: 0120412039, New York.

Barsh, G.S., Faroogi, I.S., & O'Rahilly, S. (2000). Genetics of body-weight regulation. *Nature,* Vol. 404, No. 6778, pp. 644-651.

Birch, L.L., & Fisher, J.O. (1998). Development of eating behaviors among children and adolescents. *Pediatrics,* Vol. 101(3 Pt 2), pp. 539-549.

Birch, L.L., & Fisher, J.O. (2000). Mothers' child-feeding practices influence daughters' eating and weight. *American Journal of Clinical Nutrition,* Vol. 71, No. 5, pp. 1054-1061.

Birch, L.L., & Ventura A. K. (2009). Preventing childhood obesity: what works? *International Journal of Obesity,* Vol. 33, S74-S81.

Bronfenbrenner, U. (1979). *The ecology of human development;* Cambridge, MA: Harvard University.

Burke, V., Beilin, L.J., & Dunbar, D. (2001). Family lifestyle and parental body mass index as predictors of body mass index in Australian children: a longitudinal study. *International Journal of Obesity,* Vol. 25, No. 2, pp. 147-157.

Campbell, K., Hesketh, K., Crawford, D., Salmon, J., Ball, K., & McCallum, Z. (2009. The infant feeding activity and nutrition trial (INFANT) an early intervention to prevent childhood obesity: cluster randomized controlled trial. BMC Public Health, Vol. 8, No. 103, doi:10.1186/1471-2458-8-103

Castro, F.G. (2007). Is acculturation really detrimental to health? American Journal of Public Health, Vol. 97, No. 7, p. 1162.

Centers for Disease Control and Prevention (CDC). (2007). Breastfeeding trends and updated national health objectives for exclusive breastfeeding—United States, birth years 2000-2004. *MMWR - Morbidity & Mortality Weekly Report*, Vol. 56, No. 30, pp. 760-763.

Centers for Disease Control and Prevention (CDC). (2010). Breastfeeding report card—United States, 2010. Accessed August 21, 2010, available from: http://www.cdc.gov/breastfeeding/pdf/BreastfeedingReportCard2010.pdf

Chapman, D.J., & Perez-Escamilla, R. (2000). Maternal perception of the onset of lactation is a valid, public health indicator of lactogenesis stage II. *Journal of Nutrition*,Vol. 130, No. 12, pp. 2972-2980.

Cheung, Y.B., Low, L., Osmond, C., Barker, D., & Karlberg J. (2000). Fetal growth and early postnatal growth are related to blood pressure in adults. *Hypertension*, Vol. 36, No. 5, pp. 795-800.

Chivers, P., Hands, B., Parker, H., Bulsara, M., Beilin. L.J., Kendall, G.E., & Oddy, W.H. (2010). Body mass index, adiposity rebound and early feeding in a longitudinal cohort (Raine Study). *International Journal of Obesity*, Vol. 34, No. 7 (July), pp. 1169-1176.

Corvalan, C., Kain, J., Weisstaub, G., & Uauy, R. (2009). Impact of growth patterns and early diet on obesity and cardiovascular factors in young children from developing countries. *Proceedings of the Nutrition Society*, Vol. 68, pp. 327-337.

Cottrell, E. C., & Ozanne, S.E. (2008). Early life programming of obesity and metabolic disease. *Physiology & Behavior*, Vol. 94, No. 1 (April 22), pp. 17-28.

Cuéllar, I., Arnold, B., & Maldonado, R. (1995). Acculturation Rating Scale for Mexican Americans–II: A revision of the original ARSMA scale. *Hispanic Journal of Behavioral Sciences*, Vol. 17, No. 3, pp. 275-304.

Curhan, G.C., Chertow, G.M., Willett, W.C., Spiegelman, D., Colditz, G.A., Manson, J.E., Speizer, F.E., & Stampfer, M.J. (1996a). Birth weight and adult hypertension and obesity in women. *Circulation*, Vol. 94, No. 6, pp. 1310-1315.

Curhan, G.C., Willett, W.C., Rimm, E.B., Spiegelman, D., Ascherio, A.L., & Stampfer, M.J. (1996). Birth weight and adult hypertension, diabetes mellitus, and obesity in US men. *Circulation*, Vol. 94, No. 12, pp. 3246-3250.

Dennison, B.A., Erb, M.S., & Jenkins, P.L. (2002). Television viewing and television in bedroom associated with overweight risk among low-income preschool children. *Pediatrics*, Vol. 109, No. 6, pp. 1028-1035.

Dennison, B.A., Rockwell, H.L., & Baker, S.L. (1997). Excessive fruit juice consumption by preschool-aged children is associated with short stature and obesity. *Pediatrics*, Vol. 99, No. 1, pp. 15-22.

de Onis, M., Garza, C.G., Victora, G., Onyango, A.W., Frongillo, E.A., & Martines, J., for the WHO Multicentre Growth Reference Study Group. (2004). The WHO Multicentre Growth Reference Study: Planning, study design, and methodology. *Food and Nutrition Bulletin*, Vol. 25 (Suppl. 1), pp. S3-S84.

Dietz, W.H. (1998). Health consequences of obesity in youth: Childhood predictors of adult disease. *Pediatrics*, Vol. 101, No. 3, part 2, pp. S518-S525.

Donath, S.M., & Amir, L.H. (2008). Maternal obesity and initiation and duration of breastfeeding: Data from the longitudinal study of Australian children. *Maternal & Child Nutrition*, Vol. 4, No. 3, pp. 163-170.

Druet, C., & Ong, K.K. (2008). Early childhood predictors of adult body composition. *Best Practice & Research Clinical Endocrinology & Metabolism,* Vol. 22, No. 3 (June), pp. 489-502.

Duerksen, S. C., Elder, J. P., Arredondo, E. M., Ayala, G. X., Slymen, D. J., Campbell, N. R., & Baquero, B. (2007). Family restaurant choices are associated with child and adult overweight status in Mexican-American families. *Journal of the American Dietetic Association,* Vol. 107, No. 5, pp. 849-853.

Epstein, L.H., & Wrotniak, B.H. (2010). Future directions for pediatric obesity treatment. *Obesity,* Vol. 18 (Suppl. 1), pp. s8-s12.

Eriksson, J., Forsen, T., Osmond, C., & Barker, D. (2003). Obesity from cradle to grave. *International Journal of Obesity & Related Metabolic Disorders: Journal of the International Association for the Study of Obesity,* Vol. 27, No. 6, pp. 722-727.

Eriksson, J.G., Forsen,T., Tuomilehto, J., Winter, P.D., Osmond, C., & Barker DJ. (1999). Catch-up growth in childhood and death from coronary heart disease: Longitudinal study. *BMJ,* Vol. 318, No. 7181, pp. 427-431.

Faith, M.S., Berman, N., Heo, M., Pietrobelli, A., Gallagher, D., Epstein, L.H., et al. (2001). Effects of contingent television on physical activity and television viewing in obese children. *Pediatrics,* Vol. 107, No. 5, pp. 1043-1048.

Fall, C. (2009). Maternal nutrition: effects on health in the next generation. *Indian Journal of Medical Research,* Vol. 130, No. 5, pp. 593-599.

Finkelstein, E.A., Fiebelkorn, I.C., & Wang, G. (2003). National medical spending attributable to overweight and obesity: How much, and who's paying? *Health Affairs. Suppl Web Exclusives.* W3-219-226.

Finkelstein, E.A., Trogdon, J.G., Cohen, J.W., & Dietz, W. (2009). Annual medical spending attributable to obesity: Payer- and service-specific estimates. *Health Affairs,* Vol. 28, No. 5, pp. w822-w831.

Fisher-Hoch, S.P., Rentfro, A.R., Salinas, J.J., Pérez, A., Brown, H.S., Reininger, B.M., et al. (2010). Socioeconomic status and prevalence of obesity and diabetes in a Mexican American community, Cameron County, Texas, 2004-2007. *Preventing Chronic Disease,* Vol. 7, No. 3. Available from: http://www.cdc.gov/pcd/issues/2010/may/09_0170.htm

Fogelholm, M., Nuutinen, O., Pasanen, M., Myohanen, E., & Saatela T. (1999). Parent-child relationship of physical activity patterns and obesity. *International Journal of Obesity & Related Metabolic Disorders: Journal of the International Association for the Study of Obesity,* Vol. 23, No. 12, pp. 1262-1268.

Gigante, D.P., Victora, C.G., & Barros, F.C. (2001). Breast-feeding has a limited long-term effect on anthropometry and body composition of Brazilian mothers. *Journal of Nutrition,* Vol. 131, No. 1, pp. 78-84.

Gill, S.L., Reifsnider, E., Mann, A.R., Villarreal, P., & Tinkle, M.B. (2004). Assessing infant breastfeeding beliefs among low-income Mexican Americans. *Journal of Perinatal* Education, Vol. 13, No. 33, pp. 39-50.

Gill, S.L., Reifsnider, E., & Lucke, J.F. (2007). Effects of support on the initiation and duration of breastfeeding. *Western Journal of Nursing Research,* Vol. 29, No. 6, pp. 708-723.

Griffiths, L.J., Smeeth, L., Hawkins, S.S., Cole, T.J., & Dezateux, C. (2009). Effects of infant feeding practice on weight gain from birth to 3 years. *Archives of Disease in Childhood,* Vol. 94, No. 8 (August), pp. 577-582.

Griffiths, L.J., Hawkins, S.S., Cole, T.J., & Dezateux, C. Millennium Cohort Study Child Health Group. (2010). Risk factors for rapid weight gain in preschool children: Findings from a UK-wide prospective study. *International Journal of Obesity,* Vol. 34, No. 4 (April), pp. 624-632.

Grote, V., von Kries, R., Closa-Monasterolo, R., Scaglioni, S., Gruszfeld, D., Sengier, A., Langhendries, J.P., et al. (2010). Protein intake and growth in the first 24 months of life. *Journal of Pediatric Gastroenterology & Nutrition,* Vol. 51 (Suppl. 3; December), pp. S117-118.

Hadar, E., & Yogev, Y. (2011). Obesity co-morbid conditions in pregnancy: Diabetes and hypertension. In: Pregnancy in the Obese Woman; Clinical Management, Deborah Conway, pp. 171-189, Wiley-Blackwell, ISBN 978-1-4051-9848-2, Oxford.

Hales, C.N., Barker, D.J., Clark, P.M., Cox, L.J., Fall, C., Osmond, C., & Winter PD. (1991). Fetal and infant growth and impaired glucose tolerance at age 64. *BMJ,* Vol. 303, No. 6809, pp. 1019-1022.

Harder, T., Bergmann, R., Kallischnigg, G. & Plagemann, A. (2005). Duration of breastfeeding and risk of overweight: A meta-analysis. *American Journal of Epidemiology,* Vol. 162, pp. 397-403.

Harder, T., Roepke, K., Diller, N., Stechling, Y., Dudenhausen, J. W., & Plagemann, A. (2009). Birth weight, early weight gain, and subsequent risk of type I diabetes: Systematic review and meta-analysis. *American Journal of Epidemiology,* Vol. 169(12), pp. 1428-1436. DOI:10.1093/aje/kwp065

Hawkins, S.S., & Law, C. (2006a). Timing and prevention of obesity-are there critical periods for intervention? *International Journal of Epidemiology,* Vol. 35, No. 4 (August), p. 1101; author reply, p. 1102.

Hawkins, S.S., & Law C. (2006b). A review of risk factors for overweight in preschool children: a policy perspective. *International Journal of Pediatric Obesity,* Vol. 1, No. 4, pp. 195-209.

He, Q. (2006). BMI monitoring in the management of obesity in toddlers. *American Family Physician,* Vol. 74, No. 9, pp. 1483-1484.

Hesketh, K.D., & Campbell, K.J. (2010). Interventions to prevent obesity in 0-5 year olds: An updated systematic review of the literature. Obesity, Vol. 18 (Suppl. 1), pp. s27-s35.

Heinig, M.J., Nommsen, L.A., Peerson, J.M., Lonnerdal, B., & Dewey, K.G. (1993). Intake and growth of breast-fed and formula-fed infants in relation to the timing of introduction of complementary foods: The DARLING study. Davis Area Research on Lactation, Infant Nutrition and Growth. *Acta Paediatrica,* Vol. 82, No. 12 (December), pp. 999-1006.

Holzhauer, S., Hokken Koelega, A.C., Ridder, M., Hofman, A., Moll, H.A., Steegers, E.A., Witteman, J.C., & Jaddoe, V.W. (2009). Effect of birth weight and postnatal weight gain on body composition in early infancy: The Generation R Study. *Early Human Development,* Vol. 85, No. 5 (May), pp. 285-290.

Horta, B. L., Bahl, R., Martines, J. C., & Victora, C. S. (2007). *Evidence on the long-term effects of breastfeeding*. Accessed August 21, 2011, available from: http://whqlibdoc.who.int/publications/2007/9789241595230_eng.pdf

Huh, S.Y., Rifas-Shiman, S.L., Taveras, E.M., Oken, E., & Gillman, M.W. (2011). Timing of solid food introduction and risk of obesity in preschool-aged children. *Pediatrics,* Vol. 127, No. 3 (March), pp. e544-551.

Huang, T.T-K., & Story, M.T. (2010). A journey just started: Renewing efforts to address childhood obesity. *Obesity,* Vol. 18 (Suppl. 1), pp. s1-s3.

Hurley, K.M., Cross, M.B., & Hughes, S.O. (2011). A systematic review of responsive feeding and child obesity in high-income countries. *Journal of Nutrition,* Vol. 141, pp. 495-501. ODFI: 10.3945/jn.110.130047

Inge, T., & Xanthakos, S. (2010). Obesity at the extremes: The eyes only see what the mind is prepared to comprehend. *Journal of Pediatrics,* Vol. 157, No. 1, pp. 3-4.

Institute of Medicine (IOM). (2011). *Early Childhood Obesity Prevention Policies.* Washington, D.C.: National Academies Press.

International Association for the Study of Obesity International Obesity Task Force. (n.d.). The global epidemic. Accessed August 21, 2011, available from: http://www.iaso.org/iotf/obesity/obesitytheglobalepidemic/

Jevitt, C., Hernandez, I., & Groer, M. (2007). Lactation complicated by overweight and obesity: Supporting the mother and newborn. *Journal of Midwifery & Women's Health,* Vol. 52, No. 6, pp. 606-613.

Johnson, S.L., & Birch, L.L. (1994). Parents' and children's adiposity and eating styles. *Pediatrics,* Vol. 94, No. 5, pp. 653-661.

Kac, G., Benicio, M.H., Velasquez-Melendez, G., Valente, J.G., & Struchiner, C.J. (2004). Gestational weight gain and prepregnancy weight influence postpartum weight retention in a cohort of Brazilian women. *Journal of Nutrition,* Vol. 134, No. 3, pp. 661-666.

Kaditis, A.G., Alexopoulos. E.I., Hatzi, F., Karadonta, I., Chaidas, K., Gourgoulianis, K., Zintzaras, E., & Syrogiannopoulos, G.A. (2008). Adiposity in relation to age as predictor of severity of sleep apnea in children with snoring. *Sleep & Breathing,* Vol. 12, No. 1, pp. 25-31.

Kaplowitz, P. B. (2008). Link between body fat and the timing of puberty. *Pediatrics,* Vol. 121 (Suppl. 3), pp. S208-S217. DOI: 10.1542/peds.2007-1813F

Keller, K.L., Pietrobelli, A., Johnson, S.L., & Faith, M.S. (2006). Maternal restriction of children's eating and encouragements to eat as the "non-shared environment": A pilot study using the Child Feeding Questionnaire. *International Journal of Obesity,* Vol. 30, No. 11, pp. 1670-1675.

Kitsantas, P., & Pawloski, L.R. (2010). Maternal obesity, health status during pregnancy, and breastfeeding initiation and duration. *Journal of Maternal-Fetal and Neonatal Medicine,* Vol. 23, No. 2 (February), pp. 135-141.

Koletzko, B., et al., European Childhood Obesity Trial Study Group. (2009). Infant feeding and later obesity risk. *Advances in Experimental Medicine & Biology,* Vol. 646, pp. 15-29.

Kramer, M. S. (1981). Do breast feeding and delayed introduction of solid foods protect against subsequent obesity? *Journal of Pediatrics,* Vol. 98, pp. 883-887.

Kramer, M.S. (2010). "Breast is best": The evidence. *Early Human Development,* Vol. 86, No. 11 (November), pp. 729-732.

Kramer, M. S., & Kakuma, R. (2002). The optimal duration of exclusive breastfeeding: A systematic review. *Cochrane Database of Systematic Reviews*, (1):CD003517. Accessed August 21, 2011, available from: http://www.who.int/nutrition/topics/optimal_duration_of_exc_bfeeding_review_eng.pdf

Kramer, M.S., Matush, L., Vanilovich, I., Platt, R.W., Bogdanovich N. Sevkovskaya Z. et al. (2009). A randomized breast-feeding promotion intervention did not reduce child obesity in Belarus. *Journal of Nutrition*, Vol. 139, No. 2 (February), pp. 417S-421S. DOI:10/3945/n.108.097675

Lamb, M. M., Dabelea, D., Yin, Xiang, Ogden, L. G., Klingensmith, G. J., Rewers, M., & Norris, J. M. (2010). Early-life predictors of higher body mass: Index in healthy children. *Annals of Nutrition & Metabolism*, Vol. 56, pp. 16-22. DOI:10.1159/000261899

Lauber, E., & Reinhardt, M. (1979). Studies on the quality of breast milk during 23 months of lactation in a rural community of the Ivory Coast. *American Journal of Clinical Nutrition*, Vol. 32, No. 5, pp. 1159-1173.

Levi, J., Segal, L. M., St. Laurent, R., & Kohn, D. (2011). F as in fat: How obesity threatens America's future 2011. Accessed August 21, 2011, available from: http://healthyamericans.org/reports/obesity2010/Obesity2010Report.pdf

Li, R., Fein, S.B., & Grummer-Strawn, L.M. (2010). Do infants fed from bottles lack self-regulation of milk intake compared with directly breastfed infants? *Pediatrics*, Vol. 125, No. 6, pp. e1386-e1393.

Li, R., Jewell, S., & Grummer-Strawn, L. (2003). Maternal obesity and breast-feeding practices. *American Journal of Clinical Nutrition*, Vol. 77, No. 4, pp. 931-936.

Li, R., Ogden, C., Ballew, C., Gillespie, C., & Grummer-Strawn, L. (2002). Prevalence of exclusive breastfeeding among US infants: the Third National Health and Nutrition Examination Survey (Phase II, 1991-1994). *American Journal of Public Health*, Vol. 92, No. 7, pp. 1107-1110.

Lightwood, J., Bibbins-Domingo, K., Coxson, P., Wang, Y.C., Williams, L., & Goldman, L. (2009). Forecasting the future economic burden of current adolescent overweight: An estimate of the coronary heart disease policy model. *American Journal of Public Health*, Vol. 99, No. 12, pp. 2230-2237.

Linne, Y., Dye, L., Barkeling, B., & Rossner, S. (2003). Weight development over time in parous women--the SPAWN study--15 years follow-up. *International Journal of Obesity & Related Metabolic Disorders: Journal of the International Association for the Study of Obesity*, Vol. 27, No. 12, pp. 1516-1522.

Lovelady, C.A. (2005). Is maternal obesity a cause of poor lactation performance? *Nutrition Reviews*, Vol. 63, No. 10, pp. 352-355.

Lucas, A., Boyes, S., Bloom, S.R., & Aynsley-Green, A. (1981). Metabolic and endocrine responses to a milk feed in six-day-old term infants: Differences between breast and cow's milk formula feeding. *Acta Paediatrica Scandinavica*, Vol. 70, No. 2 (March), pp. 195-200.

Magee, B.D., Hattis, D., & Kivel, N.M. (2004). Role of smoking in low birth weight. Journal of Reproductive Medicine, Vol. 49, No. 1, pp. 23-27.

Mangrio, E., Lindstrom, M., & Rosvall, M. (2010). Early life factors and being overweight at 4 years of age among children in Malmo, Sweden. *BMC Public Health,* Vol. 10:764, www.biomed central.com/1471-2458/10/764

McDowell, M. M., Wang, C., & Kennedy-Stephenson, J. (2008). *Breastfeeding in the United States: Findings from the National Health and Nutrition Examination Survey 1999-2006.* NCHS Data Brief, no. 5. Hyattsville, MD: National Center for Health Statistics. Accessed August 21, 2011, available from: http://www.flbreastfeeding.org/HTMLobj-899/db05.pdf

McCormick, D., Sarpong, K., Jordan, L., Ray, L., & Jain, S. (2010). Infant obesity: Are we ready to make this diagnosis? *Journal of Pediatrics,* Vol. 157, No. 1 (July), pp. 15-19.

Mericq, V., Ong, K.K., Bazaes, R., et al. (2005). Longitudinal changes in insulin sensitivity and secretion from birth to age three years in small- and appropriate-for-gestational-age children. *Diabetologia,* Vol. 48, pp. 2609–2614.

Metzger, M.W., & McDade, R.W. (2010). Breastfeeding as obesity prevention in the United States: A sibling difference model. *American Journal of Human Biology,* Vol. 22, pp. 291-296.

Michels, K.B., Willett, W.C., Graubard, B.I., Vaidya, R.L., Cantwell, M.M., Sansbury, L.B., & Forman, M.R. (2007). A longitudinal study of infant feeding and obesity throughout life course. *International Journal of Obesity,* Vol. 31, No. 7 (July), pp. 1078-1085.

Mizutani, T., Suzuki, K., Kondo, N., & Yamagata, Z. (2007). Association of maternal lifestyles including smoking during pregnancy with childhood obesity. *Obesity,* Vol. 15, No. 12 (December), pp. 3133-3139.

Monasta, L., Batty, G.D., Cattaneo, A., Lutje, V., Ronfani, L., Van Lenthe, F.J., & Brug, J. (2010). Early-life determinants of overweight and obesity: a review of systematic reviews. *Obesity Reviews,* Vol. 11, No. 10 (October), pp. 695-708.

Monasta, L., Batty, G.D., Macaluso, A., Ronfani, L., Lutje, V., Bacvar, A, . . . & Cattaneo, A. (2010). Interventions for the prevention of overweight and obesity in preschool children: A systematic review of randomized control trials. *Obesity Reviews,* Vol. 12, pp. e107-e118. DOI:10/1111/j.1467-2010.00774.x

Monteiro, P.O.A., & Victora, C.G. (2005). Rapid growth in infancy and childhood and obesity in later life – a systematic review. *Obesity Reviews* 6, 143-154.

Montgomery, S.M., Ehlin, A., & Ekborn, A. (2005). Smoking during pregnancy and bulimia nervosa in offspring. *Journal of Perinatal Medicine,* Vol. 33, No. 3, pp. 206-211.

Moran, O., & Phillip, M. (2003). Leptin: Obesity, diabetes, and other peripheral effects—A review. *Pediatric Diabetes,* Vol. 4, pp. 101-109.

Morrison, J.A., Glueck, C.J., Horn, P.S., Schreiber, G.B., & Wang, P. (2008). Pre-teen insulin resistance predicts weight gain, impaired fasting glucose, and type 2 diabetes at age 18–19 y: A 10-y prospective study of black and white girls. *American Journal of Clinical Nutrition,* Vol. 88, No. 3, pp. 778-788.

Morrison, J.A., Glueck, C.J., & Wang, P. (2010). Preteen insulin levels interact with caloric intake to predict increases in obesity at ages 18 to 19 years: A 10-year prospective study of black and white girls. *Metabolism: Clinical & Experimental,* Vol. 59, No. 5, pp. 718-727.

Morrow, D.A. (1976). Fat cow syndrome. *Journal Dairy Science,* Vol. 87, pp. 672-679.

Mouton, C., Calmbach, W., Dhanda, R., Espino, D., & Hazuda, H. (2000). Barriers and benefits to leisure time physical activity among older Mexican Americans. *Archives in Family Medicine,* Vol. 9, pp. 892-897.

Moynihan, A.T., Hehir, M.P., Glavey, S.V., Smith, T.J., & Morrison, J.J. (2006). Inhibitory effect of leptin on human uterine contractility in vitro. *American Journal of Obstetrics & Gynecology,* Vol. 195, No. 2, pp. 504-509.

Must, A., & Anderson, S.E. (2003). Effects of obesity on morbidity in children and adolescents. *Nutrition in Clinical Care,* Vol. 6, No. 1, pp. 4-11.

Neutzling, M. B., Hallal, P. R. C, Araujo, C. L. P., Horta, B. L., Vieira, M. F. A., Menezes, A. M. B., & Victora, C. G. (2009). Infant feeding and obesity at 11 years: Prospective birth cohort study. *International Journal of Pediatric Obesity,* Vol. 4, pp. 143-149. DOI:10.1080/17477160802453530

Oddy, W.H., Li, J., Landsborough, L., Kendall, G.E., Henderson, S., & Downie, J. (2006). The association of maternal overweight and obesity with breastfeeding duration. *Journal of Pediatrics,* Vol. 149, No. 2, pp. 185-191.

Olstad, D. L., & McCargar, L. (2009). Prevention of overweight and obesity in children under the age of 6 years.

Applied Physiology, Nutrition, & Metabolism, Vol. 34, No. 4, pp. 551-570.

Ong, K.K., & Loos, R.F. (2006). Rapid infancy weight gain and subsequent obesity: systematic reviews and hopeful suggestions. *Acta Paediatrica,* Vol. 95, pp. 904-908.

Ong, K.K., et al., ALSPAC Study Team. (2006). Dietary energy intake at the age of 4 months predicts postnatal weight gain and childhood body mass index. *Pediatrics,* Vol. 117, No.3, pp. e503-508.

Owen, C.G., Martin, R.M., Whincup, P.H., Smith, G.D., & Cook, D.G. (2005). Effect of infant feeding on the risk of obesity across the life course: A quantitative review of published evidence. *Pediatrics,* Vol. 115, pp. 1367-1377. DOI:10.1542/peds.2004-1176

Owen, C.G., Martin, R.M., Whincup, P.H., Smith, G.D., & Cook, D. G. (2006). Does breastfeeding influence risk of type 2 diabetes in later life? A quantitative analysis of published evidence. *American Journal of Clinical Nutrition,* Vol. 84, pp. 1043-1054.

Palou, A., & Picó, C. (2009). Leptin intake during lactation prevents obesity and affects food intake and food preferences in later life. *Appetite,* Vol. 52, pp. 249-252.

Pfeuffer, M., & Schrezenmeir, J. (2007). Milk and the metabolic syndrome. Obesity *Reviews, Vol. 8, No. 2, pp. 109-118.*

Plagemann, A., & Harder T. (2009). Hormonal programming in perinatal life: Leptin and beyond. *British Journal of Nutrition,* Vol. 101, No. 2, pp. 151-152.

Polhamus, B., Dalenius, K., Mackentosh, H., Smith, B., & Grummer-Strawn, L. (2009). *Pediatric Nutrition Surveillance 2008 Report.* Atlanta, GA: U.S. Department of Health and Human Services, Centers for Disease Control and Prevention.

Rasmussen, K.M. (2007). Association of maternal obesity before conception with poor lactation performance. *Annual Review of Nutrition,* Vol. 27, pp. 103-121.

Rasmussen, K.M., & Kjolhede, C.L. (2004). Prepregnant overweight and obesity diminish the prolactin response to suckling in the first week postpartum. *Pediatrics,* Vol. 113, No. 5, pp. e465-471.

Rasmussen, K., & Kjolhede, C. (2008). Maternal obesity: A problem for both mother and child. *Obesity,* Vol. 16, No. 5, pp. 929-931.

Rasmussen, K.M., Lee, V.E., Ledkovsky, T.B., & Kjolhede, C.L. (2006). A description of lactation counseling practices that are used with obese mothers. *Journal of Human Lactation,* Vol. 22, No. 3, pp. 322-327.

Reifsnider, E. (2011). Breastfeeding and contraception. In: Pregnancy in the Obese Woman; Clinical Management, Ed. Deborah Conway, pp. 217-233., Wiley-Blackwell, ISBN 978-1-4051-9848-2, Oxford.

Reifsnider, E. (1995). The use of human ecology and epidemiology in nonorganic failure to thrive. *Public Health Nursing,* Vol. 12, No. 4, pp. 262-268.

Reifsnider, E., Allan, J., & Percy, M. (2000a). Mothers' explanatory models of lack of child growth. *Public Health Nursing,* Vol. 17, No. 6, pp. 434-442.

Reifsnider, E., Allan, J, & Percy, M. (2000b). Low-income mothers' perceptions of health in their children with growth delay. *Journal of the Society of Pediatric Nurses,* Vol. 5, No. 3, pp. 122-130.

Reifsnider, E., Flores-Vela, A.R., Beckman-Mendez, D., Nguyen, H., Keller, C., & Dowdall-Smith, S. (2006). Perceptions of children's body sizes among mothers living on the Texas-Mexico border (La Frontera). *Public Health Nursing,* Vol. 23, No. 6, pp. 488-495.

Reifsnider, E., Gallagher, M., & Forgione, B. (2005). Using ecological models in research on health disparities. *Journal of Professional Nursing,* Vol. 21, No. 4, pp. 216-222.

Reifsnider, E., Gill, S., Villarreal, P., & Tinkle, M.B. (2003). Breastfeeding attitudes of WIC staff: A descriptive study. *Journal of Perinatal Education,* Vol. 12, No. 3, pp. 7-15.

Reifsnider, E., & Ritsema, M. (2008). Ecological differences in weight, length, and weight for length of Mexican American children in the WIC program. *Journal for Specialists in Pediatric Nursing,* Vol. 13, No. 3, pp. 154-167.

Risnes, K.R., Vatten, L.J., Baker, J.L, Jameson, K., Sovio, U., Kajantie, E., et al. (2011). Birthweight and mortality in adulthood: a systematic review and meta-analysis. *International Journal of Epidemiology,* Vol. 40, No. 3, pp. 647-661.

Rodriguez-Artalejo, F., Garces, C., Gorgojo, L., Lopez Garcia, E., Martin-Moreno, J.M., Benavente, M., et al. (2002). Investigators of the four provinces study: Dietary patterns among children aged 6-7 y in four Spanish cities with widely differing cardiovascular mortality. *European Journal of Clinical Nutrition,* Vol. 56, pp. 141-148.

Rutishauser, I.H., & Carlin, J.B. (1992). Body mass index and duration of breast feeding: a survival analysis during the first six months of life. *Journal of Epidemiology & Community Health,* Vol. 46, No. 6, pp. 559-565.

Rzehak, P. , Sausenthaler, S., Koletzko, S., Bauer, C.P., Schaaf, B., von Berg, et al. (2009). Period-specific growth, overweight and modification by breastfeeding in the GINI and LISA birth cohorts up to age 6 years. *European Journal of Epidemiology,* Vol. 24, No. 8, pp. 449-467.

Satcher, D. (2011). Personal commentary: The Surgeon General looks back and forward: Some progress, but not enough. Accessed August 22, 2011, available from: http://healthyamericans.org/reports/obesity2010/Obesity2010Report.pdf

Saunders, K. L. (2007). Preventing obesity in pre-school children: A literature review. *Journal of Public Health,* Vol. 29, pp. 368-375. DOI:10/1093/pubmed/fdm061

Scaglioni, S., Agostoni, C., Notaris, R., Radaelli, G., Radice, N., et al. (2000). Early macronutrient intake and overweight at five years of age. *International Journal of*

Obesity & Related Metabolic Disorders: Journal of the International Association for the Study of Obesity, Vol. 24, No. 6 (June), pp. 777-781.

Schack-Nielsen, L., Sorensen, T., Mortensen, E., & Michaelsen, K. (2010). Late introduction of complementary feeding, rather than duration of breastfeeding, may protect against adult overweight. *American Journal of Clinical Nutrition*, Vol. 91, No. 3, pp. 619-627.

Scholl, T.O. (2008). Maternal nutrition before and during pregnancy. *Nestle Nutrition Workshop Series. Paediatric Programme*, Vol. 61, pp. 79-89.

Schwarz, E., Ray, R., Stuebe, A., Allison, M., Ness, R. et al. (2009). Duration of lactation and risk factors for maternal cardiovascular disease. *Obstetrics & Gynecology*, Vol. 113, No. 5, pp. 974-982.

Seach, K.A., Dharmage, S.C., Lowe, A.J., & Dixon, J.B. (2010). Delayed introduction of solid feeding reduces child overweight and obesity at 10 years. *International Journal of Obesity*, Vol. 34, pp. 1475-1479.

Sebire, N., Jolly, M., Harris, J., Wadsworth, J., Joffe, M. et al. (2001). Maternal obesity and pregnancy outcome: A study of 287,213 pregnancies in London. *International Journal of Obesity & Related Metabolic Disorders: Journal of the International Association for the Study of Obesity*, Vol. 25, No. 8, pp. 1175-1182.

Shrago, L., Reifsnider, E., & Insel, K. (2006). The Neonatal Bowel Output Study: Indicators of adequate breast milk intake in neonates. *Pediatric Nursing*, Vol. 32, No. 3, pp. 195-201.

Simon, V., de Sousa, J., & de Sousa, S. (2008). Breastfeeding, complementary feeding, overweight and obesity in pre-school children. *Rev Saúde Pública*, Vol. 43, No. 1, pp. 1-9.

Skinner, A., Steiner, M., Henderson, F., & Perrin, E. (2010). Multiple markers of inflammation and weight status: cross-sectional analyses throughout childhood. *Pediatrics*, Vol. 125, No. 4, pp. e801-809.

Story, M., Holt, K., & Sofka, D. (2002). *Bright Futures in Practice: Nutrition* (2nd ed.). National Center for Education in Maternal and Child Health, Arlington, VA.

Sturm, R. (2002).The effects of obesity, smoking, and drinking, on medical problems, and costs. *Health Affairs*, Vol. 21, No. 2, pp. 245-253.

Summerbell, C., Waters, E., Edmunds, L., Kelly, S., Brown, T., et al. (2005). Interventions for preventing obesity in children. *Cochrane Database of Systematic Reviews* 2005, Issue 8. DOI:10.1002/14651858.CD001871.pub2

Sussner, K., Lindsay, A., & Peterson, K. (2009).The influence of maternal acculturation on child body mass index at age 24 months. *Journal of the American Dietetic Association*, Vol. 109, No. 2, pp. 218-225.

Taveras, E., Gilman, M., Kleinman, K., Rich-Edwards, J. & Rifas-Shiman, S. (2010). Racial-ethnic differences in early life risk factors for childhood obesity. *Pediatrics*, Vol. 125, No. 4, pp. 686-695. DOI:10.1542/peds.2009-2100

Toschke, A., Montgomery, S., Pfeiffer, U., & von Kries, R. (2003a). Early intrauterine exposure to tobacco-inhaled products and obesity. *American Journal of Epidemiology*, Vol. 158, No. 11 (December 1), pp. 1068-1074.

Toschke, A., Ehlin, A., von Kries, R., Ekbom, A., & Montgomery S. (2003b). Maternal smoking during pregnancy and appetite control in offspring. *Journal of Perinatal Medicine*, Vol. 31, No. 3, pp. 251-256.

Treviño, R., Fogt, D., Jordan Wyatt, T., Leal-Vasquez, L., Sosa, E., & Woods, C. (2008). Diabetes risk, low fitness, and energy insufficiency levels among children from poor families. *Journal of the American Dietetic Association,* Vol. 108, No. 11, pp. 1846-1853.

UNICEF. (n.d.) Infant and young child feeding. Accessed August 21, 2011, available from: http://www.unicef.org/nutrition/index_breastfeeding.html

Valente, T., Fujimoto, K., Chou, C., & Spruijt-Metz, D. (2009). Adolescent affiliations and adiposity: A social network analysis of friendships and obesity. *Journal of Adolescent Health,* Vol. 45, No. 2, pp. 202-204.

Walker, L., Freeland-Graves, J.H., Milani, T., Hanss-Nuss, H., George, G., et al. (2004). Weight and behavioral and psychosocial factors among ethnically diverse, low-income women after childbirth: II: Trends and Correlates. *Women & Health,* Vol. 40, No. 2, pp. 19-34.

Ward-Begnoche, W., Gance-Cleveland, B., & Portilla, M. (2009). Circumventing communication barriers with Spanish-speaking patients regarding pediatric obesity. *Journal of Pediatric Health Care,* Vol. 23, No. 4, pp. 272-280.

Wardle, J., Guthrie, C., Sanderson, S., Birch, L., & Plomin, R. (2001). Food and activity preferences in children of lean and obese parents. *International Journal of Obesity,* Vol. 25, No. 7, pp. 971-977.

Warner, M.J., & Ozanne, S.E. (2010). Mechanisms involved in the developmental programming of adulthood disease. *Biochemical Journal,* Vol. 427, No. 3 (May 1), pp. 333-347.

Wasser, H., Bentley, M., Borja, J., Davis Goldman, B., Thompson, A. et al. (2011). Infants perceived as "fussy" are more likely to receive complementary foods before 4 months. *Pediatrics,* Vol. 127, No. 2 (February), pp. 229-237.

Welsh, J.A., Cogswell, M.E., Rogers, S., Rockett, H., Mei, Z., et al. (2005). Overweight among low-income preschool children associated with consumption of sweet drinks: Missouri, 1999-2002. *Pediatrics,* Vol. 115, No. 2, pp. e223-229.

Whincup, P., Kaye, S., Owen, C., Huxley, R., Cook, D., Anazawa, S., et al. (2008). Birth weight and risk of type 2 diabetes: A systematic review. *JAMA,* Vol. 300, No. 24, pp. 2886-2897.

White House Task Force on Childhood Obesity. (2010). Early childhood: Breastfeeding, "Solving the problem of childhood obesity within a generation," an excerpt from the White House Task Force on Childhood Obesity: Report to the president, May, 2010. *Breastfeeding Medicine,* Vol. 5, No. 5 (October), pp. 205-206. DOI:10.1089/bfm.2010.9980

World Health Organization (WHO). (2006). Nutrition data banks: Global data bank on breastfeeding). Accessed August 21, 2011, available from: https://apps.who.int/nut/db_bfd.htm

World Health Organization. (n.d.[a]). Global strategy on diet, physical activity and health: Child overweight and obesity. Retrieved August 22, 2011 from http://www.who.int/dietphysicalactivity/childhood/en/

World Health Organization. (n.d.[b]) Global strategy on diet, physical activity and health: What are the causes? Reasons for children and adolescents to become obese. Accessed August 22, 2011, available from: http://www.who.int/dietphysicalactivity/childhood_why/en/index.html

Zemel, M. B. (2005). The role of dairy foods in weight management. *Journal of the American College of Nutrition, Vol. 24, No. 6 (Suppl.), pp. 537S-546S.*

Ziol-Guest, K.M., & Hernandez, D.C. (2010). First- and second-trimester WIC participation is associated with lower rates of breastfeeding and early introduction of cow's milk during infancy. *Journal of the American Dietetic Association*, Vol. 110, No. 5, pp. 702-709.

3

Can Breastfeeding Reduce the Risk of Childhood Obesity?

Laurie Twells, Leigh Anne Newhook and Valerie Ludlow
Memorial University
Canada

1. Introduction

Over the last two decades, rates of childhood obesity have increased to a point where the World Health Organization (WHO) has described it as "globesity" to indicate the "escalating global epidemic of overweight and obesity" (WHO, 2011). A number of factors have been identified that increase the risk of childhood obesity, including: high birth weight (Apfelbacher et al., 2008), mother's pre-pregnancy Body Mass Index (BMI) (Catalano et al., 2009; Gibson et al., 2007; Vos & Welsh, 2010), weight gain through pregnancy and diabetes in mother (Boney et al., 2005), mother's/father's BMI (Moens et al., 2009; Whitaker et al., 1997), early introduction of solid foods (Huh et al., 2011) and screen time (Fulton et al., 2009; Sisson et al., 2009), lower educational level, smoking in the home, and breastfeeding for less than three months (Apfelbacher et al., 2008). In some studies, low socioeconomic status (SES) and household income levels are seen as predictors (Veugelers & Fitzgerald, 2005; Vieweg et al., 2007); conversely, other studies have reported high socioeconomic status as a predictor (Cui et al., 2010). In addition, living in a single-parent family has been cited as a predictor of childhood obesity (Gibson et al., 2007), while maternal psychopathology has been shown to be an inconsistent predictor of childhood obesity (Gibson et al., 2007; McConley et al., 2011).

Childhood obesity can have very serious short and long term adverse health consequences on quality of life, performance achieved and long term health and life expectancy. It is estimated that the obesity epidemic will increase both direct and indirect costs to society and the health care and social insurance systems. One major concern is that obesity has been shown to track through the lifecycle. Obese children most often become obese adolescents (Deshmukh-Taskar et al., 2006) and obese adolescents have a 33% increase in the probability of having a life threatening event before the age of 60 (Baker et al., 2007).

There are few proven treatment options for either obese children or obese adults and those that do exist tend to be costly (Flodgren et al., 2010; Summerbell et al., 2004). Many feel the emphasis must be on the primary prevention of childhood obesity. It has been suggested that early infant nutrition may be one important factor in this pursuit. There are many well-evidenced reasons to support breastfeeding as it relates to the improved health of the mother and baby, but research that exists on breastfeedng as a public health obesity intervention is equivocal. The objectives of this chapter are to 1) describe the epidemiology of childhood obesity and its related comorbid conditions 2) discuss the biology of breastmilk and to explain how it differs in constituents and method of delivery from infant formula and 3) to summarize the high level research (i.e., systematic reviews and meta analysis) that examines the relationship between breastfeeding and childhood obesity.

1.1 Definition of obesity/childhood obesity

Obesity is defined as excessive accumulation of fatty tissue that can hinder the effective functioning of the human body (WHO, 2000). As a result, health problems may ensue, leading to a poor quality of life and decreased lifespan. When seen in childhood, the issues of obesity can be far more extensive, as health problems occur earlier in life and place a burden on the child, family, community and health care system.

The calculations that determine obesity in children are not as clear-cut as one might think. It has been suggested that the standard BMI (weight (kg)/height (m^2)) should not be used as the sole measurement, since children's height and weight vary greatly during major growth spurts (Logue & Sattar, 2011). In addition, waist circumference should be included in the calculation, as central obesity is considered a major risk factor for Type 2 Diabetes Mellitus (DM) and Coronary Artery Disease (CAD) (Kovacs et al., 2010; Steene-Johannessen et al., 2010; Stevens et al., 2010).

Currently, the classification of overweight and obesity varies among major agencies (Table 1). The US Centre for Disease Control (CDC), International Obesity Task Force (IOTF) and WHO base their determinations on different populations during different time periods. The CDC surveyed American children from 1963-1994 (National Centre for Health Statistics, 2002). In 2000, the IOTF based their criteria on children from US, Brazil, Great Britain, Hong Kong, Netherlands and Singapore (Cole et al., 2000). In comparison, in 2006, the WHO collected data on children from US, Brazil, Ghana, India, Oman and Norway (WHO Multicentre Growth Reference Study Group, 2006) who lived in optimal health conditions, and were exclusively/primarily breastfed for up to 4 months, with some breastfeeding extending until 12 months of age. Using information and extrapolating for children, the cut-off points are given below. These guidelines should be considered when reviewing data on obesity rates in various reports, as different definitions provide varying prevalence estimates. For example the CDC cut-offs tend to report a much higher prevalence of obesity compared to the other growth references (Twells & Newhook, 2011).

Another point to consider is whether or not growth charts for infants (based on age) should be modified based on infant feeding method. Formula fed children grow faster than those who are breastfed (Dewey, 1998; Kramer et al., 2004; Victora et al., 1998), possibly due to the higher protein content of formula versus breast milk, which should be considered when referring to patterns of infant growth (Alexy et al., 1999; Koletzko et al., 2005). Even with guidelines, such as those from CDC, IOTF, and WHO, it is suggested that childhood overweight and obesity are often underdiagnosed. The development of a better diagnostic tool may be beneficial, since it is within childhood that interventions might prove to be more effective (Benson, 2009).

	US CDC	IOTF	WHO
Overweight	>85th	≥91st	>84th
Obese	≥95th	≥99th	>97.7th

Table 1. Childhood obesity rankings (percentile)

1.2 Global prevalence of childhood obesity

The prevalence of obesity is increasing throughout the world, particularly among children. In 2008, 1.5 billion adults (20 and older) were overweight; comparatively in 2010, 43 million children under the age of 5 were overweight (WHO, 2011a).

Human obesity develops as a result of interactions between genes, environmental factors, and behaviour. It has been found that genetic disorders such as Bardet-Biedl and Prader-Willi syndromes can directly cause obesity and, as a result of the study of twins and adopted children, heritability estimates of 40–70% have been reported (Farooqi & O'Rahilly, 2006). The relatively recent rise in global obesity rates over the last 25 years however suggest that mainly environmental factors are involved. Current environmental and lifestyle issues (social, behavioural, cultural and community) which promote an imbalance between energy intake and energy expenditure are purported to be the main causes of increasing obesity rates. The sedentary lifestyle and high-caloric diet seen in many populations have led to alarming rates of childhood obesity. As shown in Figure 1, since 1976 the United States has seen a surge in obesity rates among all age groups of children; particularly, obesity rates among preschool children aged 2-5 increased from 5.0% to 10.4% over the 1976/1980 to the 2007/2008 time span (Ogden & Carroll, 2010). Similar increases have been reported in regional populations in Canada (Canning et al., 2007).

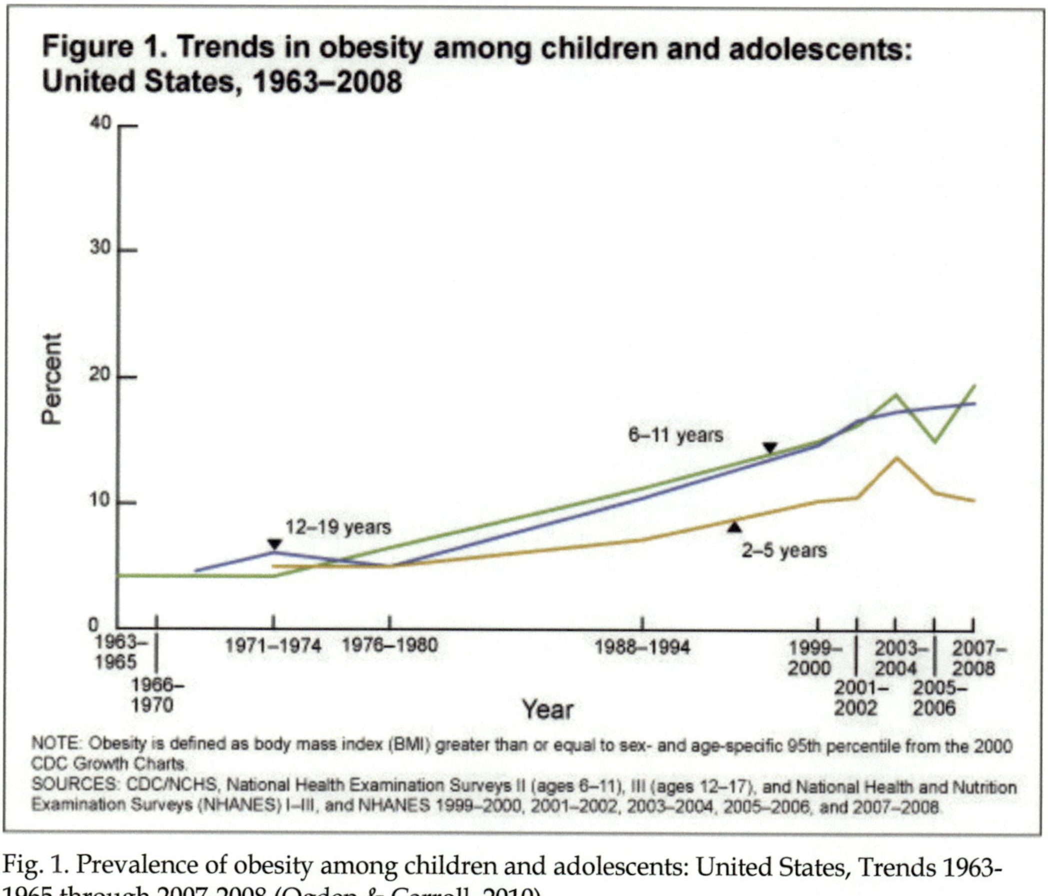

Fig. 1. Prevalence of obesity among children and adolescents: United States, Trends 1963-1965 through 2007-2008 (Ogden & Carroll, 2010).

Geographical differences in childhood obesity are also being observed. As can be seen in Figures 2 and 3, the 2010 worldwide prevalence varies among countries. Obesity rates are rising in low and middle income countries, a trend which had been previously seen in high income countries (WHO, 2011b). Although in the early 2000s Scandinavian countries had lower childhood obesity rates than Mediterranean, their rates (along with those of the US, Japan, United Kingdom, Spain, France and Greece) showed major increases throughout (Dehghan et al., 2005). Interestingly, more recent studies indicate that in France, Switzerland, Sweden, the US and UK, the childhood obesity trends appear to be stabilizing (Stamatakis et al., 2010; The Health and Social Care Information Centre, 2010). It has been suggested that in developed countries, the childhood obesity epidemic may be slowing as a result of increased awareness and policy programs that have been put in place in very recent years (Stamatakis et al., 2010).

Additionally, there is discussion regarding rural versus urban childhood obesity rates. Several authors (Bruner et al., 2008; Ismailov & Leatherdale, 2010; Simen-Kapeu et al., 2010) found that rural Canadian children were more likley to be overweight/obese; however, the WHO stated in 2011 that obesity is rising in urban settings (WHO, 2011a).

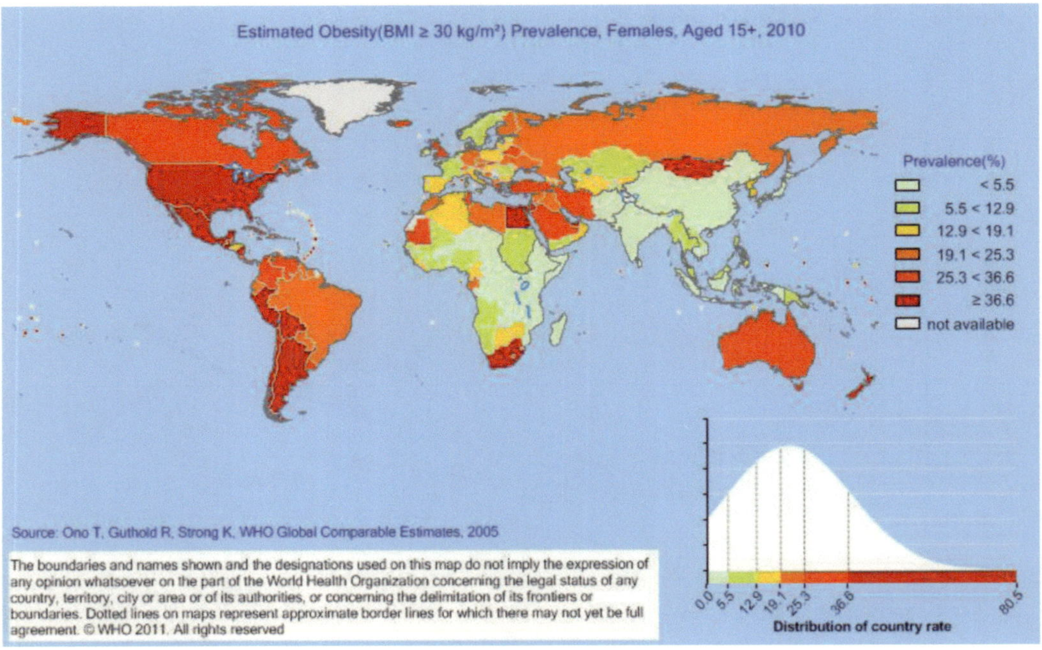

Fig. 2. Estimated Obesity Prevalence in Females 15 years and over, 2010 (WHO, 2011b).

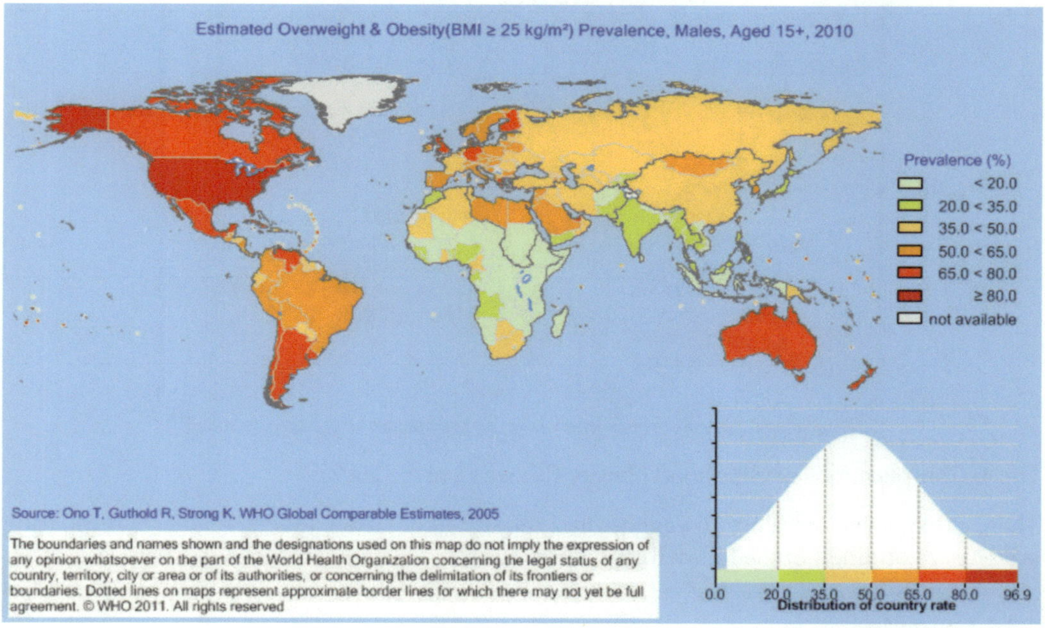

Fig. 3. Estimated Obesity Prevalence in Males, 15 years and over, 2010 (WHO, 2011b).

1.3 Health consequences of obesity

Overweight and obesity are responsible for 2.8 million adult deaths per year and add to the burden on the healthcare system, in particular, 44% of Diabetes Mellitus, 23% of Ischemic Heart Disease, and 7-41% of certain types of cancers (WHO, 2011a). Even more alarming is that childhood obesity puts the child at risk for disease in most of the body systems (see Figure 4) even before it predisposes the person to future adult obesity/ disability and premature death. As adiposity and age increase, if the child's body mass does not normalize, the obesity will track into adolescence and then adulthood (Biro, 2010). This may result in cardiovascular effects (raised systolic blood pressure and structural cardiac enlargement) (Logue & Sattar, 2011) and a potentially life threatening event. Interestingly, it was found that being an obese adolescent increased one's risk for adult morbidities, even if the person achieved normal weight during adulthood (Biro, 2010).

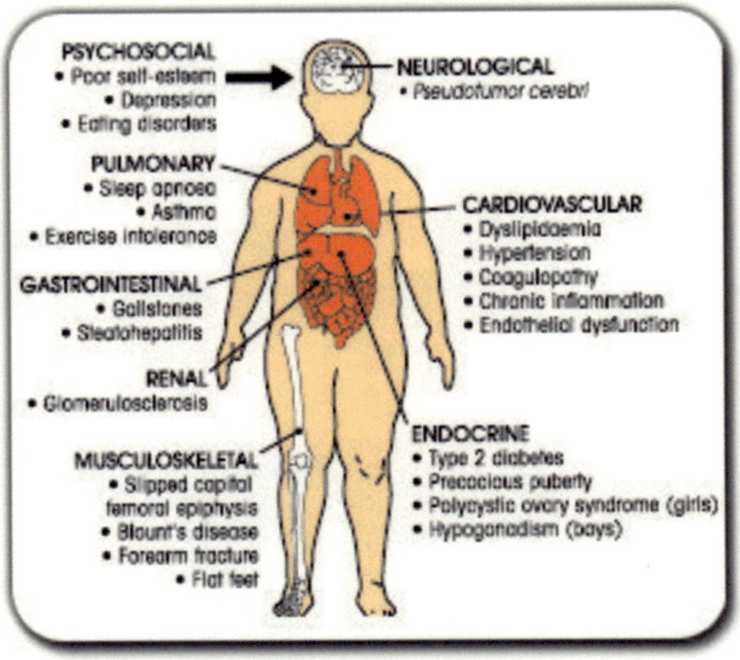

Fig. 4. Complications of childhood obesity (Ebbeling et al., 2002).

There is extensive evidence to suggest that obesity in children adversely affects most body systems, as outlined in the following sections.

1.3.1 Endocrine

Even though the definition of **Type 2 Diabetes Mellitus (DM)** has recently been updated to include an elevated glycated haemoglobin of at least 6.5 (Abrams & Levitt Katz, 2011), obese children are being treated for ketoacidosis as a result of an inadequate insulin response and before receiving a diagnosis of DM (Abrams & Levitt Katz, 2011; Stamatakis et al., 2010). When you add central abdominal obesity, hypertension, and dyslipidemia (lowered High Density Lipoproteins and raised triglycerides) to DM, a **metabolic syndrome** is identified in the child (Nyberg et al., 2011; Philippi-Hohn, 2010). This has been recognized as a predictor for higher cardiovascular morbidity/mortality in adults (Abrams & Levitt Katz, 2011).

Leukocyte telomere lengths (LTL) are DNA-protein complexes, found at the end of linear chromosomes, that protect those chromosome ends from degradation. In adults, shortened LTLs are associated with cardiovascular disease, Type 2 DM, insulin resistance, impaired glucose tolerance, and hypertension. In a large case controlled study of LTLs in obese children, prepubescent and pubescent males and females (< 9 years of age) were found to have significantly shorter lengths, putting them at greater risk to develop these health issues during adulthood (Buxton et al., 2011).

Androgen (male) hormones are present in adipose tissue. In the presence of obesity, these levels increase leading to hyperandrogenism, a medical condition characterized by excessive production and/or secretion of androgens. In women, these high levels of the male hormone, along with irregular menstruation and obesity, can lead to polycystic ovarian syndrome, which can subsquently develop into female subfertility (Abrams & Levitt Katz, 2011).

1.3.2 Renal

Obesity is linked to **end-stage renal disease (ESRD)** and **chronic kidney disease (CKD)** (Savino et al., 2011). Obese children have shown a significant positive correlation between microalbuminemia and BMI (Savino et al., 2011), waist circumference, systolic and diastolic blood pressure (Savino et al., 2011), insulin resistance and fasting glucose level (Sanad & Gharib, 2011). Subjects who had microalbuminemia were found to have a lower High Density Lipoprotein (HDL) cholesterol, and higher Low Density Lipoprotein (LDL) cholesterol and triglycerides (Sanad & Gharib, 2011). This is significantly associated with **metabolic syndrome**. Metabolic syndrome, alone, is an independent risk factor for **ESRD** and **CKD** (Sanad & Gharib, 2011; Savino et al., 2011) in adults.

Nitrous oxide (NO) is an important modulator of renal function and structure and, when impaired, renal complications may ensue. An inverse relationship was seen between NO levels and obese children (Savino et al., 2011).

1.3.3 Cardiovascular

Excessive inflammation and oxidation, which are possible biochemical links between obesity and cardiovascular events in adults, have been found in young obese children. Additionally, left ventricular (LV) mass and hypertrophy, LV dysfunction, and a three-fold higher risk of early development of arterial hypertension have been found in obese children (Philippi-Hohne, 2010). These disorders predispose obese children to future cardiovascular disease (Oliver et al., 2010).

1.3.4 Gastrointestinal

Increased Gastrointestinal (GI) disturbances such as constipation, gastroesophageal reflux (Philippi-Hohne, 2010), Irritable Bowel Syndrome, and abdominal pain (Abrams & Levitt Katz, 2011) have been found in obese children. Also, in pediatric autopsies of overweight and obese children between the ages of 2-19 years, Schwimmer et al. (Abrams & Levitt Katz, 2011) found **non-alcoholic fatty livers** in the majority of cases. Twenty-three percent of those cases had progressed to steatohepatitis, which can develop into fibrosis and cirrhosis of the liver.

1.3.5 Pulmonary

With the exception of **adeno-tonsillar** involvement, significantly more obstructive apnea/hypopnea events per hour of sleep have been found in obese children (Abrams & Levitt Katz, 2011). This chronic nocturnal hypoxemia can lead to pulmonary hypertension (Philippi-Hohne, 2010), which is a precursor to lung damage. Researchers have found a significant correlation between obesity and current asthma among children and adolescents. This relationship was stronger in nonatopic (non-allergic) children as compared to atopic (allergic - positive response to at least 1 allergen) (Stamatakis et al., 2010; Visness et al., 2010).

1.3.6 Musculoskeletal

Orthopedic complications such as poor balance, pain (especially in knee joints), impaired mobility, lower extremity malignancy, and fractures requiring surgical interventions (Abrams & Levitt Katz, 2011) have all been documented in obese children.

1.3.7 Psychosocial

Interestingly, in countries considered the 'happiest' in the world, the rates of adult and childhood obesity are low (Goran & Ventura, 2011). People in Denmark, Sweden, Norway, Finland, and the Netherlands ranked their country high in meeting their psychological, social and basic needs. Childhood overweight and obesity were 17% (combined) in these countries. In Griffith et al.'s (2010) review of 42 studies, self-esteem and quality of life were significantly lower in obese youth. Physical competence, appearance, and social functioning were also compromised (Goran & Ventura, 2011). Lower self-esteem was also found in overweight and obese children (Cornette, 2008). Females who were very overweight reported lower self-esteem than females classified as moderately overweight (Cornette, 2008). Overweight/obese children were more likely to be victims and perpetrators of bullying than 'normal' weight children. Bullying experienced by overweight/obese children was generally name-calling related to their size; however, when the overweight/obese child was the bully, racial, color or religious slurs were used against the other person (Janssen et al., 2004). As well, a lower quality of life was experienced by obese children. Schwimmer et al. (2003) found that obese children rated their quality of life to be comparable with that of young cancer patients on chemotherapy. In particular, teasing at school, difficulties playing sports, fatigue, and sleep apnea greatly decreased the quality of life in these children.

1.3.8 Cancers

Although cancers do not develop until later in life, several are more prevalent in obese individuals when compared to their normal weight counterparts. Eesophageal, thyroid, colon, and renal cancers are more prevalent in obese men while endometrial, gall bladder, esophageal, adenocarcinoma, and renal cancers are more common in obese women (Biro, 2010).

2. Biology of breastmilk

In humans, early infant nutrition appears to be critically important in determining long-term positive or negative health effects. A complex fluid, breastmilk is the optimal source of nutrition for infants and appears to be a crucial factor in determining health and preventing chronic disease. The following section reviews the process of breastmilk production, the protective components of breastmilk purported to be linked with the prevention of childhood obesity, and the relationship with metabolic programming. It also contrasts breastmilk and breastfeeding with infant formula and associated methods of feeding.

2.1 Process of production

During pregnancy, the breast prepares anatomically and physiologically for infant feeding. Lactogenesis is the the production of human milk and occurs due to a complex interplay of pituitary, ovarian, thyroid, adrenal, and pancreatic hormones. Lactogenesis occurs in stages. The initiation of lactogenesis results from a fall in plasma progesterone and high prolactin levels during the post-partum period. Lactogenesis stage 1 occurs in the latter stage of pregnancy. The breast produces thick yellow colostrum and at this stage high progesterone levels inhibit milk production. Lactogenesis 2 occurs at or soon after birth progesterone levels drop and prolactin levels remain high. This results in milk production. Upon stimulation of the breast, prolactin levels in the blood rise, peak in about 45 minutes, and return to the pre-breastfeeding state about three hours later. The release of prolactin triggers the cells in the alveoli to make milk. During lactogenesis stage 3, the more that milk is removed from the breasts, the more the breast will produce milk. Milk supply depends strongly on how often the baby feeds and how well it is able to transfer milk from the breast. At two-three days post-partum, when mothers usually feel their milk "coming in", secretion of milk rapidly increases and major changes in milk composition occur over the next ten days. The changes over this period subsequently result in the establishment of mature milk (Lawrence, 1999). The volume of milk increases gradually, starting at about 100ml/day increasing to about 600 ml/day by day four (Lawrence, 1999) adapting to the new infant's energy needs.

2.2 Nutritional components and properties

Human milk is not a uniform body fluid but a heterogeneous secretion of the mammary gland. Its composition is frequently changing throughout the day and throughout feedings. Breastmilk contains many bioactive factors (lactoferrin, oligosaccharides, long-chain polyunsaturated fatty acids, glycoproteins and antibodies) that do not function primarily as nutrients but may control nutrient use or play a role in regulating metabolic pathways(Labbok et al., 2004). Breastmilk also contains other biologically active factors, which include hormones, growth factors and cytokines. These are all involved in energy balance regulation and seem to be important for infant nutrition and growth(Savino et al., 2009).

Milk composition changes during a feeding period, as well as throughout the day. Concentrations of protein, fat, carbohydrates, and minerals change, in addition to osmolarity and pH. There are more than 200 components of human milk which include an assortment of several molecules, many of which have yet to be specifically determined. There are differences in foremilk and hindmilk, and colostrum differs from transitional and mature milks.

Colostrum is the first mammary secretion of lactation, and consists of a thick, yellowish fluid that is small in volume and is high in protein . Secretory immunoglobulin A (sIgA) is particularly plentiful and prominent. Transitional milk occurs next from approximately seven to ten days to two weeks postpartum. During this time the concentration of immunoglobulins and total protein decreases whereas lactose, fat, and total caloric content increases. In mature milk, water is the largest constituent. The main fats in human milk are triacylglycerols, phospholipids, and their component fatty acids. Fat concentration changes depending on many different factors and conditions. Fat provides about 50 percent of the infant's calories. Human milk also consists of casein and lactalbumin (whey) proteins. The principal carbohydrate in human milk is lactose. Human milk also contains minerals, electrolytes, trace elements, vitamins, enzymes, hormones, bile salts, and growth factors(Lawrence, 1999).

Other important compounds in breast milk are leptin, ghrelin, adiponectin, resistin. Synthesis of leptin occurs in adipose tissue (Zhang et al., 1994). Leptin production occurs in mammary glands, and epithelial cells secrete leptin in milk fat globules (Smith-Kirwin, 1998). Milk-borne leptin has been implicated not only in growth, but also in short-term appetite regulation in infancy, especially during lactation(Savino et al., 2009). Leptin in breastmilk could exert a long-term effect on energy balance and body weight composition(Savino et al., 2009).

Ghrelin is a protein produced primarily by the stomach, involved in both short-term regulation of feeding and the long-term regulation of weight and energy metabolism(Savino et al., 2009). It has many endocrine and non-endocrine functions, including energy balance regulation (Hellstrom, 2009). As a component of breastmilk, ghrelin plays a role in both short-term regulation of food intake (by stimulating appetite) and in long-term body-weight reduction (by inducing adiposity). Considering these effects, ghrelin could be one of the factors through which breastfeeding may influence infant behavior and body composition(Savino et al., 2009).
Adiponectin is the most abundant adipose-specific protein. It has multiple identified functions(Scherer et al., 1997) and a reduction in its expression is associated with insulin resistance(Savino et al., 1997). It has been shown that adiponectin levels correlate negatively with the degree of adiposity in children between five and ten years of age(Nader et al., 2002). It is present in human milk(Martin et al., 2006) and may influence infant growth and development.
Resistin is a cytokine that is secreted by adipocytes(Steppan, 2001). It is expressed in the human placenta and may play a role in the regulation of energy metabolism during pregnancy. It has also been identified in human milk(Ilcol et al., 2008) and may be important for the metabolic development of infants(Savino et al., 1997).

2.3 Learned self-regulation

One hypothesis regarding the association of breastfeeding and obesity prevention relates to the ability of breastfed infants to self-regulate their energy intake to match their energy needs (Owen et al., 2005). Infants fed directly at the breast must actively suckle to draw milk out, whereas infants are passive when being fed from a bottle. The control of caregivers in bottle-feeding could lead to infants' poor self-regulation on the basis of internal cues of hunger and satiety. Infants who are bottle-fed in early infancy are more likely to empty the bottle or cup in late infancy than those who are fed directly at the breast. Bottle-feeding, regardless of the type of milk, is distinct from feeding at the breast in its effect on infants' self-regulation of milk intake (Fein & Grummer-Strawn, 2010).
Infants who are fed from the breast can control milk intake, because they decide when to start and when to stop sucking. Mothers who breastfeed often develop a feeding style that is less controlling, thereby allowing their infants to maintain their natural ability to regulate their energy intake (Taveras et al., 2006). Also, infants fed at the breast need to suck nonnutritively until the milk-ejection reflex occurs, and it is known that as sucking pressure decreases, the duration of each suck lengthens, and suckling frequency decreases from nonnutritive sucking (NNS) to nutritive sucking (NS) (Richard & Alade, 1992). This transition from NNS to NS may play an important role in establishing infants' self-regulation of milk intake (Mizuno & Ueda, 2006).
The taste and smell of breastmilk changes from meal to meal, depending on what the mother has consumed, which exposes the breastfed infant to a wider array of sensory experiences than the formula- fed infant. It is possible that the breastfed infant may be programmed to accept a different food selection which may affect dietary habits later in life(Koletzko, 2009). These factors regarding taste and smell remain constant during bottle-feeding. For example, breast milk fat content toward the end of the feeding episode is much higher than that at the start of the feeding, which might signal to the infant that the feeding episode is coming to an end. In contrast, bottle-fed infants are not exposed to such

"physiologic signaling" during the feeding episode. Research on regulation of food intake by chemosensory receptors suggests that bottle-fed infants who had no exposure to the varied flavors of breast milk may miss the important oropharyngeal sensory experience that is needed for the development of physiologic regulation of food intake later in life (Poothullil, 1995).

2.4 Differences from formula

Infant formula tends to have a higher average caloric density compared to breast milk with higher energy supplies per kilogram of bodyweight (Heinig et al., 1993). It has been suggested that a higher protein intake in formula-fed infants could increase the risk of obesity later in life by causing an earlier adiposity rebound(Taylor et al., 2005). Adiposity rebound refers to the period of increasing body mass index after the early childhood nadir, usually at about 6 years old (Medlexicon International Limited, 2011).

Also, a higher protein intake during infancy may promote the stimulation of insulin release and the programming of higher long-term insulin concentrations. Consistent with this occurence, formula-fed infants have been found to have higher plasma insulin levels and insulin-like growth factor 1, than those who were breastfed(Lucas et al., 1981). The growth acceleration hypothesis suggests that the protective benefits of breastfeeding on the development of long-term obesity may be due to a slower pattern of growth in breastfed infants when compared with formula-fed infants(Singhal & Lucas, 2004).

3. Breastfeeding as a prevention strategy for childhood obesity

It has been suggested that the choice of early infant feeding method may impact the growth trajectory of an infant and how that infant develops through childhood, adolescence and into adulthood. A large number of primary studies and several systematic reviews and meta-analyses have compared breastfeeding to formula feeding and the subsequent development of overweight and/or obesity overtime. Many of these studies have reported an inverse relationship between breastfeeding and childhood obesity. The prevalence of childhood obesity continues to increase in most developed countries and there is evidence it tracks through the life cycle. As there are a very limited number of effective treatment options available for either obese children or adults, the emphasis must be put on identifying, evaluating and implementing effective methods of primary prevention for obesity.

Due to the nature of the relationship and the inability to feasibly or ethically assign infant feeding choice via a randomization process, researchers have had to rely on observational studies to provide empirical evidence for what may be a causal protective relationship. The previous section described the plausible mechanisms by which breastfeeding can influence early growth and development. The final section in this chapter will summarize the systematic reviews and meta-analyses on breastfeeding and obesity conducted over the last 10 years and provide some thoughts on future research.

The protective effect of breastfeeding against childhood obesity was initially proposed by Kramer in 1981 (Kramer, 1981) and since then numerous studies have been conducted in order to examine the relationship between breastfeeding and childhood overweight and obesity (Twells & Newhook, 2010; Bergmann et al., 2003; Hediger et al., 2001, Buyken et al., 2008; Dewey, 1998; Kramer et al., 2007; Metzger & McDade, 2010; Savino et al., 2009; Singhal

& Lanigan, 2007; Victora et al., 1998; Araujo et al., 2006; Burdette et al., 2006; Gummer-Strawn & Mei, 2004). More recently, a number of systematic reviews and meta-analyses on this topic have been conducted (Arenz et al., 2004; Harder et al., 2005; Owen et al., 2005; Owen et al., 2005, Horta et al., 2007). Four of these reviews suggest that breastfeeding provides a small but significant protective effect (Arnez et al., 2004; Harder et al., 2005, Owen et al., 2005, Horta et al., 2007) against the development of overweight and/or obesity while one study suggests there is no effect of breastfeeding on differences in mean BMI between groups that were breastfed compared to those formula- fed (Owen et al., 2005).

3.1 Evidence from observational studies

The first systematic review and meta-analysis on the association of breastfeeding and childhood obesity was conducted by Arenz et al. in 2004. This review included studies published in English, French, Italian, Spanish and German from 1966 to December 2003. The researchers examined the relationship between breastfeeding and childhood obesity in children at least one year of age. Obesity was defined as a BMI greater than the 90th, 95th or 97th percentile(s). Only studies that adjusted for at least three potential confounding or interacting factors (e.g., birth weight, parental overweight, parental smoking, dietary factors, physical activity and socioeconomic status (SES) or parental education) and reported an odds ratio (OR) or relative risk (RR) with the last follow-up between 5 and 18 years of age were included in the meta-analysis. Nine of 28 eligible studies met the inclusion criteria including two prospective cohort studies and seven cross-sectional studies totalling more than 69,000 children from developed countries.

The meta-analysis used both fixed and random effects models and pooled crude and adjusted odds ratios (AOR) from the individual studies. Definitions of breastfeeding and other infant feeding methods were not always consistent across studies, especially the definition of exclusive breastfeeding. Sensitivity analyses were carried out to identify potential sources of heterogeneity by testing the strength of the findings stratified by study design, exposure ascertainment and the selection of study participants.

The combined crude odds ratio comparing any breastfeeding to no breastfeeding was calculated for six of the nine studies and was 0.67 (95%CI 0.62-0.73). The AOR calculated for the nine studies was 0.78 (95% CI 0.71-0.85) for both fixed and random effects models. The protective effect of breastfeeding was more pronounced in studies with adjustment for less than seven potential confounding factors (AOR 0.69 95%CI 0.59-0.81) compared to adjustment for seven or more potential confounding factors (AOR 0.78 95%CI 0.70-0.87). The evidence for duration of breastfeeding was inconsistent. Four studies demonstrated an inverse association between breastfeeding duration and the prevalence of obesity in the crude and adjusted analysis. One study reported a dose-response relationship in the crude analysis that lost significance after adjustment. Three studies reported no significant effect of duration of breastfeeding.

These results suggest a significant protective effect of breastfeeding against obesity. Although there was no indication of heterogeneity between the individual studies and several confounders were adjusted for in the analysis, there was some evidence of publication bias with smaller studies tending to report higher protection against obesity. Residual confounding could not be ruled out.

The second systematic review and meta-analysis was published by Owen et al. in 2005 who also published another meta-analysis in the same year. The first of Owen et al.'s two meta-analyses included studies from the same time period as Arenz et al., (1966-2003) but involved a broader search strategy. The objective was to examine the relationship between breastfeeding and obesity assessed at any age. The definition of obesity was flexible, although most studies used a cut-off of >95th or 97th percentiles. Only those studies that reported crude OR's were included. Of 61 studies reviewed, 28 provided 29 AOR's including a total of 298,900 subjects aged 0.5-33 years of age. A fixed effects model was used and meta regression and sensitivity analysis examined the influence of a number of confounding factors that included parental body size, SES, and maternal smoking.

Twenty-eight of the 29 studies reported that breastfeeding was associated with a lower risk of obesity including four estimates for infants, 23 for children and two for adults. The fixed effects model indicated that breastfed infants were less likely to be obese than those formula-fed: OR 0.87 (95% CI 0.85-0.89). Six studies allowed for the adjustment of the following confounders: SES, parental BMI, and current maternal smoking or maternal smoking in early life. The pooled OR in these studies was reduced but breastfeeding remained a significant protective factor. Adjusting for birth weight in ten studies had no real effect on the OR and there was no clear evidence that the protective effect of breastfeeding changed with increasing age of outcome assessment.

In 14 studies that provided data on breastfeeding duration, the protective effect of breastfeeding over formula-feeding was greater among subjects breastfed for at least 2 months OR 0.81 (95% CI 0.77-0.84), compared with those never breastfed. The smaller studies reported a greater protective effect (OR 0.43 95% CI 0.33–0.55) and the larger studies reported a less protective effect (OR 0.88 95%CI 0.86–0.90) providing some evidence for publication bias and selective reporting. There was evidence of heterogeneity among the studies ($p<.001$) and residual confounding could not be ruled out.

Although the results demonstrated a protective effect of breastfeeding against the development of later obesity, the authors suggested that a protective effect may be due to confounding by SES and parental body composition and suggested that a further review was required that included large unpublished studies (the subject of the second Meta-analysis by Owen et al).

Harder et al. (2005), published a third systematic review and meta-analysis in the same year. Unlike the previous two reviews, Harder et al., attempted to assess the effect of *duration* of breastfeeding on the risk of overweight in order to examine whether a dose-response relationship existed. Study eligibility included any original report comparing breastfed subjects with exclusively formula-fed subjects at any age. Studies were included if the findings used OR's and/or contained data for the calculation of an OR for the risk of overweight with reference to feeding history. In addition information on the *duration* of breastfeeding had to be reported. All definitions of overweight and obesity were included. At risk of overweight was defined most often as BMI > than the 85th and >90th percentiles and obesity was defined most often as BMI > 90th, 95th and 97th percentiles.

The final analysis included 17 studies published between 1966 and December 2003 including 120,831 subjects from Great Britain, United States, Canada, Germany, Australia, New Zealand and Czechoslovakia. Fourteen studies provided results on more than one category of breastfeeding duration.

Using a random effects model, the duration of breastfeeding was inversely associated with the risk of overweight: OR 0.94 (95% CI 0.89-0.98). The odds of overweight were reduced by 6% per month of breastfeeding. In addition, a pooled OR for overweight calculated for five time

periods (<1, 1-3, 4-6, 7-9 and >9months) indicated that the risk of overweight continued to decrease by breastfeeding duration reaching a plateau at 9 months. For nine months or more of breastfeeding the OR was 0.68 (95%CI 0.50-0.91). A supplementary trend analysis of 11 studies demonstrated that a dose-response relationship existed between breastfeeding duration and the risk of overweight with an OR of 0.96(95%CI 0.94-0.98) per month of breastfeeding.
The age at examination had little influence on the effect of breastfeeding duration on the risk of overweight. The pooled OR from five studies that investigated subjects up to five years of age was 0.97 (95% CI 0.94-0.99) while for six studies on subjects six years of age or older, was 0.96 (95% CI 0.93-0.99). A sub-group analysis demonstrated that varying definitions of overweight and obesity influenced the estimate of the OR only marginally.
The authors reported that the duration of breastfeeding was inversely and linearly associated with the risk of overweight. In addiition the risk of overweight was reduced by 4% for each month of breastfeeding up to a duration of breastfeeding of 9 months. This finding was independent of the definition of overweight and obese and age at follow-up, suggesting a dose-response relationship. The authors concluded that although the result was relatively small in size, the association, if causal, may be an important factor from a population health perspective. There was no evidence of publication bias.
A critique of this meta-analysis was published as a letter (Quigley, 2006) suggesting a number of methodological concerns existed that included: non-consideration of ethnic background or SES as confounders, inconsistent definitions of both breastfeeding and overweight/obesity, and the reliance on crude OR's. A response was published by the authors (Harder & Plagemann, 2006) suggesting that irrespective of how the subgroups were defined as overweight, the pooled adjusted OR's did not differ from the unadjusted OR inferring a high stability of effect size despite heterogeneity in exposure and/or outcome definition, thus strengthening even more the validity and conclusions of the study.
In 2007, the USA Department of Health and Human Services Office on Women's Health requested that the Agency for Healthcare Research and Quality (AHRQ) summarize the literature and report on the relationship of breastfeeding and various infant and maternal health outcomes including childhood obesity (Ip et al., 2007). Due to restrictions of resources and time, the AHRQ relied primairly on a review of the exiting systematic reviews and meta-analyses, and based on a scoring system (discussed below), provided a grade for each review that assessed the strength of methodological rigor. A, B or C grades were given. Studies given an A grade (good) were described as those having the least bias and consequently results that were considered valid. A grade A study was considered high in quality in that it included; a rigorous systematic review and/or meta-analysis; a clear description of the population, setting, interventions and comparison groups; a clear description of the content of the comparison groups; appropriate measurement of outcomes; appropriate statistical assumptions and analytic methods. In addition the study authors demonstrated; appropriate consideration and adjustment for potential confounders; rigorous assessment of individual study quality; no reporting errors; and well-reasoned conclusions based on the data reported.
Studies given a B grade (fair/moderate) were considered susceptible to some bias, but not sufficient to invalidate the results. B grade studies did not meet all the criteria in category A because of some deficiencies. Grade B studies for example may have demonstrated suboptimal adjustment for potential confounders and be missing information, making it difficult to assess limitations and potential problems.

Studies given a C grade (poor) had significant biases that could invalidate the results. The study either did not consider potential confounders or adjust for them properly. Grade C studies had serious errors in design and analysis and had large amounts of missing information and discrepancies in reporting.

The AHRQ scheme for grading reviews was supplemented with the MOOSE guideline (Meta-analysis of Observational Studies in Epidemiology) and an additional checklist of items that were used to evaluate the quality of the systematic reviews specific to observational studies (Stroup et al., 2000; Ip et al., 2007).

Based on the search criteria by the AHRQ, the meta-analyses by Arenz, Harder and the first of two by Owen were reviewed. After careful appraisal and evaluation Arenz et al., was given an A grade and both the meta-analyses by Harder et al. and Owen et al. were given B grades, primarily due to the suboptimal consideration for potential confounding.

The fourth and second meta-analysis by Owen et al. was also published in 2005 and included both published studies from the previous meta-analysis and unpublished data. In contrast to the previous analyses, studies were included that examined the influence of infant feeding on obesity measured as *mean BMI* throughout life from 6 weeks after birth. Observational studies of cross-sectional and longitudinal cohort design were included and case-control studies that could not provide reliable data for comparisons based on mean BMI were excluded. Seventy studies were reviewed providing a total of 414,750 subjects in the age range from 1 to 70 years of age. Mean differences in BMI were required for analysis. Using a fixed effects model, the mean difference in BMI between those initially breastfed and those formula-fed was examined. Meta-regression was used to examine: influence of study size, quintiles of age at outcome measurement, year of birth and the collection method of infant feeding status on the study outcome. Meta-regression and sensitivity analyses were also used to examine the influence of exclusive feeding, or duration of breastfeeding adjusting for study size.

In this meta-analysis, breastfeeding was associated with a slightly lower BMI compared with formula- feeding; mean difference -0.04 (95%CI -0.05, -0.02). The mean difference was larger for small studies: -0.12 (95%CI -0.29, 0.04) and smaller for larger studies: mean difference -0.03 (95%CI -0.04,-0.01) suggesting some publication bias. If the meta-analysis was restricted to 11 studies that adjusted for age, SES, maternal smoking and maternal BMI, the mean difference was reduced to non-significance between the groups from a mean difference of -0.12 (95% CI: -0.16, -0.08) to a mean difference of -0.01 (95%CI -0.05,0.03) demonstrating both the impact and the need to adjust for relevant confounders.

The authors concluded that the potential effect of breastfeeding on mean BMI was small and non-significant after controlling for confounding factors. Differences in BMI may be strongly influenced by publication bias. Therefore in contrast to the three previous meta-analyses, Owen et al. concluded that the promotion of breastfeeding although important for other reasons was not likely to reduce mean BMI.

In 2007, the WHO published a report summarizing the literature on the "Evidence of the Long-Term Effects of Breastfeeding: Systematic Reviews and Meta-Analysis" (http://www.ahrq.gov/downloads/pub/evidence/pdf/brfout/brfout.pdf) conducted by Horta et al. This report included a section on the long-term effects of breastfeeding on obesity. Previous published meta-analyses were briefly summarized and a new meta-analysis was conducted that considered all the papers included in previously published meta-analyses, and those papers newly identified by two independent literature searches at the WHO. The analysis included 33 studies providing 39 estimates on the effect of breastfeeding on the prevalence of overweight/obesity with follow-up from 1 to 66 years of age. In a random effects model, breastfed individuals were less likely to be considered overweight/obese OR 0.78 (95% CI 0.72-0.84). In spite of the evidence of publication bias, a protective effect of breastfeeding was observed among the larger studies (>1500 participants). Studies that controlled for SES and parental weight reported that breastfeeding was associated with a lower prevalence of obesity. Therefore, according to Horta et al., the evidence suggested that breastfeeding may have a *small protective effect* on the prevalence of obesity.

In 2008, Cope and Allison published a critical review of the WHO report (Cope & Allison, 2008). The authors argued that due to the limitations of the empirical evidence currently available and the major shortcomings of these studies (e.g., publication bias, confounding, residual confounding, self-selection) there was insufficient evidence at this time to suggest that breastfeeding protects against either obesity in childhood or adulthood. The authors questioned the overall conclusion of the WHO report and concluded that "while breastfeeding may have benefits beyond any putative protection against obesity, and benefits of breastfeeding most likely outweigh any harms, any statement that a strong, clear or consistent body of evidence shows that breastfeeding causally reduces the risk of overweight or obesity is unwarranted at this time" (pp.594).

In summary, four of the five meta-analyses published in the last 10 years demonstrate a modest protective effect of breastfeeding against the risk of overweight and obesity. These analyses conducted by different groups of investigators using different inclusion criteria and varying methodologies demonstrated independently a significant association. The findings have remained consistent despite the different settings and populations studied, the use of crude and adjusted data and the varying definitions of infant feeding and overweight. In addition the evidence of a dose-response relationship was observed in some analyses. As a result, there is evidence to support a causal protective relationship between breastfeeding and later risk of overweight; however these conclusions must be placed in the context of the limitations of the study designs currently being used to examine this relationship. There are several weaknesses that limit the validity of meta-analyses of observational studies on the association between breastfeeding and risk of overweight and obesity. Tthese include: publication bias, heterogeneity between studies, the lack of adjustment of confounders and issues of residual confounding. Breastfeeding is associated with many other factors that can influence a child's weight status (e.g., maternal BMI, education, and smoking during pregnancy) and other family lifestyle habits that may be difficult to assess and adjust for in non-experimental study designs. It must be acknowledged that failing to limit the impact of these factors may result in spurious conclusions. (Berylein & Von Kries, 2011).

3.2 Randomized controlled trials

The doubled-blinded randomized controlled trail (RCT) is the gold standard in study design for minimizing biases and increasing the internal validity of the research (Sackett et al., 1991). Although interventional or experimental studies based on random assignment of the mother–infant pair to infant meeting method (breastfeeding or formula-feeding) would provide strong evidence for the association between breastfeeding and risk of overweight/obesity, they are for obvious reasons not feasible or ethical. However, one large RCT conducted in Belarus in 1996-1997 randomized mother-infant pairs to a breastfeeding promotion intervention(Kramer et al., 2001). The Promotion of Breastfeeding Intervention Trial (PROBIT) was a cluster-randomized trial in which a total of 16,491 healthy mothers of full-term singletons with birth weights ≥ 2500g were randomly assigned to a breastfeeding promotion intervention and followed for 12 months. A total of 13,889 children were followed up at 6.5 years. The intervention based on the Baby Friendly Hospital Initiative (BFHI) and developed by the World Health Organization and the United Nations Children's fund was to promote and support breastfeeding, especially in mothers who have chosen to initiate breastfeeding. The control maternity hospitals and polyclinics continued the practices and policies in effect at the time of randomization (Kramer et al., 2001).

The intervention was successful in increasing the breastfeeding rates in the intervention group compared to the control group (43.3% versus 6.4%, $P < 0.001$), duration and exclusivity of breastfeeding; however evidence from the PROBIT study failed to demonstrate an effect of a breastfeeding promotion intervention on children's BMI. For children followed up at 6.5 years, there were no significant differences in mean BMI (i.e., 15.6kg/m^2 in both arms of the trial) or in the prevalence of overweight; OR 1.1(95%CI 0.8-1.4) or obesity; OR 1.2 (95%CI 0.8-1.6) between the two groups. (Kramer et al., 2007). The authors concluded that the PROBIT trial did not provide conclusive evidence for or against a potential effect of breastfeeding on body composition.

There have been a number of limitations of the PROBIT trial discussed regarding its ability to draw conclusions on the relationship between breastfeeding and childhood overweight and obesity. First, the study was not designed to study childhood overweight/obesity directly but rather to study the effects of the BFHI on breastfeeding exclusivity and duration. It may be that the study had insufficient statistical power to assess the outcome of childhood obesity. Second, only women who initiated breastfeeding were enrolled in the study and therefore there was no comparison group of formula-feeding mothers, therefore a self-selection bias existed. Third, the authors examined mean BMI and differences in mean BMI between the intervention and control groups but did not examine any changes in percentage overweight or obese (Berylein, 2011). If breastfeeding is affecting mainly the tail end of the distribution and not the mean BMI as has been suggested it might have been useful to examine the percentages of overweight and obese in both groups(Grummer-Strawn, 2004).

3.3 Future research

Observational studies will remain the primary study design used to collect information on the relationship between breastfeeding and obesity. As has been discussed, challenges arise in that observational or non-experimental studies (i.e., cohort, case-control and cross--sectional) are inherently biased with issues of misclassification of exposure (i.e., self-reported breastfeeding duration), confounding (i.e., mothers/family lifestyle, SES, maternal smoking), residual confounding and self-selection that are difficult to fully adjust for in analysis. However, the validity and reliability of these studies can be improved significantly by: defining careful subject selection criteria; using common and consistent definitions of infant feeding especially that of "exclusive" breastfeeding; ensuring the reliable collection of duration of infant feeding data by trained research personnel; guaranteeing the use of standard cut-off criteria for measuring childhood overweight and obesity such as the WHO criteria (WHO Multicentre Growth Reference Study Group, 2006) as well as blinding assessment of the outcome. A well-designed observational study should provide high quality evidence upon which to draw valid conclusions.

In the context of these limiations, future prospective cohort studies may attempt to include, if data is available, a sibling analysis that provides an opportunity to control for hereditary and confounding factors (e.g., household/family/environmental factors) that are often difficult to adjust for in other studies (Metzger & McDade, 2010). In addition although RCT's are unlikely to be conducted in this area, there is the opportunity to randomize and evaluate the effectiveness of breastfeeding promotion interventions such as the one conducted in Belarus. A well-designed and performed RCT that includes randomization, allocation concealment, clear definitions of breastfeeding exposure compared with non-breastfeeding, and blinded assessment of outcomes could provide the best evidence in supporting the causality of breast milk in affecting the risk overweight and obesity. Analysing the differences in the degree of breastfeeding between the two groups as a result of the intervention will provide researchers with the opportunity to investigate differences in health outcomes such as the development of childhood overweight or obesity between the two groups. This may be the strongest study design available assuming the study is sufficiently powered to evaluate this secondary outcome.

3.4 Conclusion

In conclusion, the prevalence of childhood obesity has increased dramatically in many developed countries over the last few decades and its association with increased morbidity and mortality is of great public health concern. The tracking of childhood obesity and the lack of available effective treatment options suggest that areas of primary prevention must be the focus if we want to curb and reduce this epidemic. Although there are many limitations of the type of study design currently used to explore this relationship, the research evidence that does exist supports a modest but significant protective effect of breastfeeding against the development of obesity with some evidence of a dose-response relationship. It is recognized that breastfeeding is only one of many factors that impact body composition, but as the many benefits of breastfeeding are well-evidenced, continuing to promote and encourage breastfeeding may have the additional benefit of helping to protect against the obesity epidemic.

4. References

Abrams, P. & Levitt Katz, L. E. (2011). Metabolic effects of obesity causing disease in childhood. *Current Opinion in Endocrinology, Diabetes & Obesity,* Vol. 18, No. 1, (February 2011), pp. (23–27), ISSN 1531- 7064

Alexy, U., Kersting, M., Sichert-Hellert, W., Manz F., & Schoch G. (1999). Macronutrient intake of 3- to 36- month-old German infants and children: results of the DONALD Study. *Annals of Nutrition and Metabolism,* Vol. 43, No. 1, (June 1999), pp. (14–22), ISSN 1421-9697

Apfelbacher, C. J., Loerbroks, A., Cairns, J., Behrendt, H., Ring, J., & Kramer, U. (2008). Predictors of overweight and obesity in five to seven-year-olds in Germany: Results from cross-sectional studies. *BMC Public Health,* Vol. 8, No. 171, (September – December 2008), ISSN 1471-2458

Araujo, C.L., Victora, C.G., Hallal, P.C., & Gigante, D.P. (2006). Breastfeeding and overweight in childhood: evidence from the Pelotas 1993 birth cohort study. *International Journal of Obesity,* Vol. 30, (2006), pp. (500-506), ISSN 0307-0565

Arenz, S., Ruckerl, R., Koletzko, B., & Von Kries, R. (2004). Breastfeeding and childhood obesity--a systematic review. International Journal of Obesity Related Metabolic Disorders, Vol. 28, No. 10, (October 2004), pp. (1247- 1256), ISSN 0307-056

August, G.P., Caprio, S., Fennoy, I., Freemark, M., Kaufman, F.R., Lustig, R.H., Silverstein, J.H., Speiser, P.W., Styne, D.M., Montori, V.M.; Endocrine Society. (2008). Prevention and treatment of pediatric obesity: an Endocrine Society clinical practice guideline based on expert opinion. *The Journal of Clinical Endocrinology and Metabolism,* Vol. 93, No. 12, (December 2008), pp. (4576–4599), ISSN 1945- 7197

Baker, J.L., Olsen L.W., Sorensen, T.I. (2007). Childhood Body-Mass Index and the Risk of Coronary Heart Disease in Adulthood. *New England Journal of Medicine,* Vol. 357, No. 23, (December 2007), pp. (2329-2337), ISSN 1533- 4406

Bassali, R., Waller, JL., Gower, B., Allison, J, & Davis, C.L. Utility of waist circumference percentile for risk evaluation in obese children. *International Journal of Pediatric Obesity,* Vol. 5, No. 1, (January 2010), pp. (97 – 101), ISSN 1747- 7174

Benson, L., Baer, H. J., & Kaelber, D. C. (2009). Trends in the diagnosis of overweight and obesity in children and adolescents: 1999-2007. *Pediatrics,* Vol. 123, No. 1, (January 2009), pp. (e153-158), ISSN 0031- 4005

Bergmann, K.E., Bergmann, R.L., Von Kries, R., Bohm, O., Richter, R., Dudenhausen, J.W. & Wahn, U. (2003). Early determinants of childhood overweight and adiposity in a birth cohort study: role of breastfeeding. *International Journal of Obesity Related Metabolic Disorders,* Vol. 27, No. 2, (February 2003), pp. (162-172), ISSN 0307-0565

Beyerlein, A., & Von Kries, R. (2011). and body composition in children: will there ever be conclusive empirical evidence for a protective effect against overweight? *American Journal of Clinical Nutrition,* Epub ahead of print, (April 2011), ISSN 1938-3207

Biro, F. M. & Wien, M. (2010). Childhood obesity and adult morbidities. *American Journal of Clinical Nutrition,* Vol. 91, No. 5, (May 2010), pp. (1499S–1505S), ISSN 1938-3207

Boney, C. M., Verma, A., Tucker, R., & Vohr, B. R. (2004). Metabolic syndrome in childhood: Association with birth weight, maternal obesity, and gestational diabetes mellitus. *Pediatrics,* Vol. 115, No. 3, (March 2005), pp. (e290-e296), ISSN: 0031-4005

Bosma, J.F., Hepburn, L.G., Josell, S.D., & Baker, K. (1990). Ultrasound demonstration of tongue motions during suckle feeding. *Developmental Medicine and Child Neurology,* Vol. 32, No. 3, (March 1990), pp. 223-229, ISSN 1469-8749

Bruner, M. W., Lawson, J., Pickett, W., Boyce, W., & Janssen, I. (2008). Rural canadian adolescents are more likely to be obese compared with urban adolescents. *International Journal of Pediatric Obesity,* Vol. 3, No. 4, (January 2008), pp. (205-211), ISSN 1747- 7174

Burdette, H.L., Whitaker, R.C., Hall W.C., & Daniels, S.R. (2006). Breastfeeding, introduction of complementary foods, and adiposity at 5 y of age. *The American Journal of Clinical Nutrition,* Vol. 83, (2006), pp. (550- 558), ISSN 1938-3207

Buxton, J. L., Walters, R. G., Visvikis-Siest, S. & Meyre, D., Froguel, P., & Blakemore, A. (2011). Childhood obesity is associated with shorter leukocyte telomere length. *The Journal of Clinical Endocrinology and Metabolism,* Vol. 96, (February 2011), pp. (1500–1505), ISSN 1945-7197

Buyken, A.E., Karaolis-Danckert, N., Remer, T., Bolzenius, K., Landsberg, B., & Kroke, A. (2008). Effects of breastfeeding on trajectories of body fat and BMI throughout childhood. *Obesity,* Vol. 16, No. 2, (February 2008), pp. (389-395), ISSN: 1930-7381

Canning, P., Courage M.L., Frizzell L.M., & Seifert T. (2007). Obesity in a provincial population of Canadian preschool children: Differences between 1984 and 1997 birth cohorts. *International Journal of Pediatric Obesity,*Vol. 2, No. 1, (January 2007), pp. (51-57), ISSN 1747- 7174

Catalano, P.M., Farrell, K., Thomas, A., Huston-Presley, L., Mencin P., Hauguel de Mouzon, S., & Amini, S.B. (2009). Perinatal risk factors for childhood obesity and metabolic dysregulation. *American Journal of Clinical Nutrition,* Vol. 90, No. 5, (2009), pp. (1303–1313), ISSN 1938-3207

Cole, T., Bellizzi, M., Flegal, K., Dietz, W. Establishing a standard definition for child overweight and obesity worldwide: National Survey. *British Medical Journal,* Vol. 320, No. 7244, (May 2000), pp. (1240-1243), ISSN 09598138

Connelly, J.B., Duaso, M.J. & Butler, G. (2007). A systematic review of controlled trials of interventions to prevent childhood obesity and overweight: a realistic synthesis of the evidence. *Public Health,* Vol. 121, No. 7, (July 2007), pp. (510–517), ISSN 0033-3506

Cope, M.B., & Allison, D.B. (2008). Critical review of the World Health Organization's (WHO) 2007 report on evidence of the long-term effects of breastfeeding: systematic reviews and meta-analysis' with respect to obesity. *Obesity Review,* Vol. 9, No. 6, (November 2008), pp. 594-605, ISSN 1467-789X

Cornette, R. The emotional impact of obesity on children. *Worldviews on Evidence-Based Nursing,* Vol. 5, No. 3, (September 2008), pp. (136–141), ISSN 1741-6787

Cui, Z., Huxley, R., Wu Y., & Dibley, M. J. Temporal trends in overweight and obesity of children and adolescents from nine Provinces in China from 1991 - 2006. *International Journal of Pediatric Obesity,* Vol. 5, No. 5, (October 2010), pp. (365–374), ISSN 1747- 7174

Dehghan, M., Akhtar-Danesh, N., & Merchant, A. T. Childhood obesity, prevalence and prevention. *Nutrition Journal,* Vol. 4, No 24, (September 2005), ISSN 1541-6100

Deshmukh-Taskar P., Nicklas T.A., Morales M., Yang S.J., Zakeri I., & Berenson G.S. (2006). Tracking of overweight status from childhood to young adulthood: the Bogalusa Heart Study. *The European Journal of Clinical Nutrition,* Vol. 60, No. 1, (January 2006), pp. 49-57, ISSN 0954-3007

Dewey, K.G. Growth characteristics of breast-fed compared to formula-fed infants. (1998). *Biology of the Neonate,* Vol. 74, No. 2, (1998), pp. (94-105), ISSN 1421-9727

Ebbeling, C. B., Pawlak, D. B., & Ludwig, D. S. (2002). Childhood obesity: Public-health crisis, common sense cure. *The Lancet,* Vol. 360, (2002), pp. (473-482), ISSN 0140-6736

Farooqi, S. & O'Rahilly, S. (2006). Genetics of obesity in humans. *Endocrine Reviews,* Vol. 27, No. 7, (December 2006), pp. 710-718, ISSN 0163-769X

Flodgren, G., Deane, K., Dickinson, H.O., Kirk, S., Alberti, H., Beyer, F.R., Brown, J.G., Penney, T.L., Summerbell, C.D., & Eccles, M.P. (2010). Interventions to change the behaviour of health professionals and the organisation of care to promote weight reduction in overweight and obese adults. *The Cochrane Library,* No. 8, (2010), ISSN 1464-780X

Fulton, J.E., Wang, X., Yore, M.M., Carlson S.A., Galuska, D.A., & Caspersen C.J. (2009). Television viewing, computer use, and BMI among US children and adolescents. *Journal of Physical Activity and Health,* Vol. 6(suppl 1), (2009), pp. (S28–S35), ISSN 1543-5474

Gibson, L. Y., Byrne, S. M., Davis, E. A., Blair, E., Jacoby, P., & Zubrick, S. R. The role of family and maternal factors in childhood obesity. *Medical Journal of Australia,* Vol. 186, No. 11, (2007), pp. (591–595), ISSN 0025-729X

Goran, M. I. & Ventura, E. E. International journal of pediatric obesity: Year in review 2010. *International Journal of Pediatric Obesity,* Vol. 6, (2011), pp. (163–168), ISSN 1747- 7174

Griffiths, L.J., Parsons, T.J., Hill, A.J. (2010). Self-esteem and quality of life in obese children and adolescents: a systematic review. International Journal of Pediatric Obesity, Vol. 5, No. 4, (2010), pp. 282-304, ISSN 1747- 7174

Gummer-Strawn, L., & Mei, Z. (2004). Does Breastfeeding Protect Against Pediatric Overweight? Analysis of Longitudinal Data From the Centers for Disease Control and Prevention Pediatric Nutrition Surveillance System. *Pediatrics,* Vol. 113, No. 2, (February 2004), ISSN 1347-7358

Harder, T., Bergmann, R., Kallischnigg, G., & Plagemann, A. (2005). Duration of breastfeeding and risk of overweight: a meta-analysis. *American Journal of Epidemiology, Vol. 162, No. 5, (September 2005), pp. 397-403, ISSN* 1476-6256

Harder, T., & Plagemann, A. (2006). Two of the authors reply. *American Journal of Epidemiology,* Vol. 163, No. 9, (May 2006), pp. (872-873), ISSN 1476-6256

Hediger, M.L., Overpeck, M.D., Kucznarsjum R.J., & Ruan W.J. (2001). Association between infant breastfeeding and overweight in young children. *Journal of the American Medical Association,* Vol. 285, No. 19, (May 2001), pp. (2453-2460), ISSN 1538-3598

Heinig, M.J., Nommsen, L.A., Peerson, J.M., Lönnerdal, B., & Dewey, K.G. (1993). Energy and protein intakes of breast-fed and formula-fed infants during the first year of life and their association with growth velocity: the DARLING Study. *American Journal of Clinical Nutrition,* Vol. 58, No. 2, (1993), pp. (152-61), ISSN 1938-3207

Hellstrom, P.M. (2009). Faces of ghrelin-research for the 21st century. *Neurogastroenterology and Motility,* Vol. 21, No. 1, (January 2009), pp. 2-5, ISSN 1365-2982

Horta, B.L., Bahl, R., Martines, J.C., & Victora, C.G. (2007). Evidence on the long-term effects of breastfeeding: Systematic Reviews and Meta-analyses, *World Health Organization,* August 20, 2011, Available from:
http://www.who.int/child_adolescent_health/documents/9241595230/en/index.html

Huh, S. Y., Rifas-Shiman, S. L., Taveras, E. M., Oken, E., & Gillman, M. W. Timing of solid food introduction and risk of obesity in preschool-aged children. *Pediatrics,* Vol. 127, No. 3, (March 2011), pp. (e544- e551), ISSN 1347- 7358

Ilcol, Y.O., Hizli, Z.B., & Eroz, E. (2008). Resistin is present in human breast milk and it correlates with maternal hormonal status and serum level of C-reactive protein. *Clinical Chemistry and Laboratory Medicine,* Vol. 46, No. 1, (2008), pp. (118-124), ISSN 1437-4331

Ip, S., Chung, M., Raman, G., Chew, P., Magula, N., DeVine, D., Litt, M., Trikalinos, T., & Lau, J. (2007). Breastfeeding and Maternal and Infant Health Outcomes in Developed Countries. In *AHRQ Evidence Report/Technology Assessment No. 153.* August 20, 2011. Available From:

http://www.ahrq.gov/downloads/pub/evidence/pdf/brfout/brfout.pdf

Ismailov, R. M., & Leatherdale, S. T. (2010). Rural-urban differences in overweight and obesity among a large sample of adolescents in Ontario. *International Journal of Pediatric Obesity*, Vol. 5, No. 4, (August 2010), pp. (351-360), ISSN 1747- 7174

Janssen, I., Craig, W. M., Boyce, W. F. & Pickett, W. (2004). Association between overweight and obesity with bullying behaviours in school-aged children. *Pediatrics*, Vol. 113, No. 5, (May 2004), pp. (1187- 1194), ISSN 1347-7358

Koletzko, B., Decsi, T., Molnár, D., & Hunty, A. (2009). Early nutrition programming and health outcomes in later life: obesity and beyond. Advances in Experimental Medicine and Biology, Vol. 646, (2009), pp. (15-29), ISSN 0065-2598

Koletzko, B., Broekaert, I., Demmelmair, H., et al. Protein intake in the first year of life: a risk factor for later obesity? The EU Childhood Obesity project. In: Koletzko, B. Dodds, P.F., Akerblom, H., Ashwell, M., eds. Early nutrition and its later consequences: new opportunities. Dordrecht, Netherlands: Kluwer Academic, (2005), pp. (69–79)

Kovacs, V.A., Gabor, A., Fajcsak, Z., & Martos, E. (2010). Role of waist circumference in predicting the risk of high blood pressure in children. *International Journal of Pediatric Obesity*, Vol. 5, No. 2, (2010), pp. (143 - 50), ISSN 1747- 7174

Kramer, M.S. (1981). Do breastfeeding and delayed introduction of solid foods protect against subsequent obesity? *The Journal of Pediatrics*, Vol. 98, No. 6, (June 1981), pp. (883-887), ISSN 10976833

Kramer M.S., Guo, T., Platt, R.W., Vanilovich, I., Sevkovskaya, Z., Dzikovich, I., Michaelsen K.F., Dewey, K for the promotion of Breastfeeding Intervention Trial Study Group (2004). Feeding effects on growth during infancy. *Journal of Pediatrics*, Vol. 145, (2004), pp. (600–605), ISSN 1347-7358

Kramer, M.S., Chalmers, B., Hodnett, E.D., Sevkovskaya, Z., Dzikovich, I., Shapiro, S., Collet, J.P., Vanilovich, I., Mezen, I., Ducruet, T., Shishko, G., Zubovich, V., Mknuik, D., Gluchanina, E., Dombrovskiy, V., Ustinovitch, A., Kot, T., Bogdanovich, N., Ovchinikova, L.,& Helsing, E (2001). Promotion Of Breastfeeding Intervention Trial (PROBIT): a randomized trial in the Republic of Belarus. *Journal of the American Medical Association*, Vol. 285, No. 4, (January 2001), pp. 413-420, ISSN 1538-3598

Kramer, M.S., Matush, L., Vanilovich, I., Platt, R.W, Bogdanovich, N., Sevkovskaya, Z., Dzikovich, I., Shishko, G., Collet, J.P., Martin, R.M., Davey Smith, G., Gillman, M.V., Chalmers, B., Hodnett, E., & Shapiro, S. (2007). Effects of prolonged and exclusive breastfeeding on child height, weight, adiposity, and blood pressure at age 6.5 y: evidence from a large randomized trial. *American Journal of Clinical Nutrition*, Vol. 86, No. 6, (December 2007), pp. 1717-1721, ISSN 1938-320

Lawrence R.A. (1999). *Breastfeeding: A guide for the medical profession*, (5th edition), Mosby, Inc., St. Louis, MO

Labbok, M.H., Clark, D., Goldman, A.S. (2004). Breastfeeding: maintaining an irreplacable immunological resource. *Nature Review Immunology*, Vol. 4, No. 7, (July 2004), pp. (565-72), ISSN 1474-1741

Li, R., Fein, S.B., & Grummer-Strawn, L.M. (2010). Do infants fed from bottles lack self-regulation of milk intake compared with directly breastfed infants? *Pediatrics*, Vol. 125, No. 6, (June 2010), pp. 1386- 1393, ISSN 0031-4005

Logue, J. & Sattar, N. Childhood obesity: A ticking time bomb for cardiovascular disease? *Clinical pharmacology & Therapeutics*, Vol. 90, No. 1, (July 2011), pp. (174-178), ISSN 0009-9236

Logue, J., Thompson, L., Romanes, F., Wilson, D.C., Thompson, J. & Sattar, N. (2010). Guideline development group. Management of obesity: summary of SIGN guideline. *British Medical Journal*, Vol. 24, No. 340, (February 2010), pp. (c154), ISSN 09598138

Lucas, A., Boyes, S., Bloom, R., & Aynsley-Green, A. (1981). Metabolic and endocrine responses to a milk feed in six-day-old term infants: differences between breast and cow's milk formula feeding. *Acta Paediatrica Scandinavica*, Vol. 70, No. 1, (March 1981), pp. (195-200), ISSN 0001-656X

Martin, L.J., Woo, J.G., Geraghty, S.R., Altaye, M., Davidson, B.S., Banach, W., Dolan, L.M., Ruiz-Palacios, G.M., & Morrow, A.L. (2006). Adiponectin is present in human milk and is associated with maternal factors. *American Journal of Clinical Nutrition*, Vol. 83, No. 5, (2006), pp. 1106-1111, ISSN 938-3207

Mathew, O.P. & Batia, J. (1989). Suckling and breathing patterns during breast and bottle-feeding in term neonates. Effects of nutrient delivery and composition. *American Journal of Diseases in Children*, Vol. 143, No. 5, (1989), pp. (588-592), ISSN 0002-922X

Medilexicon International Limited. (2011) July 28, 2001. Available from: www.medilexicon.com/medicaldictionary.php?t=76341

McConley, R., Mrug, S., Gilliland, M. J., Lowry, R., Elliott, M. L., Schuster, M. A., et al., Mediators of maternal depression and family structure on child BMI: Parenting quality and risk factors for child overweight. *Obesity*, Vol. 19, No. 2, (2011), pp. (345–352), ISSN 1930-739X

Metzger, M.W., & McDade, T.W. (2010). Breastfeeding as obesity prevention in the United States: a sibling difference model. *American Journal of Human Biology*, Vol. 22, No. 3, (May-June 2010), pp. (291-296), ISSN 1520-6300

Mizuno, K., & Ueda, A. (2006). Changes in sucking performance from non-nutritive sucking to nutritive sucking during breast- and bottle-feeding. *Pediatric Research*, Vol. 59, No. 5, (May 2006) pp. (728- 731), ISSN 1530-0447

Moens, E., Braet, C., Bosmans, G., & Rosseel, Y. Unfavourable family characteristics and their associations with childhood obesity: A cross-sectional study. *European Eating Disorders Review*, Vol. 17, No. 4 (July/August 2009), pp. (315–32), ISSN 1099-0968

National Centre for Health Statistics (2002). Centre for Disease Control: CDC Growth charts. June 5, 2011. Available from: http://www.cdc.gov/GROWTHCHARTS/

Nyberg, G., Ekelund, U., Yucel-Lindberg, T., Mode, T., & Marcus, C. Differences in metabolic risk factors between normal weight and overweight children. *International Journal of Pediatric Obesity*, Vol. 6, No. 3-4, (August 2011), pp. (244–252), ISSN 1747-7174

Ogden, C., & Carroll, M. (2010). Prevalence of obesity among children and adolescents: United States, Trends 1963-1965 through 2007-2008. July 7th, 2011. Available from: http://www.cdc.gov/nchs/data/hestat/obesity_adult_07_08/obesity_adult_07_08.pdf

Oliver, S. R. Rosa, j. S., Milne, G. L., Pontello, A. M., Borntrager, H. L., Heydari, S. & Galassetti, P. R. (2010). Increased oxidative stress and altered substrate metabolism in obese children. *International Journal of Pediatric Obesity*, Vol. 5, No. 5, (October 2010), pp. (436–444), ISSN 1747-7174

Owen, C.G, Martin, R.M., Whincup, P.H., Davey-Smith, G., Gillman, M.W, & Cook, D.G. (2005). The effect of breastfeeding on mean body mass index throughout life: a quantitative review of published and unpublished observational evidence. The American Journal of Clinical Nutrition, Vol. 82, No. 6, (December 2005), pp. (1298-1307), ISSN 1938-3207

Owen C.G., Martin, R.M., Wincup, P.H., Davey Smith, G., & Cook, D.G. (2005) Effect of infant feeding on the risk of obesity across the life course: a quantitative review of published evidence. *Pediatrics,* Vol. 115, No. 5, (May 2005), pp. 1367–1377, ISSN 1538-3628

Philippi-Hohne, C. (2010). Anaesthesia in the obese child. *Best practice & research in Clinical Anaesthesiology*, Vol. 25, No. 1, (Match 2010), pp. (53-60) ISSN 1521-6896

Poothullil, J.M. (1995). Regulation of nutrient intake in humans: a theory based on taste and smell. *Neuroscience and Biobehavioural Reviews,* Vol. 19, No. 3, (Fall 1995), pp. 407-412, ISSN 1873-7528

Quigley, M.A. (2006). Re: "Duration of breastfeeding and risk of overweight: a meta-analysis". *American Journal of Epidemiology*, Vol. 163, No. 9, (May 2006), pp. (870-872), ISSN 1476-6256

Righard, L. & Alade, M.O. (1992). Sucking technique and its effect on success of breastfeeding. *Birth,* Vol. 19, No. 4, (December 1992), pp. (185–189), ISSN 1523-536X

Sackett, D., Haynes, R.B., Guyatt, G.H., & Tugwell, P. (January 1991), *Clinical Epidemiology: A Basic Science for Clinical Medicine,* (2nd edition), ISBN 0316765996

Sanad, M., & Gharib, A. (2011). Evaluation of microalbuminuria in obese children and its relationship to metabolic syndrome, *Pediatric Nephrology*, Epub ahead of print, (June 2011), ISSN 1432-198X

Savino, F., Fissore, M.F., Liguori, S.A., & Oggero R. (2009) Can hormones contained in mothers' milk account for the beneficial effect of breast-feeding on obesity in children? *Clinical Endocrinology*, Vol. 71, No. 6, (December 2009), pp. (757-765), ISSN 1365-2265

Savino, A., Pelliccia, P., Giannini, C., de Giorgis, T., Cataldo, I., Chiarelli, F. & Mohn, A. (2011). Implications for kidney disease in obese children and adolescents. *Pediatric Nephrology*, Vol. 26, No. 5, (May 2011), pp. (749-758), ISSN 1432-198X

Scherer, P.E., Williams, S., Fogliano, M., Baldini, G., & Lodish, H. (1995). A novel serum protein similar to C1q, produced exclusively in adipocytes. The Journal of Biological Chemistry (November 1995) Vol. 270, pp. (26746-26749), ISSN 1083-351X

Schwimmer, J. B., Burwinkle, T. M., & Varni, J. W. (2003). Health-related quality of life of severely obese children and adolescents. *Journal of the American Medical Association*, Vol. 289, No. 14, (2003), pp. (1813-1819), ISSN 0098-7484

Simen-Kapeu, A., Kuhle, S. & Veugelers, P. J. (2010). Geographical differences in childhood overweight, physical activity, nutrition and neighbourhood facilities: Implications for prevention. *Canadian Journal of Public Health*, Vol. 101, No. 2, (March-April 2010), pp. (128-132), ISSN 0008-4263

Singhal, A., & Lanigan, J. (2007). Breastfeeding, early growth and later obesity. *Obesity Reviews*, Vol. 8, Supplement 1, (March 2007), pp. 51-54, ISSN 1467-789X

Singhal, A., & Lucas, A. (2004). Early origins of cardiovascular disease: is there a unifying hypothesis? *The Lancet*, Vol. 363, No. 9421, (May 2004), pp. (1642-1645), ISSN 0140-6736

Sisson, S.B., Church, T.S., Martin, C.K.,Tudor-Locke, C., Smith, S.R., Bouchard, C., Earnest, C.P., Rankinen, T., Newton, R.L., & Katzmarzyk, P.T. (2009). Profiles of sedentary behavior in children and adolescents: the US National Health and Nutrition Examination Survey, 2001–2006. *International Journal of Pediatric Obesity,* Vol. 4, No. 4, (2009), pp. (353–359), ISSN 1747-7174

Smith-Kirwin, S.M., O'Connor, D.M., De Johnston, J., Lancey, E.D., Hassink, S.G., & Funanage, V.L. (1998). Leptin expression in human mammary epithelial cells and breast milk. *Journal of Clinical Endocrinology and Metabolism,* Vol. 83, No. 5, (May 1998), pp. 1810-1813, ISSN 1945-7197

Stamatakis, E., Zaninotto, P., Falaschetti, E., Mindell, J., & Head, J. (2010). Time trends in childhood and adolescent obesity in England from 1995 to 2007 and projections of prevalence to 2015. *Epidemiological Community Health,* Vol. 64, No. 2, (February 2010), pp. (167e-174), ISSN 1470-2738

Steene-Johannessen, J., Kolle, E., Reseland, J.E., Anderssen, S.A., & Andersen, L.B. (2010). Waist circumference is related to low-grade inflammation in youth. *International Journal of Pediatric Obesity,* Vol. 5, No. 4, (August 2010), pp. (313–319), ISSN 1747-7174

Stefan, N., Bunt J.C., Salbe, A.D., Funahashi, T., Matsuzawa, Y., & Tataranni, P.A. (2002). Plasma adiponectin concentrations in children: relationships with obesity and insulinemia. *Journal of Clinical Endocrinology and Metabolism,* Vol. 87, No. 10, (October 2002), pp. 4652-4656, ISSN 1945-7197

Steppan, C.M., Bailey, S.T., Bhat, S., Brown, E.J., Banerjee, R.R., Wright, C.M., Patel, H.R., Ahima, R.S., & Lazar, M.A.(2001).The hormone resistin links obesity to diabetes. *Nature,* Vol. 409, No. 6818, (January 2001), pp. 307-312, ISSN 476-4687

Stevens, J. (1995). Obesity, fat patterning and cardiovascular risk. *Advances in Experimental Medicine and Biology,* Vol. 369, (1995), pp. (21-27), ISSN 0065-2598

Stroup, D., Berlin, J., Morton, S., Olkin, I., Williamson, G.D., Rennie, D., Moher, D., Becker, B., Sipe, T.A., & Thacker, S. (2000). Meta-analysis of observational studies in epidemiology: a proposal for reporting. *Journal of the American Medical Association,* Vol. 283, No. 15, (April 2000), pp. (2008-2012), ISSN 1538-3598

Taveras E.M., Rifas-Shiman S.L., Scanlon K.S., Grummer-Strawn L.M., Sherry B., & Gillman M.W. (2006). To what extent is the rotective effect of breastfeeding on future overweight explained by decreased maternal feeding restriction? *Pediatrics,* Vol. 118, No. 6, (December 2006), pp. 2341–2348, ISSN 10984275

Taveras, E.M., Scanlon, K.S., Birch, L., Rifas-Shiman, S.L., Rich-Edwards, J.W.,& Gillman, M.W. (2004). Association of breastfeeding with maternal control of infant feeding at age 1 year. *Pediatrics,* Vol. 114, No. 5, (November 2004), pp. (e577-e583), ISSN 10984275

Taylor, R.W., Grant, A.M, Goulding, A., & Williams, S.M. (2005). Early adiposity rebound: review of papers linking this to subsequent obesity in children and adults. *Clinical Endocrinology,* Vol. 71, No. 6, (November 2005), pp. 757-765, ISSN 1365-2265

The Health and Social Care Information Centre (2010). Health Survey for England. March 2011. Available from:

http://www.ic.nhs.uk/statistics-and-data-collections/health-and-lifestylesrelated-surveys/health-survey-for-england

Twells, L. & Newhook, L.A. (2010). Can exclusive breastfeeding reduce the likelihood of childhood obesity in some regions of Canada? *Canadian Journal of Public Health,* Vol. 101, No. 1, (January-February 2010), pp. (36-39), ISSN 0008-4263

Twells, L. & Newhook, L. A.(2011). Obesity prevalence estimates in a Canadian regional population of preschool children using variant growth references, *BMC Pediatrics,* Vol. 11, No. 21, (February 2011), pp. (21), ISSN 1471-2431

Veugelers, P. J., & Fitzgerald, A. L. (2005). Prevalence of and risk factors for childhood overweight and obesity. *Canadian Medical Association Journal,* Vol. 173, No. 6, (September 2005), pp. (607-613), ISSN 1488-2329

Victora, C.G., Morris, S.S., Barros, F.C., Horta, B.L., Weiderpass, E., & Tomasi, E. (1998). Breast-feeding and growth in Brazilian infants. *American Journal of Clinical Nutrition,* Vol. 67, No. 3, (March 1998), pp. (452–458), ISSN 1938-3207

Vieweg, V. R., Johnston, C. H., Lanier, J. O., Fernandez, A. & Pandurangi, A. K. (2007). Correlation between high risk obesity groups and low socioeconomic status in school children. *Southern Medical Journal,* Vol. 100, No. 1, (January 2007), pp. (8-13), ISSN 0038-4348

Visness, C. M., London, S. J., Daniels, J. L., Kaufman, J. S., Yeatts, K. B., Siega-Riz, A., Calatroni, A. & Zeldin, D. C. (2010). Association of Childhood Obesity with Atopic and Non-Atopic Asthma: Results from the National Health and Nutrition Examination Survey 1999-2006. *Journal of Asthma,* Vol. 47, No. 7, (September 2010), pp. (822–829), ISSN 0277-0903

Vos, M. B., & Welsh, J. (2010). Childhood obesity: update on predisposing factors and prevention strategies. *Journal of Current Gastroenterology Reports,* Vol. 12, No. 4, (August 2010), pp. (280–287), ISSN 1534- 312X

Whitaker, R.C., Wright, J.A., Pepe, M.S., Seidel, K.D., & Dietz, W.H. (1997). Predicting obesity in young adulthood from childhood and parental obesity. *New England Journal of Medicine,* Vol. 337, No. 13, (September 1997), pp. (869-73), ISSN 1533-4406

World Health Organization (2000). WHO Technical Report Series no.894. Obesity: Preventing and managing the global epidemic. Geneva: World Health Organization.

World Health Organization (WHO). (2011a). World Health Organization: obesity and overweight fact sheet. July 28, 2011. Available from: http://www.who.int/mediacentre/factsheets/fs311/en/index.html

World Health Organization (WHO). (2011b) Global Info Base (maps). July 28, 2011. Available from: https://apps.who.int/infobase/Index.aspx

World Health Organization (WHO). (2011c). Nutrition: Controlling the global obesity epidemic. July 28, 2011. Available from:
http://www.who.int/nutrition/topics/obesity/en

World Health Organization Multicentre Growth Reference Study Group. (2006). WHO Child Growth Standards based on length/height, weight and age. *Acta Paediatrica,* Vol. 450 (suppl), (April 2006), pp. (76-85), ISSN 1651-2227

Zhang, Y., Proenca, R., Maffei, M., Barone, M., Leopold, L., & Friedman, J.M. (1994). Positional cloning of the mouse obese gene and its human homologue. *Nature,* Vol. 372, No. 6506, (December 1994), pp. 425-432, ISSN 1476-4687

4

Waist Circumference in Children and Adolescents from Different Ethnicities

Peter Schwandt and Gerda-Maria Haas
Arteriosklerose- Präventions – Institut München-Nürnberg, Germany

1. Introduction

In their Bulletin 2001; 79 the World Health Organisation (WHO) had published: "The last two decades have witnessed the emergence and consolidation of an economic paradigm which emphasizes domestic deregulation and the removal of barriers to international trade and finance. If properly managed, such an approach can lead to perceptible gains in health status."

Globalization in the last two decades influenced lifestyle and especially food patterns all over the world (Bauchner H, 2008 and Hu FB, 2008). In a "Nutrition transition" the consumption of dietary fat and/ or high -caloric meals and sweetened drinks has been increased, in developed countries as well as in developing ones (Hawkes C, 2006). At the same time overweight and obesity just as increased and diet- related chronic diseases like diabetes mellitus II, hypertension or lipid disorders or cardiovascular diseases known from elder adults are observed in children and adolescents.

Waist circumference (WC) is a generally accepted measure of central obesity that is a traditional risk factor for cardiovascular disease (CVD). A worldwide standardization of WC is warranted because of considerable differences between different ethnicities. For adults pragmatic ethnic-specific cut-off values for WC were defined between >85 cm and >94 cm for men and between >80 cm and >90 cm for women (Alberti et al., 2005). For children and adolescents from different ethnicities no uniform definition of WC cut-offs exists because of physiological growth and development.

The aim of this study is to develop age- and gender-specific reference curves of WC for German children and adolescents, to define cut-off values, to collect percentile curves from other ethnicities, and to compare global findings. Calculation of our cut-off values is based on conventional anthropometric and non-anthropometric cardiovascular risk factors.

WC is obligate for the definition of the metabolic syndrome already in youths. Early detection and intervention by lifestyle change are mandatory to prevent adult adiposity and its multiple complications. Thus, precise diagnosis is prerogative for the estimation of the worldwide prevalence of the metabolic syndrome and global intervention.

2. Subjects and methods

For the PEP Family Heart Study representative samples of 3531 German children (1788 boys, 1743 girls) aged 3-11 years and of 3024 German adolescents (1633 males, 1391 females) aged 12–18 years participating in yearly cross-sectional surveys between 1994 and 2004 respectively between 2000 and 2007 were studied (Schwandt et al., 2008; Haas et al., 2011). The CASPIAN Study was performed in 2003-2004 and contributes representative samples of 1616 Iranian children (757 boys and 859 girls) and of 2608 Iranian adolescents (1216 males and 1392 females) in these age groups. The Belo Horizonte Heart Study contributes 464 Brazilian children (241 boys and 223 girls) and 545 Brazilian adolescents (255 males and 290 females) to this large data set of the BIG study consisting of 11,788 youths from three continents. All the three studies followed the Declaration of Helsinki and the same methodology.

The ethical committee of the medical faculty of the Ludwig- Maximilians- University Munich, the Bavarian Ministry of Science and Education, and the local school authorities approved the Prevention Education Program (PEP). Written informed consent together with oral consent from children and adolescents was obtained from all parents, assessment of the pubertal status was not accepted. Exclusion criteria of the PEP Family Heart Study were non-German ethnicity (2.6% of children from 17 non-German ethnicities to avoid ethnic bias), incomplete data sets, apparent cardiovascular, metabolic, endocrine and malignant diseases, extreme physical activities, special nutrition habits and taking any medication.

Continuously trained research assistants performed all measurements along the study manual as previously described (Schwandt et al., 1999, 2009, 2010). Physical examination included measurements of weight, height, body mass index (BMI), waist circumference (WC), waist-to-height ratio (WHtR), skin fold thickness (SFT), percent body fat (%BF) and blood pressure (BP). Lipids, lipoproteins and glucose were measured in fasting venous blood samples, processed and stored at -20°C every year during November and December. Definition of risk factors is shown in Table 1.

Overweight:	85th to 95th percentile of BMI (kg/m^2)
General obesity:	≥95th percentile of BMI (kg/m^2)
Central obesity:	WC≥ 90th and/or waist to height ratio ≥0.5
Hypertension: SBP and/or DBP	≥95th percentile
Fasting hyperglycemia:	≥100 mg/dL plasma glucose
Hypertriglyceridemia:	≥150 mg/dL
Increased LDL-Cholesterol:	≥130 mg/dL
Decreased HDL-Cholesterol:	<40 mg/dL
Increased Non HDL-Cholesterol:	≥123 mg/dL
Increased ratio of LDL-C/HDL-C:	≥ 3.0
Increased ratio of TG/HDL-C	≥3.5

Table 1.

Statistical analyses were performed with PASW 17.0 version for Windows (SPSS, Illinois, USA) according to a predefined analysis plan and program. Continuous variables are presented as the mean ± standard deviation (SD). Smoothed age- and gender-specific curves were constructed for WC, WHtR, SFT and BMI (Schwandt et al., 2008; Haas et al., 2011) using the software package LMS Chart Maker Pro, version 2.3. The associations between anthropometric measurement and cardiovascular risk factors were calculated by multivariate logistic regression using the backward Likelihood Quotient Model. All of the tests were 2-sided, and *p* values of <0.05 were considered to be statistically significant.

3. Results

3.1 Age- and gender-specific percentiles of waist circumference in German children and adolescents

The anthropometric characteristics of healthy German children are demonstrated in Table 2

Age (years)	Number (n)	Weight (kg)	Height (cm)	WC (cm)	BMI (kg/m³)	HC (cm)	WHR	WHtR
Boys								
3	95	15.7±2.19	100.61±4.61	50.93±3.24	15.44±1.35	55.37±3.51	0.92±0.05	0.51±0.03
4	164	17.86±2.14	107.31±4.46	52.85±2.82	15.50±1.51	57.58±3.45	0.92±0.05	0.50±0.03
5	101	19.59±3.11	113.18±5.30	53.57±4.28	15.22±1.58	59.58±4.86	0.90± 0.05	0.50±0.03
6	670	23.77±4.17	122.40±5.42	56.55±4.98	15.79±1.96	64.23±5.36	0.88± 0.05	0.46±0.04
7	447	25.12±4.37	125.30±5.34	57.81±5.60	15.93±2.10	65.60±5.87	0.88±0.08	0.45±0.04
8	80	29.09±5.23	132.24±6.45	59.79±6.50	16.61±2.86	68.68±6.23	0.87±0.04	0.45±0.05
9	104	31.69±5.55	138.68±6.25	61.13±5.47	16.39±2.09	71.45±5.64	0.86±0.04	0.44±0.03
10	77	37.75±8.18	144.60±5.53	65.69±8.00	17.93±3.04	76.30±7.74	0.86±0.06	0.45±0.05
11	60	38.95±8.37	147.27±6.75	65.67±7.63	17.85±2.88	77.18±7.03	0.85±0.05	0.45±0.04
Total	1788	24.74±7.32	123.33±11.87	57.19±6.66	15.98±2.28	64.84±7.76	0.88±0.06	0.47±0.04
Girls								
3	91	14.58±1.60	99.09±4.56	49.88±2.74	14.84±1.21	54.87±3.07	0.91±0.05	0.50±0.03
4	133	17.23±2.53	106.53±5.61	52.00±4.31	15.16±1.73	57.43±3.64	0.91±0.06	0.49±0.04
5	98	19.64±2.78	112.45±4.70	53.71±3.93	15.60±1.77	60.18±4.12	0.89±0.04	0.48±0.03
6	702	23.10±3.79	121.43±5.40	55.45±4.74	15.60±1.82	64.28±5.38	0.86±0.04	0.46±0.03
7	410	24.82±4.67	124.27±5.25	56.63±5.63	15.99±2.30	66.23±6.13	0.86±0.05	0.46±0.04
8	87	29.29±6.12	132.63±6.69	58.72±6.46	16.54±2.61	69.94±6.74	0.84±0.05	0.44±0.04
9	90	30.93±6.20	137.13±6.57	58.98±6.13	16.32±2.23	71.66±6.38	0.82±0.05	0.43±0.04
10	77	36.86±9.29	143.96±7.11	62.70±8.06	17.65±3.52	76.78±7.92	0.82±0.06	0.44±0.05
11	55	41.18±8.78	149.09±7.69	64.36±7.69	18.41±3.10	81.27±6.88	0.80±0.06	0.43±0.05
Total	1743	24.31±7.21	122.53±12.05	56.02±6.04	15.88±2.23	65.25±7.81	0.86±0.05	0.46±0.04

Table 2. Weight, height, waist circumference (WC), hip circumference (HC), body mass index (BM), waist to hip ratio (WHR) and waist to height ratio (WHtR) by age and sex in 3531 German boys and girls (mean± SD) (Schwandt et al 2008)

Among boys and girls, WC increased continuously from 3 years to 11 years at all percentiles, steepest at the 97th percentile in both genders (Figure 1). At the 50th percentile, this corresponds to an increase of WC by 14 cm in boys and by 13 cm in girls from age 3 years to age 11 years (Table 2). However, in adolescents WC increased less, by 11 cm in males and only by 5 cm in females with even slight decreases between 15 years and 18 years (Table 3).

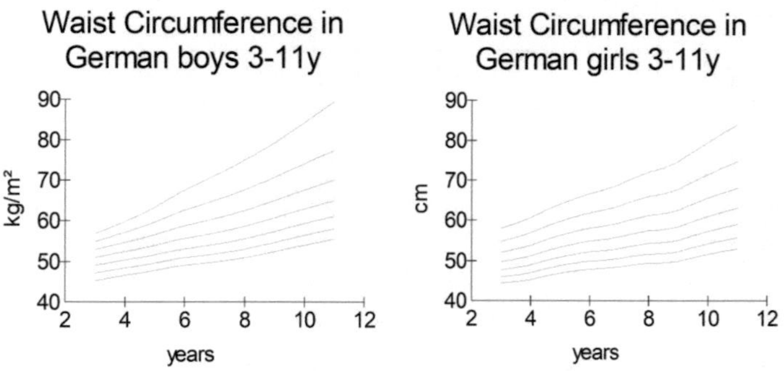

Fig. 1. Smoothed reference curves for the 3rd, 10th, 25th, 50th, 75th and 97th percentiles for waist and body mass index in 3 years to 11-years old German boys and girls (Schwandt et al. 2008)

Age	n	3rd	10th	25th	50th	75th	90th	97th
Boys								
3	95	45.4	47.2	49.0	50.9	52.9	54.9	57.0
4	154	46.7	48.5	50.4	52.5	54.8	57.2	60.1
5	101	47.9	49.7	51.7	54.0	56.7	59.8	63.6
6	670	49.1	51.0	53.1	55.7	58.8	62.6	67.6
7	447	49.9	51.9	54.2	57.0	60.5	64.9	71.0
8	80	50.9	53.1	55.6	58.6	62.5	67.5	74.6
9	104	52.5	54.7	57.4	60.7	65.0	70.6	79.0
10	77	54.1	56.6	59.4	62.9	67.6	74.0	84.0
11	60	55.5	58.0	61.0	64.8	69.8	77.1	89.2
Girls								
3	91	44.2	45.8	47.5	49.7	52.1	55.0	58.5
4	133	45.4	47.2	49.1	51.4	54.1	57.3	61.3
5	98	46.8	48.7	50.8	53.3	56.2	59.6	64.1
6	702	47.9	49.9	52.2	54.8	58.0	61.8	66.7
7	410	48.6	50.7	53.1	55.9	59.4	63.7	69.2
8	87	49.3	51.5	54.1	57.2	61.0	65.8	72.1
9	90	50.2	52.6	55.4	58.7	62.9	68.2	75.4
10	77	51.5	54.1	57.1	60.7	65.3	71.3	79.7
11	55	52.9	55.6	58.8	62.8	67.9	74.7	84.6

Table 3. Age- and sex-specific WC percentile values (cm) for German children 3-11 years of age in the PEP Family Heart Study (Schwandt et al. 2008)

The prevalence of severe obesity (WC>97th percentile) was significantly ($p<0.05$) higher in boys than in girls (4.1% vs. 2.8%) corresponding to similar gender differences for BMI >97th percentile (6.3% vs. 4.9%) in this cohort children.

Age (y)	n	Weight (kg)	Height (cm)	Waist (cm)	BMI (kg/m²)	Hip (cm)	WHR	WHtR
Boys								
12y	361	46.4±9.8	155.3±7.6	69.3 ±8.4	19.1±3.0	82.0±7.8	0.84*±0.05	0.44*±0.05
13y	317	51.8±10.6	162.0±8.1	71.3 ±8.2	19.6±3.1	85.2±7.6	0.84*±0.05	0.44±0.05
14y	277	58.2*±11.0	169.1*±8.2	73.8*±8.7	20.3±3.0	89.2±7.7	0.83*±0.05	0.44±0.05
15y	222	64.4*±11.4	174.7*±7.7	70.1 ±8.9	21.0±2.9	92.1±7.4	0.83*±0.05	0.44±0.05
16y	186	68.6*±10.7	177.9*±6.6	77.6*±8.6	21.6±2.9	94.6±6.9	0.82*±0.05	0.44±0.05
17y	162	70.8*±11.8	178.8*±7.0	79.1*±8.4	22.1±3.3	96.2±7.5	0.82*±0.05	0.44±0.05
18y	108	72.3*±12.0	179.5*±8.2	80.4*±8.6	22.3±2.9	97.0±7.2	0.83*±0.05	0.45±0.04
Total	1633	58.5*±14.2	168.1*±11.8	74.0*±9.3	20.5±3.2	89.0±9.2	0.83*±0.05	0.44±0-05
Girls								
12y	315	47.4*±10.4	156.5*±7.4	68.0±8.9	19.2±3.4	84.9*±8.5	0.80±0.06	0.43±0.05
13y	269	52.6±10.6	161.0±6.8	70.2±8.9	20.2±3.6	89.4* ±8.0	0.78±0.06	0.44±0.05
14y	231	54.8±8.8	163.9±6.7	70.9±8.5	20.4±2.9	91.6*±6.6	0.77±0.06	0.43±0.05
15y	197	58.5±11.2	165.7±6.5	73.5*±9.8	21.3±3.7	94.3*±7.6	0.78±0.07	0.44±0.05
16y	144	58.7±11.9	165.6±6.5	73.9±8.3	21.1±2.8	95.0 ±7.9	0.78±0.06	0.45*±0.05
17y	131	59.2±8.7	166.3±6.4	74.4±8.0	21.4±2.9	95.3±6.4	0.78±0.06	0.45±0.05
18y	104	58.9±7.0	166.1±6.2	73.7±8.1	21.4±2.4	95.3±5.6	0.77±0.07	0.44±0.05
Total	1391	54.3±11.0	162.5±7.7	71.4±9.2	20.5±3.4	91.0*±8.5	0.78±0.06	0.44±0.05

Table 4. Age dependent mean values (SD) of waist circumference, body mass index, hip circumference, waist-to-hip ratio and waist-to-height ratio in male (n=1633) and female (n=1391) adolescents aged 12-18 years; *$p<0.05$ between genders

Females were significantly taller and heavier than males at age 12 y, whereas from age 14 to 18 years males were significantly taller and heavier than females. Female adolescents reached their maximal weight and height at age 17 years one year earlier than males.
As demonstrated in **Table 5** the increase of WC in males was twice of that in females (11.4 cm respectively 6.0 cm)

Males (n=1634)	Age	-2.0001 3rd	-1.3334 10th	-0.6667 25th	0 50th	0.6667 75th	1.3334 90th	2.0001 97th
	12	56.6	59.7	63.4	67.8	73.3	80.4	90.2
	13	58.9	62.0	65.7	70.1	75.7	82.9	92.7
	14	61.0	64.2	67.9	72.5	78.1	85.3	95.0
	15	62.8	66.1	70.0	74.6	80.3	87.4	96.7
	16	64.3	67.7	71.7	76.4	82.1	89.1	98.0
	17	65.9	69.3	73.3	78.0	83.7	90.6	99.5
	18	67.2	70.6	74.6	79.2	84.9	91.8	100.8
Females (n=1392)								
	12	51.4	57.0	62.6	68.2	73.8	79.4	85.0
	13	52.8	58.5	64.3	70.0	75.8	81.5	87.2
	14	53.7	59.5	65.4	71.2	77.0	82.9	88.7
	15	54.9	60.9	66.8	72.8	78.8	84.7	90.7
	16	55.6	61.7	67.7	73.8	79.8	85.9	91.9
	17	55.8	61.8	67.9	74.0	80.0	86.1	92.2
	18	55.3	61.3	67.3	73.3	79.3	85.4	91.4

Table 5. Percentile values of waist circumference in 3026 German adolescents aged 12-18 years

3.2 Cut-off points of waist circumference in adolescents

Since the International Diabetes Federation (IDF) proposed that the metabolic syndrome should not be diagnosed in children younger than age 10 years (Zimmet et al. 2007) we calculated cut-off points only for the group of adolescents.

3.2.1 Cut-off points in terms of seven anthropometric variables

Receiver operating characteristic (ROC) curves were calculated from <90th percentiles of skin fold thickness (SFT) from biceps, triceps and sub-scapular areas, SFT sum, percent body fat, waist-to-height ratio and waist-to-hip ratio. In both genders WHtR at the >90th percentile was closest to 1 in terms of an area under the curve (AUC) of 0.974 in males and 0.986 in females, followed by BF% (0.937) in males respectively by WHR (0.935) in females. (**Figure 2**).

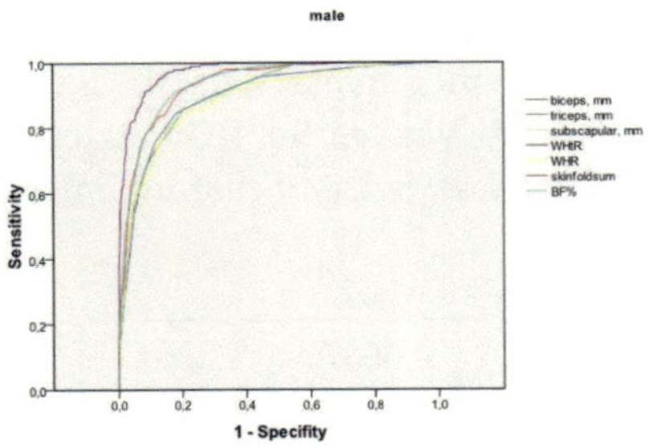

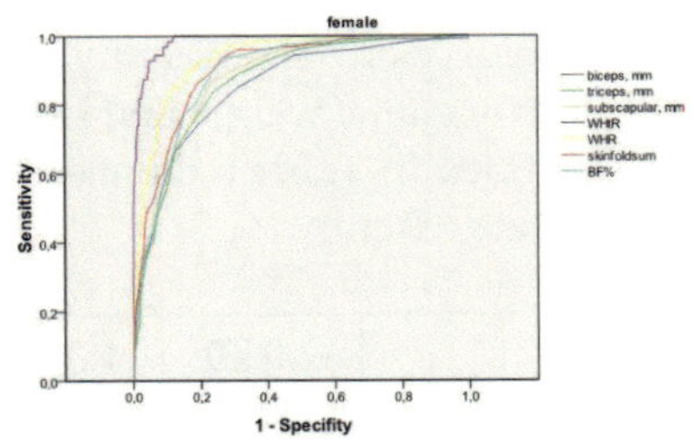

AUC (Waist Circumference >90th percentile)

Variables	area	SE	Significance asymptotic	CI 95% (asymptotic) Lower Limit	Upper Limit
Biceps SFT, mm	.896	.012	.000	.872	.920
Triceps SFT, mm	.903	.010	.000	.883	.924
Subscapular SFT, mm	.936	.008	.000	.921	.952
Sum SFT, mm	.934	.008	.000	.918	.950
WHtR	.974	.004	.000	.966	.982
WHR	.885	.013	.000	.859	.912
BF%	.937	.008	.000	.922	.953

AUC (Waist Circumference >90th percentile)

Variables	area	SE	Significance asymptotic	CI 95% (asymptotic) Lower Limit	Upper Limit
Biceps SFT, mm	.853	.018	.000	.818	.888
Triceps SFT, mm	.868	.015	.000	.839	.898
Subscapular SFT, mm	.884	.013	.000	.858	.910
Sum SFT, mm	.903	.013	.000	.878	.928
WHtR	.986	.003	.000	.981	.991
WHR	.935	.009	.000	.917	.954
BF%	.891	.013	.000	.865	.916

Fig. 2. ROC curves and AUC values calculated at and above the 90th percentile in 3026 German adolescents

3.2.2 Cut-off points in terms of eight non-anthropometric CVD risk factors

The WC cut-off points in children were 93.5 cm for hypertension, increased LDL-Cholesterol, low HDL-Cholesterol, increased triglycerides (TG), non-HDL-Cholesterol and TG/ HDL-Cholesterol ratio and not different for boys and girls except for fasting hyperglycaemia and an increased LDL-Cholesterol/HDL-Cholesterol ratio (Table 6). However, in adolescents the age-adjusted cut-off values were much more different between males and females than among children..

	Boys 6 - 11y	Girls 6 - 11 y	Boys 12 - 18y	Girls 12 - 18 y
Hypertension ≥ 95th percentile	93,5	93,5	93,5	82,5
LDL ≥ 130 mg/dL	93,5	93,5	93,5	62,5
HDL ≤ 40 mg/dL	93,5	93,5	93,5	93,5
TG ≥ 150 mg/dL	93,5	93,5	82,5	93,5
Non HDL ≥ 123 mg/dL	93,5	93,5	62,5	93,5
Glucose ≥ 150 mg/dL	62,5	93,5	82,5	93,5
Increased LDL/HDL-C ratio ≥ 3.0	82,5	62,5	82,5	62,5
Increased LDL/HDL-C ratio ≥ 3.0	93,5	93,5	93,5	93,5

Table 6.

3.3 Comparison with other ethnicities

3.3.1 Iranian and German children

The study population comprised 2076 (991 boys) Iranian and 1721 (851 boys) German children aged 6-11 years (Kelishadi et al 2008). Except height, the Iranian children had higher anthropometric measures than German children did (Table 7).

	Girls		Boys	
	Iranian	German	Iranian	German
Height (cm)	123.15±10.45	124.90±11.35	124.57±11.54	125.62±11.48
Weight (kg)	26.81 ±7.64	25.29±7.29	27.08 ± 7.12	25.51±7.03
Body mass index (kg/m²)	17.28±2.81	15.93±2.28	17.35± 2.84	15.89±2.08
Waist circumference (cm)	58.14 ±8.32	56.55±6.19	58.72± 8.34	57.46±6.20
Hip circumference (cm)	69.25± 9.12	66.17±7.78	68.81± 9.8	65.53±7.30
Waist-to-hip ratio	0.86±0.05	0.72± 0.06	0.88±0.07	0.71± 0.006

Table 7.

The age-specific reference curves of WC demonstrate a continuous increase in Iranian children from 6 years to 11 years whereas at 9 years the increase levelled off in German children (Figure 3).

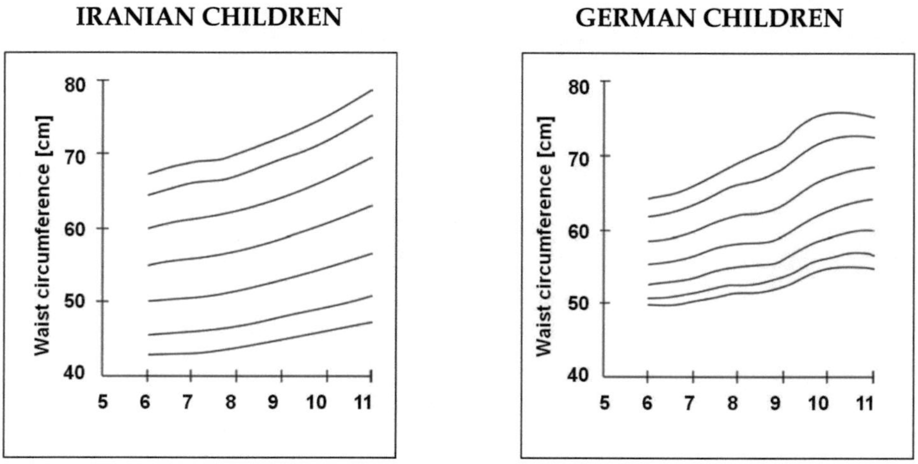

Fig. 3. LMS percentile curves of Iranian and German children (age 6-11)

The comparison of increased WC in German and Iranian adolescents mean age 12.2± 1.7 respectively 12.6±1.7 years reveals a significantly ($p<0.05$) higher prevalence in Iranian subjects than in German adolescents (Table 8).

Accordingly, the prevalence of the metabolic syndrome as defined by IDF was higher in Iranian (2.1%) adolescents than in German adolescents (0.5%).

German Total	n 3647	High WC	Iranian Total	n 2728	High WC
10 y	742	6.1	10 y	215	4.4
11 y	715	5.7	11 y	237	6.8
12 y	677	3.5	12 y	273	9.4
13 y	586	4.3	13 y	254	11.6
14 y	508	4.3	14 y	281	15.9
15 y	419	4.8	15 y	225	16.9

Table 8. Prevalence (percentage) of increased waist circumference in German and Iranian adolescents

3.3.2 Comparisons of Bazilian Iranian and German (BIG study)

The Brazilian-Iranian-German (BIG) Study compared 4473 children (6 to <10 years) and 6800 adolescents (10 to <16 years) participating in the Belo Horizonte Heart Study in Brazil, the CASPIAN Study in Iran and the PEP Family Heart Study in Germany (Schwandt et al. 2010). Table 9 shows the mean values of WC and the prevalence of increased WC (>90th percentile) for males and females of these age groups. Males from the three countries had higher mean values of WC than females. Iranian children and adolescents had lower mean values compared with Brazil and Germany. The prevalence of increased WC was lowest in Brazilian children but highest in Brazilian adolescents.

	Brazil		Iran		Germany	
	Males	Females	Males	Females	Males	Females
Age 6-<10 y						
N	241	223	757	859	1220	1173
Mean age	7.9±1.0	7.9±0.9	7.7±1.0	7.7±1.0	7.6±1.1	7.7±1.1
Mean WC cm	59.2±7.2	58.0±6.8	58.6±7.3*	57.0±7.2	59.3±6.0*	58.3±6.2
WC >90th percentile	4.4%*†	0.9%†	10.9*¶	8,0%¶	8,7%†	9.3%†
Age 10-<16 y						
N	255	290	1216	1392	1938	1709
Mean age	13.0±1.7	13.2±1.7	12.6±1.7	12.6±1.7	12.2±1.7	12.2±1.7
Mean WC cm	68.4±10.0*	65.7±8.1	67.5±9.8*	66.3±9.1	69.9±8.9*	68.0±9.1†
WC >90th percentile	16.1%*	8,9%	10.5%¶	9,0%	8.8%	9,7%

Legend *p<0.05 for gender, †p<0.05 for Germany vs. Iran, ¶p<0.05 for Iran vs. Brazil

Table 9. Comparison of WC values and prevalence of increased WC in children and adolescents from Brazil, Iran and Germany

3.3.3 Turkish and German children

Comparing 2473 Turkish and German first graders (mean age 6.4 years) participating in the PEP Family Heart Study in Nuremberg Turkish boys (58.5±8.9 vs. 56.9±6.1) and Turkish girls (57.6±9.2 vs. 55.8±5.8) girls had significantly higher values than German children did although living in the same town. These differences might be due to different lifestyle as well as to genetic factors (Haas et al. 2008).

Age- and gender-specific percentile values are shown in table 10 and table 11 for 320 Turkish (155 boys and 165 girls) and 3531 German (1788 boys and 1743 girls) children participating in the PEP Family Heart Study.

	Age (y)	3rd perc	10th perc	25th perc	50th perc	75th perc	90th perc	97th perc
German Boys	3	45,42125	47,18961	49,02191	50,92029	52,88695	54,92416	57,03426
	4	46,69526	48,46758	50,39043	52,48431	54,77372	57,28811	60,06324
	5	47,85518	49,65204	51,67864	53,98907	56,65722	59,7872	63,53141
	6	49,09508	50,96856	53,13880	55,69791	58,78483	62,62184	67,59351
	7	49,85503	51,85384	54,19979	57,01334	60,48490	64,93884	70,98889
	8	50,92392	53,05610	55,58078	58,64386	62,48325	67,52202	74,61327
	9	52,45929	54,71848	57,41692	60,72932	64,95015	70,62830	78,95486
	10	54,13066	56,50359	59,36617	62,92871	67,56040	73,99220	83,97658
	11	55,52872	57,99448	60,99931	64,79309	69,83402	77,09267	89,19402
Turkish Boys	3	45,13165	46,56837	48,16657	49,95961	51,99147	54,32160	57,03266
	4	46,62536	48,22576	50,02131	52,05606	54,38956	57,10463	60,32063
	5	47,56840	49,31606	51,29320	53,55601	56,18229	59,28349	63,02618
	6	48,74434	50,64942	52,82218	55,33326	58,28282	61,81867	66,17017
	7	49,72113	51,77748	54,14133	56,89969	60,17884	64,17075	69,18511
	8	50,84256	53,05759	55,62350	58,64620	62,28308	66,78065	72,55271
	9	52,21283	54,59960	57,38526	60,69772	64,73153	69,80078	76,45477
	10	53,61329	56,17588	59,18871	62,80458	67,26134	72,95489	80,60757
	11	54,60335	57,32400	60,54554	64,44736	69,31509	75,63903	84,35397

Table 10. Percentiles for waist circumference in 3 – 11 y old boys

	Age (y)	3rd perc	10th perc	25th perc	50th perc	75th perc	90th perc	97th perc
German Girls	3	44,19034	45,79188	47,60676	49,68840	52,11125	54,98302	58,46667
	4	45,43920	47,16375	49,12995	51,40178	54,07009	57,26926	61,20855
	5	46,84072	48,68316	50,79415	53,24795	56,15164	59,66655	64,05009
	6	47,94398	49,90333	52,16059	54,80217	57,95469	61,81306	66,69706
	7	48,59970	50,68025	53,09390	55,94300	59,38086	63,65009	69,16380
	8	49,32377	51,53956	54,12971	57,21650	60,98747	65,74889	72,04508
	9	50,22757	52,59150	55,37626	58,72775	62,87536	68,20625	75,44123
	10	51,51220	54,04821	57,05925	60,71992	65,31187	71,32723	79,72974
	11	52,86370	55,58198	58,83524	62,83172	67,91631	74,71423	84,51890
Turkish Girls	3	43,04967	45,53947	48,01737	50,48407	52,94023	55,38641	57,82314
	4	44,66278	47,35326	50,16913	53,11458	56,19386	59,41132	62,77140
	5	46,14307	48,96775	52,07110	55,49183	59,27567	63,47701	68,16096
	6	46,92607	49,79550	53,07608	56,86617	61,29882	66,55875	72,91049
	7	47,60613	50,46602	53,83657	57,88478	62,86421	69,18208	77,54257
	8	50,24199	53,19411	56,74006	61,11031	66,68391	74,13976	84,85235
	9	52,82375	55,86301	59,55225	64,16765	70,18581	78,52220	91,24661
	10	54,14897	57,17937	60,89252	65,60252	71,87704	80,88622	95,61519
	11	54,88581	57,84137	61,50332	66,22778	72,69708	82,45647	100,2245

Table 11. Percentiles for waist circumference in 3 – 11 y old Girls

The WC differences between Turkish and German boys decreases from age 3 to age 11 whereas the mean differences in girls increases from age 3 to age 11 years.
Figure 4 and Figure 5 demonstrate the importance of choosing the percentile for comparisons. At the 50th percentile the difference of increasing WC between years 3 and 11 in German and Turkish children is only slight whereas the curve in Turkish girls is much more steeper compared with the other three curves.

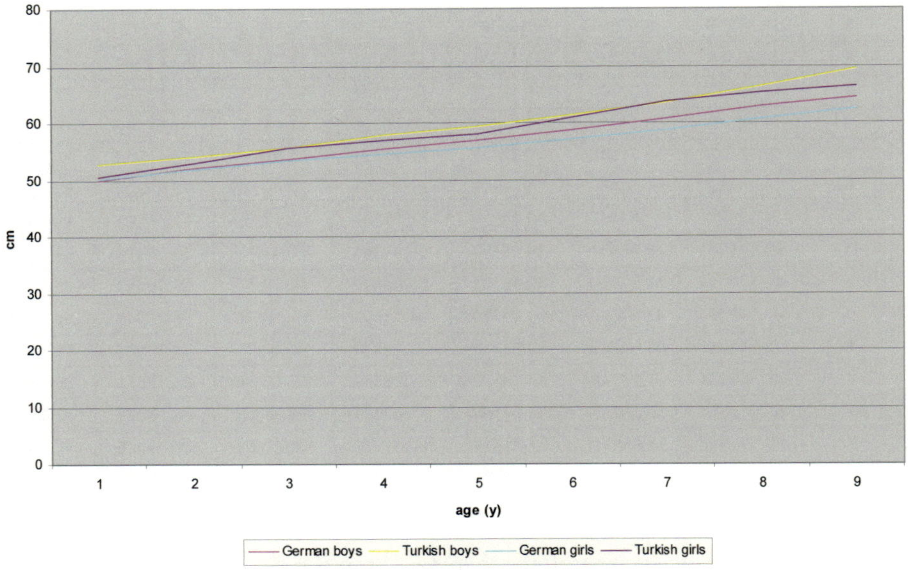

Fig. 4. 50th percentile of LMS waist circumference for German and Turkish children 3 – 11 y

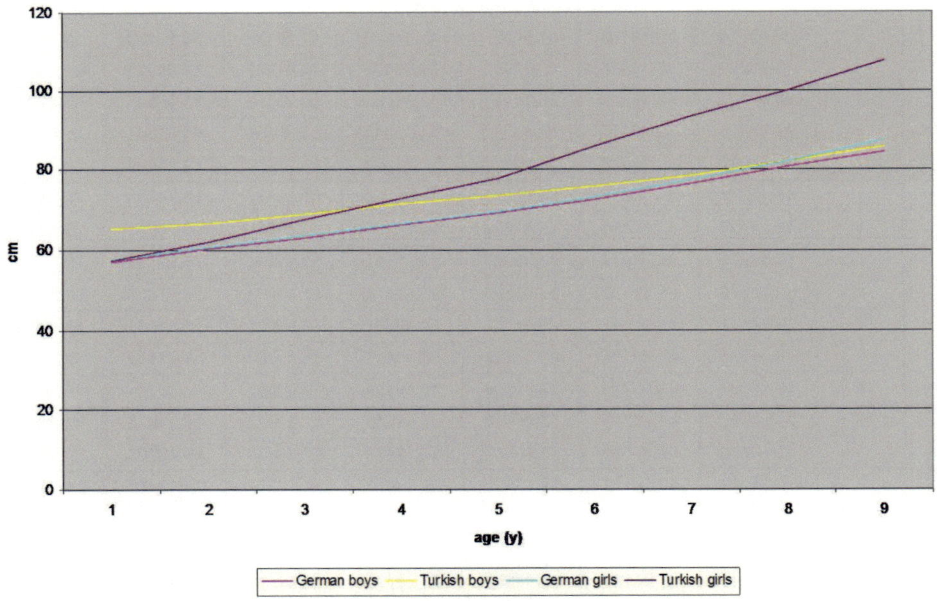

Fig. 5. 90th percentile of LMS waist circumference for German and Turkish children 3 – 11 y

Figure 6 demonstrates these differences at four different percentiles

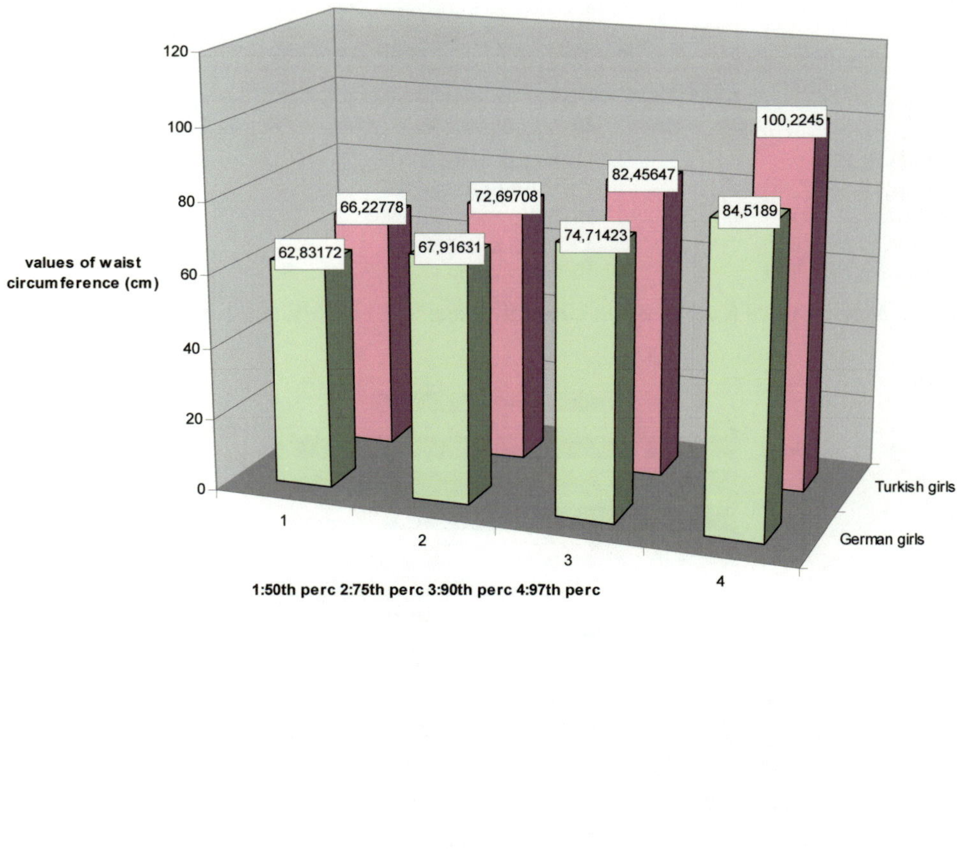

Fig. 6. 50th , 75th , 90th and 97th percentiles of waist circumference in 11 y old Turkish and German girls participatin in the PEP Family Heart Study

3.3.4 Ethnic comparisons of WC form children from literature

Table 12 and Table 13 compare the mean WC values from 6 respectively 11 years old children from 11 countries in boys and in girls. The continuous increase of waist circumference in these countries is shown in figure 5 and figure 6 (Schwandt et al. 2008).

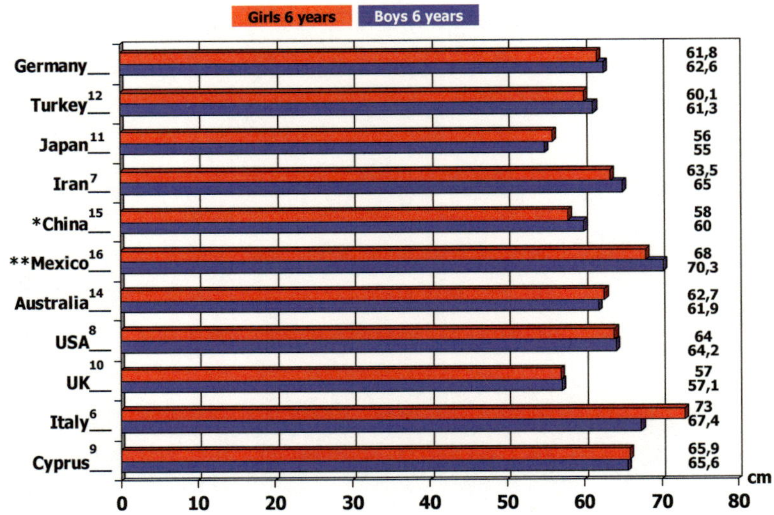

6. Zannolli R, 1996
7. Kelishadi R, 2007
8. Fernandez JR, 2004
9. Savva SC, 2001
10. McCarthy HD, 2001
11. Inokuchi M, 2007
12. Hatipoglu N, 2007
14. Eisenmann JC: 2005
15. Sung RY, 2007
16. Gómez-Diaz RA, 2005

Table 12. Mean values (cm) of waist circumference in 6 years old children from 11 countries

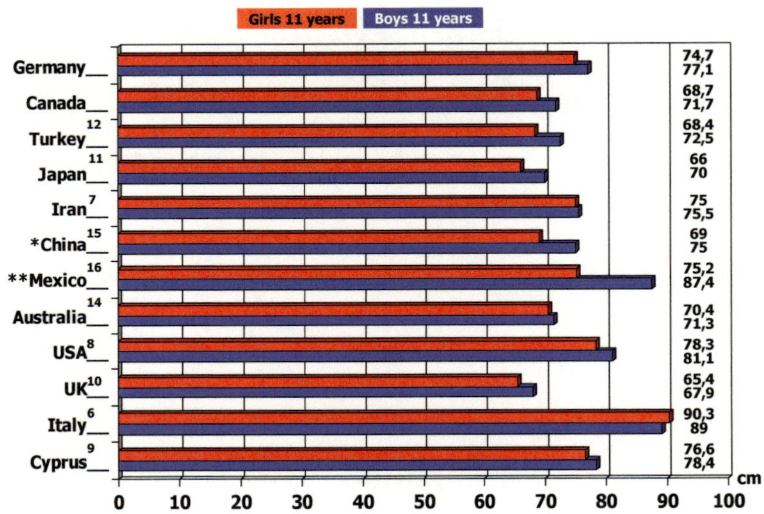

* by curve ** Mexico (10 years)

6. Zannolli R, 1996
7. Kelishadi R, 2007
8. Fernandez JR, 2004
9. Savva SC, 2001
10. McCarthy HD, 2001
11. Inokuchi M, 2007
12. Hatipoglu N, 2007
14. Eisenmann JC: 2005
15. Sung RY, 2007
16. Gómez-Diaz RA, 2005

Table 13. Mean values (cm) of waist circumference in 11 years old children from 11 countries

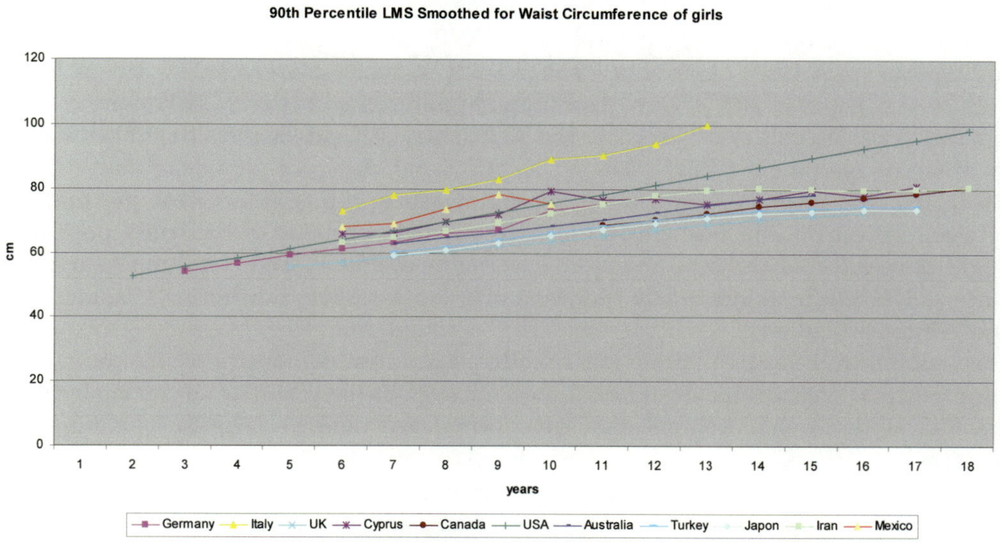

Fig. 7. Waist circumference (cm) at the 90th percentile in girls from 11 countries

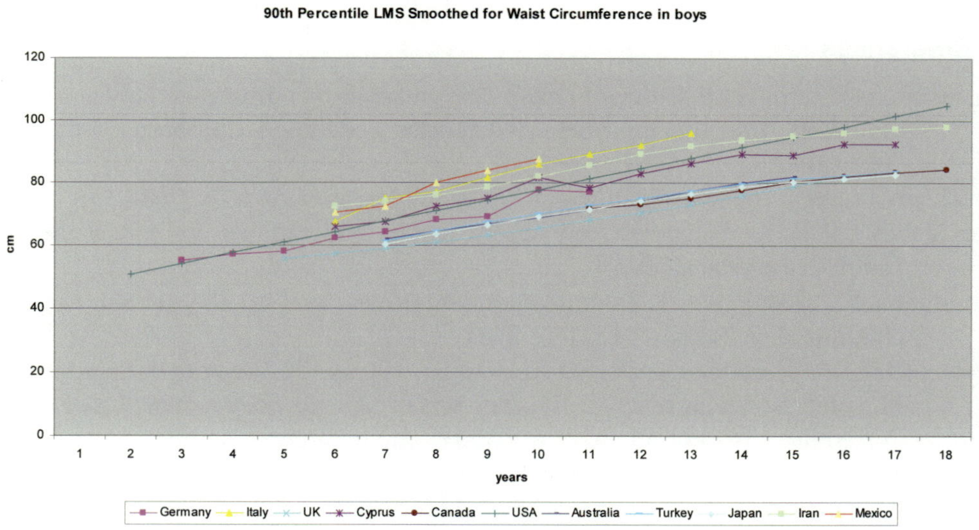

Fig. 8. Waist circumference (cm) at the 90th percentile in boys from 11 countries

4. Conclusions

In 4473 children and 6829 adolescents from Germany, Iran and Brazil the mean prevalence of increased waist circumference (≥ 90th percentile) was 7.0% respectively 10.5%. Increased waist circumference (≥ 90th percentile) is a clinically accessible diagnostic tool and a measure of central obesity that is essential for the global IDF definition of the metabolic syndrome (Zimmet et al. 2007). For adolescents aged 10 years and older increased WC and two or more other features like hypertension, hyperglycaemia, hypertriglyceridemia, and low HDL-Cholesterol are diagnostic.

The relatively homogeneous WC mean values in adolescents of the three different ethnicities in the BIG Study (Schwandt et al., 2010) are far lower than WC mean values of adolescents from USA describing 79.6±12.5 cm in males and 78.8±11.7 cm in females (Jolliffe and Janssen, 2007). These considerable differences between 2906 male and 3116 female US adolescents and 3409 male and 3328 female BIG adolescents might be explained by different age ranges (12-20 years vs. 10-<16 years), different periods of data collection (1988-2002 vs. 2000-2008) and/or different measure points (iliac crest vs. mid-point between lowest rib and iliac crest). Furthermore, heterogeneity of the study populations might have affected the outcome since The National Health and Nutrition Examination Surveys NHANES are nationally representative cross-sectional including Hispanic, Black and White participants.

This comparison of two large cross-sectional studies demonstrates the outstanding importance of comparable design and methodology of the studies. The main strength of the BIG study is that original data of a very large number (11,273) of children and adolescents from Germany, Iran and Brazil of youths from three continents were measured and evaluated by the same methodology. One limitation of the study is that genetic and environmental effects (e.g. physical activity, nutrition and second hand tobacco smoke exposition respectively active smoking) on anthropometric measures are not included.

5. References

Alberti KGMM, Zimmet P & Shaw J (2005) .The metabolic syndrome – a new world-wide definition from the International Diabetes Federation Consensus. *Lancet*, 366: 1059 - 1062.

Bauchner H (2008). The globalization of child health research. *Arch Dis Child*, 93:1

Cornia GA (2001). Globalization and health: results and options. *Bulletin of the World Health Organisation,2001*:79

Eisenmann JC. (2005) .Waist circumference percentiles for 7-to 15-year-old Australian children. *Acta Paediatr*, 94:, 1182 - 1185

Gómez-Diaz RA, Martinez-Hernández AJ, Aguilar-Salinas CA, Violante R, López-Alarcón M, Jiménez-Viallarruel M, Wacher-Rodarte.N, & Solozano-Santos F (2005). Percentile distribution of the waist circumference among Mexican pre-adolescents of a primary school in Mexico City. *Diabetes Obes Metab*; 7; 716 - 721

Haas GM, Liepold E & Schwandt P. (2008) Hypertension in Turkish and German first graders participating in the PEP Family Heart Study. *Atherosclerosis* Suppl.; 9: 95

Haas, GM, Liepold E & Schwandt P. (2008) Age- and gender-specific waist circumference in Turkish and German children participating in the PEP Family Heart Study. Oral presentation at the 77th European Atherosclerosis Society Congress, Istanbul, Turkey

Haas GM, Liepold E & Schwandt P. (2011) Percentile curves for fat pattering in German adolescents. *World J Pediatr*; 7: 16-23

Hatipoglu N, Ozturk A, Mazicioglu MM, Kurtoglu S, Seyhan S & Lokoglu F. (2007) Waist circumference percentiles for 7-17-year-old Turkish children and adolescents. *Eur J Pediatr*; published online 9 May

Hawkes C (2006) Uneven dietary development: linking the policies and processes of globalization with the nutrition transition, obesity and diet-related chronic diseases *www.globalizationandhealth.com/content/2/1/4*

Hu FB (2008) Globalization of Food Patterns and Cardiovascular Disease Risk. *Circulation; 118:*1913-1914

Inokuchi M, Matsuo N, Anzo M, Takayama JI & Hasegawa T. (2007) Age dependent percentile for waist circumference for Japanese children based on the 1992-1994 cross-sectional national survey data. *Eur J Pediatr*;166: 655-661

Jolliffe CJ and Janssen I. (2007) Development of age-specific adolescent metabolic syndrome criteria that are linked to the Adult Treatmen Panel III and International Diabetes Federation criteria. *JACC*; 49: 891-898

Katzmarzyk PT. (2004) Waist circumference percentiles for Canadian youth 11-18y of age. *Eur J Clin Nutr*; 58: 1011-1015

Kelishadi R, Schwandt P, Haas GM, Hosseini M & Mirmoghtadaee P. (2008) Reference curves of anthropometric indices and serum lipid profiles in representative samples of Asian and European children. *Arch Med Sci*; 4: 329-335

McCarthy HD, Jarrett KV & Crawley HF. (2001) The development of waist circumference percentiles in British children aged 5.0-16.9y. *Eur.J.Clin*; 55: 902-907

Savva SC, Kourides Y, Tornaritis M, Epiphanious-Savva M, Tafouna P & Kafatos A. (2001) Reference growth curves for Cypriot children 6-17 years of age. *Obes Res*; 9: 754 - 762

Schwandt P, Geiss HC, Ritter MM, Üblacker C, Parhofer KG, Otto C, Laubach E, Donner MG, Haas GM & Richter WO. (1999) The prevention education program (PEP). A prospective study of the efficacy of family-oriented life style modification in the reduction of cardiovascular risk and disease: design and baseline data. *J Clin Epidemiol*. 52: 791-800

Schwandt P, Kelishadi R & Haas GM. (2008) First Reference curves of waist: Circumference for German children: The PEP Family Heart Study. *World J Pediatr*; 4: 259-266

Schwandt P, Bischoff-Ferrari HA, Staehelin HB & Haas GM. (2009) Cardiovascular risk screening in schoolchildren predicts risk in parents. *Atherosclerosis*; 205: 626-631

Schwandt P, Bertsch T & Haas GM. (2010) Anthropometric screening for silent cardiovascular risk factors in adolescents: The PEP Family Heart Study. *Atherosclerosis*; 211: 667-671

Schwandt P, Kelishadi R, Ribeiro RQC, Haas GM & Poursafa P. (2010) A three-country study on the components of the metabolic syndrome in youths: The BIG Study. *Intern Journal of Pediatric Obesity*; 5: 334-341

Sung RY, Yu CC, Choi KC, McManus A, Li AM, Xu SL, *et al* . (2007) Waist circumference and body mass index in Chinese children: cut off values for predicting cardiovascular risk factors. *Int J Obes (Lond)*; 31: 550-558

Wang J, Thornton JC, Bari S, Williamsson B, Gallagher D, Heymsfield SB, *et a*l. (2003) Comparisons of waist circumferences measured at 4 sites. *Am J Clin Nutr*; 77: 379-384

Zimmet P, Alberti G, Kaufman F, Tajima N, Silink M, Arsolanian S, Wong G, Bennett P, Shaw J & Caprio S, (2007) on behalf of the International Diabetes Federation Task Force on Epidemiology and Prevention of Diabetes. The metabolic syndrome in children and adolescents. *Lancet*; 369: 2059-2061

5

Critical Periods for the Development of Obesity

C. Campoy[1], T. Anjos[1] and E. Martín-Bautista[2]
[1]*Department of Paediatrics. School of Medicine. Excellence Centre for Paediatric Research EURISTIKOS. University of Granada*
[2]*Progress and Health Foundation. Andalusian Regional Ministry of Health*
Spain

1. Introduction

The mother's nutritional and metabolic environment is critical in determining not only the success of reproduction but also for the future health of the newborn. Maternal genetics, maternal diet during pregnancy, lactation and infant feeding in the early stages of life can have long-term effects on children's health and may predispose to diseases such as obesity. The term "*programming*" has been used to describe the process by which stimuli or manipulations applied during critical or sensitive periods of development and organogenesis can cause changes in the long term in structures and functions of the body, compromising the future health of the individual (Barker, 1994; Lucas, 1994; Symonds et al., 2007). The concept "*programming*" defines the genetic, diet, nutrition and habits in the early stages of life for the pregnant mother and child, which are main factors influencing the optimal neurological and psychological development of children (Dunstan et al., 2008; Helland et al., 2003; Hibbeln et al., 2005; Wells, 2007) and the development of diseases in adulthood (Lucas, 2005; Wells, 2007) such as diabetes (Fernández-Twinn & Ozanne, 2006), obesity (Budge et al., 2005; Koletzko, 2006), cardiovascular disease (Feldt et al., 2007), some types of cancer (Key et al., 2004) and bone diseases (Sayer & Cooper, 2005) (Figure 1).

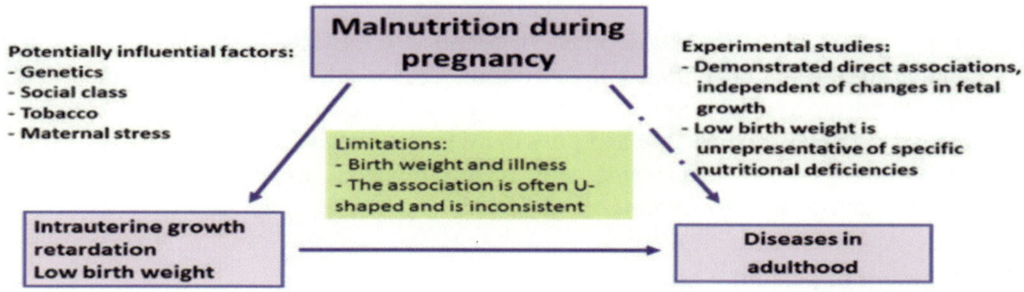

Fig. 1. The different factors that can affect the long-term health of the newborn

Studies have shown that maternal nutrition during pregnancy (Krauss-Etschmann et al., 2007; Lucas, 2005), breastfeeding (Koletzko, 2006) and complementary feeding can influence children's development and long-term health (Demmelmair et al., 2006). It has also been demonstrated that birth weight can have a significant effect on the interaction between fat and muscle metabolism (Symonds et al., 2006).

2. Programming of obesity from early stages in life

In the early 50's, Widdowson & McCance, 1963, began to study in animal models the influence of pre- and postnatal diet on the development of obesity. These researchers found that rats born with low weight and subsequently overfed during postnatal life, developed a large size and body weight in adulthood; the rats overfed during early lactation, showed high concentrations of insulin and cholesterol. Since then, numerous studies have shown that obesity, a plague in Western countries, may have its roots before birth (Cottrell & Ozanne, 2008). However, much remains to be elucidated about how the human body records these impressions. Given that obesity is primarily a disorder of energy balance, where energy intake exceeds energy expenditure, its mechanisms may involve the regulation of appetite and a disruption of energy expenditure together with an alteration of tissue metabolism and physical activity (Taylor & Poston, 2007).

Currently there is scientific evidence from both epidemiological and animal studies suggesting that programming of obesity is caused by environmental influences that occur from the embryonic stage to neonatal life and childhood. Studies in animal models show that the foetus and newborn may be receiving different hormonal and dietary insults that converge in a common phenotype of hyperphagia, obesity, impaired adipocyte function and alteration of physical activity. Although the programming of obesity is clearly a multifactorial process, the diversity of models with a common goal allows suggesting some common metabolic pathways. The change in adipocyte development and the stimulation of the secretion of glucocorticoids seems to play an important role in the plasticity of the hypothalamus at the end of gestation and early postnatal life and is also clearly involved in programming appetite and metabolism to establish a higher body weight, which may or may not be adjusted over time (Taylor & Poston, 2007).

Different mechanisms during critical stages of development may be involved in the early programming of adult obesity, including:

1. Impairment of placental function,
2. Formation of foetal adipose tissue and regulation of leptin synthesis and secretion before birth (McMillen et al., 2006; Singhal et al., 2002),
3. Some genes related to the development of obesity: FTO, INSIG 2, MC4R, Pro12AlA and PPARγ2 Ala12Ala, LEP, POMC polymorphisms C8246T and C1032G, ... (Creemers et al., 2008; Hinney et al., 2007; Loos et al., 2008) and epigenetic alteration of the foetal genome,
4. Prenatal nutrition, birth weight and growth rate in postnatal life (McMillen et al., 2006).
5. Programming the neuroendocrine network that regulates appetite (Breier et al., 2001; López-Soldado et al., 2006; Ozanne & Hales, 2002).

2.1 Impairment of placental function

The placenta is the first of the foetal organs to develop and has several fascinating and critical functions by which it plays a direct part in foetal programming. Pre-pregnancy obesity is related to established hypertension and in some cases undiagnosed type 2 diabetes (*"Diabesity"*) and it is associated with increased risk of placental dysfunction and foetal death as gestation advances. Epidemiological evidence has linked low birth weight and low placental weight to foetal programming. So, foetal growth and the long-term determination of the future offspring are intimately linked to the regulation of the main functions of the placenta.

There is some evidence which suggest that a child of an obese or diabetic mother may suffer from exposure to a sub-optimal in uterus environment and that these early life adversities may extend into adulthood. Also, the development of gestational diabetes (GDM) is associated with a shift in the concentration of several hormones, cytokines, metabolites, and growth factors that may subsequently alter placental morphology and function with very serious consequences (Hiden & Desoye, 2010). One primary mechanism that linked maternal nutritional status and the predisposition of metabolic disease is related to altered placental functionalities (Farley et al., 2009). Maternal obesity in humans determines an increase of placental and adipose tissue macrophage infiltration, and also an increase of CD14+ expression in maternal peripheral blood mononuclear cells (PBMC) and maternal hyperleptinemia. It seems that chronic inflammation state of pre-gravid obesity is extending to in uterus life with accumulation of a heterogeneous macrophage population and pro-inflammatory mediators in the placenta (Challier et al., 2008). The resulting inflammatory milieu in which the foetus develops may have critical consequences for short and long term programming of obesity (Farley, 2009).

Foetal nutrient delivery depends on the complex interaction of maternal uterine and foetal umbilical blood flow, nutrient supply, placental microstructure and transport capacity.

The placenta is an important regulator of foetal growth, due to its roles in nutrient supply to the foetus, removal from the foetus of metabolic waste and hormone production (Higgins et al., 2011). The role of the trophoblast (both amount and function), in placental transporter activity, hormone production and substrate metabolism is being recently investigated. There is evidence that changes in the activity and expression of trophoblast nutrient and ion transporters are fundamental in determining foetal growth and the molecular mechanisms regulating trophoblast transporters, which are directly related to the development of pregnancy complications and foetal programming of cardiovascular and metabolic disease (Roberts et al., 2009). The concept of the placenta as a "*nutrient sensor*" has been reported by Jansson and Powell, 2007, introducing the idea about how the placenta coordinates nutrient transport functions with maternal nutrient availability. Thus the ability of the maternal supply line to deliver nutrients (i.e. placental blood flow, maternal nutrition, substrate and oxygen levels in maternal blood, etc.) regulates key placental nutrient transporters. With this perspective, placental transport alterations represent a mechanism to match foetal growth rate to a level which is compatible with the amount of nutrients that can be provided by the maternal supply line, making the placenta a *key player* in the regulation of foetal growth and, as a consequence, foetal programming.

2.2 Foetal adipose tissue formation

The period covering uterine implantation and rapid placental growth is a critical window of organogenesis. During this period there is a marked cell division within developing organelles preceding the structural development of many foetal tissues. Adipogenesis, which begins in uterus and accelerates in the neonatal period, is the leading candidate for the development of programming. In humans, after a short period of fat deposition during childhood, there is a rapid acceleration around 6 years, which will be relevant in case of a premature development of fatty tissue mass (before 5.5 years) in children, because it is associated with an increased adult obesity (Eriksson et al., 2002).

Currently there is evidence from studies both in humans and in sheep, that the synthesis and secretion of hormones produced by adipocytes such as leptin already have regulatory mechanisms in foetal life (Symonds et al., 2003). Small perturbations in the foetal adipose tissue growth and endocrine sensitivity may have important long-term effects (Symonds et al., 2004). The magnitude of these and subsequent changes in adipose tissue are determined by the maternal and foetal nutritional environment. The consequences depend on the stage where the change occurs, either in embryogenesis, the formation of the placenta or during foetal development. All three are critical windows and it has been shown that neural development and cardiovascular function are more sensitive to the influences during the embryonic period, whereas the renal system is more affected during placental development and adipose tissue is more affected in the stage of foetal development (Symonds et al., 2007). In humans, adipose tissue has its origin during the early stages of foetal life; during normal foetal development two adipocyte cell lines, white and brown (brown) will develop (Moulin et al., 2001). Foetal fat exhibits characteristics of both cell lines, showing an ontogenetic increase of the specific uncoupled protein (UCP-1) of brown adipose tissue (Clarke et al., 1997), along with a modest increase in leptin synthesis, produced primarily by white adipocytes. Foetal adipose tissue is formed by the combination of multilocular and unilocular cells (Yuen et al., 2003), of which the latter have few/ no mitochondria (Figure 2).

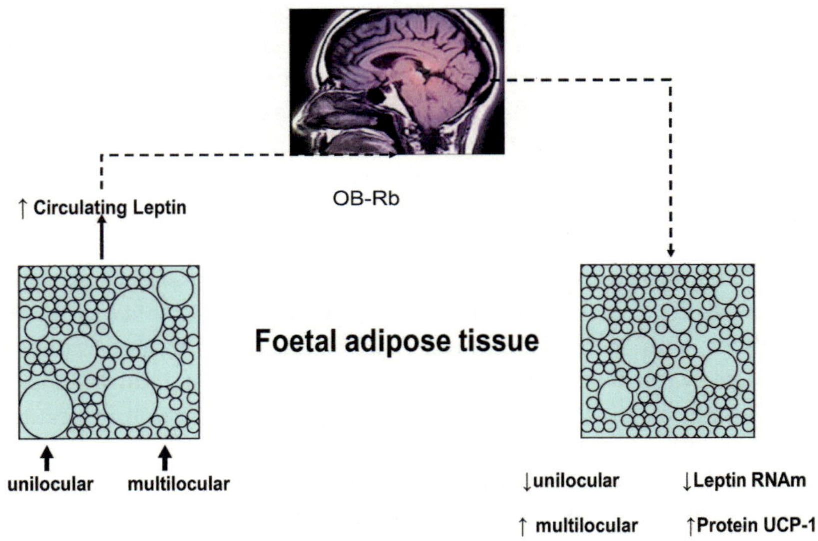

Fig. 2. Schematic diagram with a summary of the potential effects of increased circulating leptin concentrations on the structural and functional characteristics of foetal adipose tissue (modified from Yuen et al., 2003).

However, the proportional concentration increases after birth to have white adipose tissue as dominant. In lambs, after birth, there is an important endocrine stimulation that inhibits the synthesis of UCP-1 to undetectable levels at a month of life (Symonds et al., 2004). The decrease in UCP-1 is parallel to an increase in plasma leptin and the mRNA for the leptin synthesis for around the first week of life (Bispham et al., 2002) (Figure 3). The increased deposition in adipose tissue after the first week takes place independently of any change in leptin.

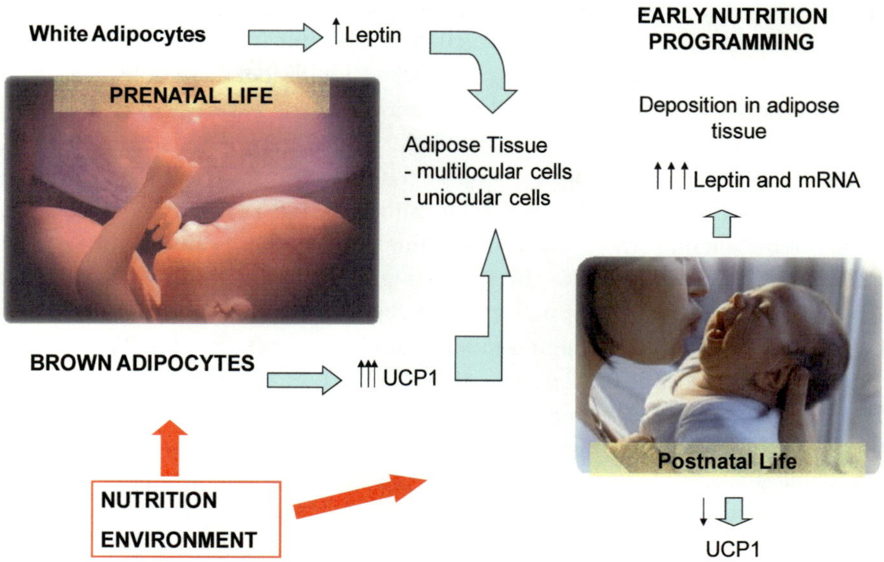

Fig. 3. Changes in the production of UCP1 and leptin during foetal and postnatal life.

It has been observed in sheep that a reduction in caloric intake of 50% during the period of implantation and placental development profoundly affects placental growth and morphology to a reduction of placental weight (Clarke et al., 1998). This takes place together with a low capacity for inactivation of maternal cortisol by the enzyme 11 hydroxysteroid dehydrogenase type 2 (11 β -HDS-2) (Whorwood et al., 2001), which occur in response to declining maternal plasma cortisol (Bispham et al., 2003). Gene expression in the placenta of both glucocorticoid receptors and uncoupled mitochondrial protein 2 (UCP-2) increases and this could partly contribute to the reduction that accompanies the decreased proliferation of placental cells after nutritional restriction (Gnanalingham et al., 2007). Birth weight, however, is not altered by this dietary manipulation and, although it has more fat, this adaptation does not persist into adulthood even though obesity is developed. It is unclear how the mother may influence foetal adipogenesis and determine the time of the "*fat rebound,*" but there is evidence of programming of the morphology and metabolism of the adipocyte. Like many other type of tissues, adipose tissue has the potential to grow limitlessly. But this diet-induced growth increases the number of fat cells in an apparently irreversible manner (Corbett et al., 1986). It should be expected a direct influence on the development of hyperplasia or fat hypertrophy in the baby after a maternal hipernutritive diet, because glucose is the major metabolic precursor of lipid synthesis; the direct infusion of glucose in the foetus is accompanied by a parallel increase in fat mass (Stevens et al., 1990), but the persistence of this effect into adulthood is not defined. Adipocyte hypertrophy also occurs in rats after weaning when the mothers were subject to pleasant diets during pregnancy and lactation (Bayol et al., 2005).

2.3 Genetic factors

Any molecular mechanism that justifies the programming of obese adult phenotype development must explain how early environmental stress can determine persistent molecular changes that give rise to profound damage that will affect health in adulthood.

2.3.1 Epigenetic programming of mitochondrial and nuclear genome

One of the molecular mechanisms by which maternal nutrition and metabolic status can influence foetal programming is the epigenetic alteration of foetal genome. These alterations may involve chromatin remodelling and regulation of gene expression. The characteristics of mitochondria in development are particularly suited to translate the early stress associated with development programming in the form of cellular dysfunction that can be observed in later periods of life. The levels of mitochondrial DNA (mtDNA) are exquisitely sensitive to environmental stress, and a suboptimal environment can produce a reduction in the quantity and quality of mtDNA by increasing the rate of mutations (Graziewicz et al., 2006; Taylor et al., 2005). Recent publications from human studies (Ruiz-Pesini et al., 2004; Wilson et al., 2004) and in experimental models of obesity and diabetes (Wisloff et al., 2005) imply that altered mitochondrial function at least contributes to the development of obesity and related conditions. MtDNA mutations are tolerated for many years before exceeding the threshold level of damage (Chinnery et al., 2002), which would explain the long-term influence of mitochondrial function with implications, in particular, on energy expenditure (Taylor et al., 2007; Wisloff et al., 2005).

2.3.2 Altered state of methylation

Persistent epigenetic changes in methylation status of nuclear DNA (nDNA) can deeply influence the programming of obesity (Blewitt et al., 2006; Lillycrop et al., 2005; Ollikainen et al., 2010; Waterland, 2006). In addition, the potential neurotrophic action of leptin can programme the genes involved in regulating centres of appetite and energy expenditure in the developing hypothalamus (Bouret et al., 2004). The alteration of methylation status in very early embryonic development may also contribute to the obese phenotype observed in embryo transfer and cloning processes. (Sakai et al., 2005). There is evidence that early nutrition has an effect on DNA methylation. Studies have shown that promoter DNA methylation of *PPARGC1A*, *PPARG*, and *Tfam* genes may be associated with newborns' anthropometric and laboratory variables, and with their mothers' pre-pregnant BMI. This suggests that maternal obesity may influence the offsprings' metabolism throughout several mechanisms, among them epigenetic regulation of many genes, such as *PPARGC1A* promoter methylation, and so the baby might be at risk of becoming obese in later life (Gemma et al., 2009). Early malnutrition (both under nutrition and overweight) with respect to methyl donors can cause what is known as *"epigenetic aging"*, contributing to increased susceptibility to diseases present in adult life (Waterland & Jirtle, 2004). There is convincing data from animal models (Champagne et al., 2006; Lillycrop et al., 2008) and experimental data in human studies (Bjornsson et al., 2008; Christensen et al., 2009). The results of human studies strongly suggest an effect of prenatal exposure to adverse environments (such as exposure to famine or dietary supplementation) in determining the level of DNA methylation present in the offspring, specifically at imprinted genomic regions implicated in regulating foetal growth (Tobi et al., 2009). Rapid growth may lead to postnatal changes in programming the expression of some genes that had been predetermined in uterus. It has been shown that increased expression of insulin receptors is present in the offspring of rodents subjected to protein restriction (Martin-Gronert & Ozanne, 2005). The genetic susceptibility to insulin resistance or β cell dysfunction causes changes in foetal growth mediated by insulin, which results in a low birth weight and increased risk of developing type 2 diabetes in adulthood (Hattersley & Tooke, 1999). Insulin is a hormone promoter of foetal growth; insulin concentrations are positively related to glucose

levels in the foetus and birth weight. Since insulin acts both as a signal for normal energy balance and as antilipolytic agent, changes in the signs of insulin may have an effect on appetite and obesity. Three genes or DNA common loci have been identified and can be replicated as candidate genes regulators in the development of obesity: FTO, INSIG 2, MC4R (Hinney et al., 2007). Still, 4 of the most studied genes are involved in the development of foetal and postnatal adipose tissue, of which two are receptors, glucocorticoid receptor - GR, and the activated receptor for proliferation of peroxisome - PPAR (Robitaille et al., 2004), and two are metabolic enzymes, the 11 *β-dehydrogenase* type I hidroesteroide or 11 *β-HSD-1* (Itoh et al., 2004) and 11 *β-dehydrogenase* type II hidroesteroide - 11 *β-HSD-2* (Nuñez et al., 1999).
Persistent alteration in the expression of any of the many proteins that influence the development of adipocytes and lipolysis (i.e. *PPAR-γ*) can exert a permanent influence on adipocyte proliferation and cell hypertrophy processes. PPAR-*γ* proteins are the main regulators of adipocyte differentiation and have been considered important factors in controlling insulin sensitivity throughout the body. The PPAR-*γ* 1 and PPAR-*γ* 2 are generated from the same gene by alternative promoter usage and mRNA (Fajas et al., 1997). However, little is known about the regulation of PPAR-*γ* gene expression in human tissues (Rosado et al., 2006). The PPAR-*γ* are members of a nuclear receptor super family that heterodimerize with acid receptor 9-cis-retinoic acid (RXR) and is linked to specific response elements in promoter regions of target genes to change their rate of transcription (Kliewer et al., 2001). In humans, it can be differentiated in 28 amino terminals, but have the same binding domain. PPAR-*γ* 1 is preferentially expressed in adipocytes, but also in other cell types and tissues such as colon, epithelial cells of the gastrointestinal tract (Lefebvre et al., 1999), kidney, macrophages (Ricote et al., 1998) and, at a smaller extent, in skeletal muscle. In contrast, the expression of PPAR-*γ* 2 mRNA is largely restricted to adipocytes. PPAR-*γ* proteins are the main regulators of adipocyte differentiation (Lowell, 1999) and have been considered important factors in controlling insulin sensitivity throughout the body. The altered expression of adipocyte proteins has been demonstrated in mothers suffering from malnutrition {(adipocytes of lambs subject to a restrictive diet in prenatal life show an increase in the expression of 11 *β-HSD-1* and GR}, which leads to increased exposure to cortisol and increased proliferation of adipocytes (Reynolds et al., 2001; Gnanalingham et al., 2005). Human studies have shown that the expression of 11 *β-HSD-1* in subcutaneous fat is correlated with BMI, suggesting a potential therapeutic role of selective antagonists in humans (Wake &Walker, 2004). The programming of PPAR-*γ* has been demonstrated in the liver of children exposed to a diet deficient in protein during foetal life and has been linked to an altered state of methylation (Lillycrop et al., 2005). These are potentially important molecular targets in programming the development of obesity and have yet to be explored in depth.

2.3.3 Mutation in the leptin gene.

Leptin is an adipocyte-derived hormone that suppresses food intake and increases energy expenditure by binding to and activating its specific receptor in the hypothalamus. Monogenic mutations in the leptin gene (LEP) and the leptin receptor gene (LEPR) have been shown to cause morbid obesity in mice (Oswal & Yeo, 2007) and humans (Beckers et al., 2009). The leptin gene is positioned in the chromosome 7q22-35 and is the most prominent candidate gene linked to body mass index (BMI). The leptin receptor, also identified as the diabetes gene product, is a single transmembrane protein that is established in many tissues and has several alternatively spliced isoforms.

There is little epidemiological evidence for an association between circulating leptin and obesity. It has been shown that small-for-gestational age and preterms have lowered leptin levels. Family history of obesity has been correlated with high umbilical cord levels of leptin (Hanley et al., 2010). Several studies investigated the impact of single nucleotide polymorphisms (SNPs) in the LEP or LEPR genes on adiposity markers, but the results are not conclusive (Paracchini et al., 2005). In addition, the association between these SNPs and body size at birth has been little studied (Souren et al., 2008), and whether body size at birth interacts with LEP and LEPR polymorphisms and later adiposity is unknown. There are however some SNPs of LEP gene involved in obesity physiopathology, such as A19G, A2548G in LEP gene, and Q223R in LEPR gene. It seems that mutations in the leptin gene lead to defective leptin production and cause recessively inherited early onset obesity (Mammes et al., 1998). Obese individuals homozygous for the G-allele showed significantly lower leptin concentration compared to obese patients either heterozygous or homozygous for the A-allele after correction for BMI (Jiang et al., 2004). Recently, it has been shown that LEP -2548GG genotype appears to be important in regulating leptin levels, whereas the LEPR 223R allele might predispose healthy subjects to develop metabolic disturbances (Constantin et al., 2010). Mutations of the promoter or the regulatory sites could affect the expression of LEP and explain the linkage of obesity with the microsatellite markers (Mammes et al., 1998). The frequencies of the LEP G/G homozygote (with Mendelian recessive and codominant models) were showed to be higher in the extremely obese subjects (BMI >35 kg/m^2) (Wang et al. 2006). The common G allele of G-2548A is overtransmitted in the obese offspring (Jiang et al. 2004b). G-2548A was associated with a difference in BMI reduction following a low calorie diet in overweight women (Mammes et al., 1998). The G−2548A substitution either is located in a regulating site specific for LEP and a mutation created probably correlates with regulating of the promoter regions. It must be confirmed that genetic variations at the *LEP* locus induce changes in leptin levels or metabolism, and that these changes are associated with differences in the predisposition to obesity or in the response to a low-calorie diet. None of these variants were associated with BMI in subjects on spontaneous diet (Mammes et al., 1998). The protein encoded by LEPR gene belongs to the gp130 family of cytokine receptors that are known to stimulate gene transcription via activation of cytosolic STAT proteins. This protein is a receptor for leptin and is involved in the regulation of fat metabolism, as well as in a novel hematopoietic pathway that is required for normal lymphopoiesis. Mutations in this gene have been associated with obesity and pituitary dysfunction. Alternatively spliced transcript variants encoding different isoforms have been described for this gene. In the 223 codon in mRNA sequences the mutation CAG→CGC was detected, that corresponds to Gln→Arg change in peptide molecule. In humans, Gln223Arg polymorphisms of LEPR have been associated with higher blood pressure levels, hyperinsulinaemia, glucose intolerance and higher BMI. Gln223Arg polymorphism is within the region encoding the extracellular domain of the leptin receptor and may change functional characteristics of this molecule This mutation results in abnormal splicing of leptin-receptor transcripts and generates a mutant leptin receptor that lacks both transmembrane and intracellular domains. The mutant receptor circulates at high concentrations, binding leptin and resulting in very elevated serum leptin levels (Lahlou et al., 2000). The association of the LEPR p.Q223R polymorphism with obesity was related to the co-dominant and dominant model, but not with the recessive model. There is the hypothesis that the p.Q223R LEPR variant is associated with a BMI increase. It has been proposed the hypothesis that variation of LEPR is participating in the union with leptin and influence on leptin serum levels. Therefore, leptin levels can influence on iron metabolism.

2.4 Impact of prenatal nutrition and birth weight on programming and the development of obesity

Changes in nutritional intake for both mother and foetus may have a profound effect on a range of metabolically important tissues. These mechanisms have the potential to protect the newborn against the adverse effects on the development of later obesity and its accompanying complications (Sébert et al., 2008). There is a potential impact of the prenatal nutritional experience on the development of endocrine and neuroendocrine systems that regulate energy balance, with particular emphasis on the role of hormones produced by adipocytes, especially leptin. In rodents, maternal leptin exerts a strong influence on the development of the appetite-regulating neural network and the consequent regulation of leptin synthesis and the risk of obesity in children. Recently, there is evidence, both in humans as in lambs, that the synthesis and secretion of the hormones produced by adipocytes like leptin already have regulatory mechanisms in foetal life (Symonds et al., 2003). Furthermore, hypothalamic neuropeptides that regulate food intake and energy expenditure in adulthood, are also present in the foetal brain and may regulate, through maternal reference levels, the foetal nutrient uptake and hormonal signals, including leptin. These results are important to determine what mechanisms are developed in the "*fat tissue-brain axis*' at the beginning of life, which will precede the development of adult obesity (McMillen et al., 2006).

The effect of maternal diet on the basal metabolism of children is still largely unknown and it has only been studied superficially in models of malnutrition. Yura et al., 2005, have demonstrated conclusively the dietary induction of thermogenesis in adult mice born from mothers with nutritional restriction during gestation (Yura et al., 2005), verifying a reduction in oxygen consumption and carbon dioxide production compared with control animals when a diet high in fat is maintained. The administration of leptin during pregnancy and lactation in pregnant rats subjected to protein restriction determines offspring with increased metabolic rate resistant to obesogenic diets (Stocker et al., 2004). It has also been shown in lambs that protein restriction during pregnancy program abnormal thyroid function in the offspring, which influences basal metabolic rate (Rae et al., 2002). In addition, this animal model has also shown that changes occur in fat mass and mitochondrial function in foetal adipose tissue, associated with an alteration of thermogenesis (Symonds et al., 2004). Polyunsaturated fatty acids of the n-3 series, especially docosahexaenoic acid (C22: 6 n-3, DHA), play an important role in the prevention of certain diseases including type 2 diabetes, insulin resistance, hypertension, cardiovascular disease, and so on. (Simopoulos, 1999). The n-3 fatty acids ingested in diet can alter the composition of the phospholipids of the cell membrane, determining the synthesis of eicosanoids and regulate their activity. Recent studies suggest that these fatty acids are important mediators of gene expression through activation of PPARs by controlling the expression of genes involved in lipid metabolism, glucose and adipogenesis (Jump, 2002; Lombardo et al., 2006). The increase of palmitic acid and saturated fatty acids in plasma triglycerides in newborns of diabetic mothers, along with the decrease in polyunsaturated fatty acids n-3 series and n-6, suggest metabolic pathways in this population may program obesity.

It has been seen in studies with pigs that birth weight has important implications on the development of skeletal muscle and adipose tissue (Mostyn et al., 2005). An important regulator of the metabolism of these tissues is the transport of fatty acids from the plasma membrane to intracellular organelles. This process of fatty acid utilization is carried out by the family of fatty acid binding proteins (FABP) that regulate the range of cellular processes. It has been observed a profound alteration of gene expression of FABP4 and FABP3 in adipose tissue and skeletal muscle between normal newborns and small and large for gestational age, indicating impaired fatty acid utilization. These adaptations are related to differences in the size of adipocytes and could be indicators of the degree of metabolic disease appearing in adult life due to differences in deposition and fat metabolism in infants that are not in the normal weight percentiles for gestational age (Sébert et al., 2008). Moreover, few studies have investigated the activity of newborns prenatally exposed to maternal obesity or a state of over nutrition; however malnutrition during gestation followed by a nutritionally rich postnatal state, determines the children's programming appetite showing hyperphagia and reduced locomotor activity, associated with obesity (Vickers et al., 2000, 2003). An animal model where mice were fed a diet rich in polyunsaturated fatty acids through gestation determined an increase in motor activity in the offspring (Raygada et al., 1998). In another animal model in which mothers were fed a diet saturated in fats, it was observed the programming of reduced locomotor activity (Khan et al., 2003). These studies suggest that the fatty acid composition of maternal diet is crucial in programming activity levels and therefore energy expenditure.

2.4.1 Birth weight and obesity in adults

The relationship between birth weight and adiposity, measured in childhood and adulthood, is generally positive, although some studies have shown a parabolic relationship with J or U shape between birth weight and adult fat mass, with high prevalence of obesity that would occur in individuals with low or high birth weight (Parsons et al., 2001). A determinant factor for health and longevity is the index "placenta / foetal size". Foetuses with a placenta disproportionately large or small have increased standardized mortality rates. In newborns it has been demonstrated the presence of a positive correlation between plasma leptin concentrations in cord blood and birth weight or neonatal adiposity. In pregnancies complicated by maternal diabetes, the foetus is hyperglycemic and hyperinsulinemic and hiperleptinémic (Cetin et al., 2004). Alterations in the programming of leptin synthesis, its secretion or its mechanisms of action, may be decisive in the early origins of obesity on nutritional exposure after both above and below the requirements in the foetal or neonatal early life. It has been suggested that the influence of maternal weight on the relationship between birth weight and increased BMI may operate through the impact of high maternal nutrient intake and high foetal uptake.

The hypothesis of teratogenesis mediated by the passage of energy substrates to the foetus (Freinkel, 1980), suggests that in women with gestational diabetes, uterine foetal exposure to excess energy nutrients such as glucose will determine a permanent change in foetal metabolism, causing malformations, increased birth weight (macrosomy or neonatal obesity), and an increased risk of developing type 2 diabetes in adulthood (Boney, 2005; Silverman et al., 1995). However, despite considering the theory of excess maternal nutritional intake as a cause of foetal macrosomy in children of diabetic mothers, the current diagnostic criteria for gestational diabetes may not be sufficient to differentiate between diabetogenic and non-diabetogenic pregnancies (Simmons et al., 2002). In the case of *obese mothers with glucose intolerance,* especially in *diabetics,* the maternal and foetal plasma levels of glucose are higher, causing higher birth weight in children and higher BMI in adulthood with a high risk of developing obesity and glucose intolerance (King, 2006; McMillen et al. 2006) (Figure 4). Therefore, the genetic base and the intrauterine/neonatal nutritional environment will condition a hormonal response that can lead to the development of morbidity from overweight.

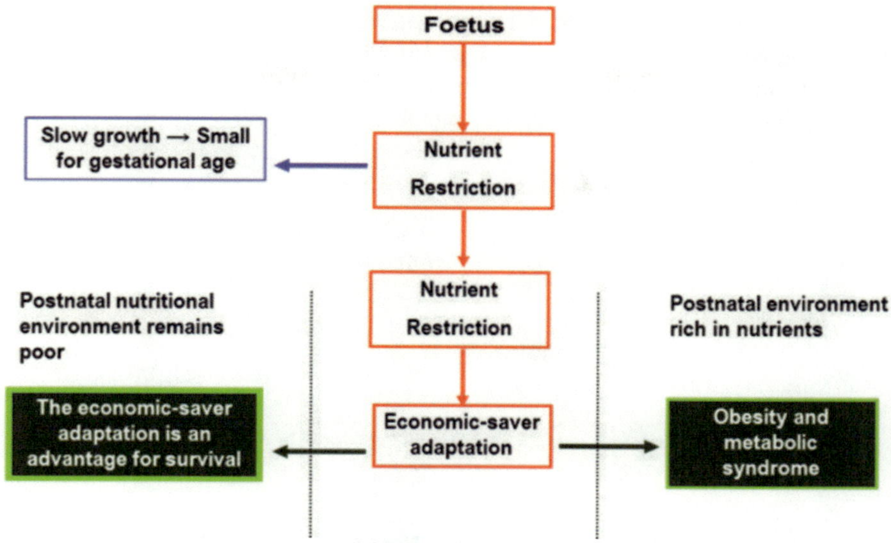

Fig. 4. Potential mechanisms explaining the relationship between high birth weight and adult obesity (Modified from McMillen, 2006).

The manipulation of both metabolic and hormonal environment in the mother as a result of decreased dietary intake at the end of pregnancy may act by determining the reduction of adipose tissue deposition in the foetus. Exposure to a reduced supply of nutrients during the first trimester of pregnancy, as occurred in the Dutch Winter Famine in 1944-1945, also determines an increase in fat mass in adulthood (Ravelli et al., 1976). Infants born small for gestational age (SGA) also show a marked reduction in body fat mass at birth, which mainly reflects the decrease in lipid accumulation in adipocytes (Levy-Marchal et al., 2004). While plasma leptin concentrations are low at birth in infants with intrauterine growth retardation, it increases to a high level compared with infants with normal birth weight (Jaquet et al., 1999). Children with low birth weight and malnourished at birth, and subsequently experience a period of very rapid growth during the first months of life, are more vulnerable to developing obesity, insulin resistance and cardiovascular disease (Eriksson et al., 2002) (Figure 5). Newborns with low birth weight for gestational age tend to have a lower BMI in adulthood than those who were large at birth; furthermore, the latter show a more central distribution of obesity, a significantly reduced muscle mass and a high body fat in adolescence and adulthood (Loos et al., 2001, 2002).

It is now known that infants with low birth weight are candidates for the development of obesity from age five. This fact directly related to a relative oversupply of nutrients in the neonatal period "*economic-saver phenotype*" of Barker (Gluckman et al., 2004; Hales & Barker et al., 2001). As a result, small perturbations in the foetal adipose tissue growth and endocrine sensitivity can have important long-term consequences. When in uterus, the foetus has been subjected to nutritional restriction and postnatal exposed to an obesogenic environment the baby will show an amplified insulin response that is not accompanied by other physiological or metabolic adverse responses for the development of obesity; It has even been observed that the kidneys seem to be protected against the adverse effects after induced obesity like glomerulosclerosis (Williams et al., 2007). One of the factors that seem to be important in renal protection is the magnitude of cellular adaptation to the cell stress of the perivisceral fat, which is upregulated in newborns of mothers who had nutritional restriction during gestation. However, during adolescence, fat mass increases and these children are insulin resistant even though basal insulin is not impaired (Mostyn et al., 2005). Potentially adverse effects do not seem to be amplified after exposure to an obesogenic environment.

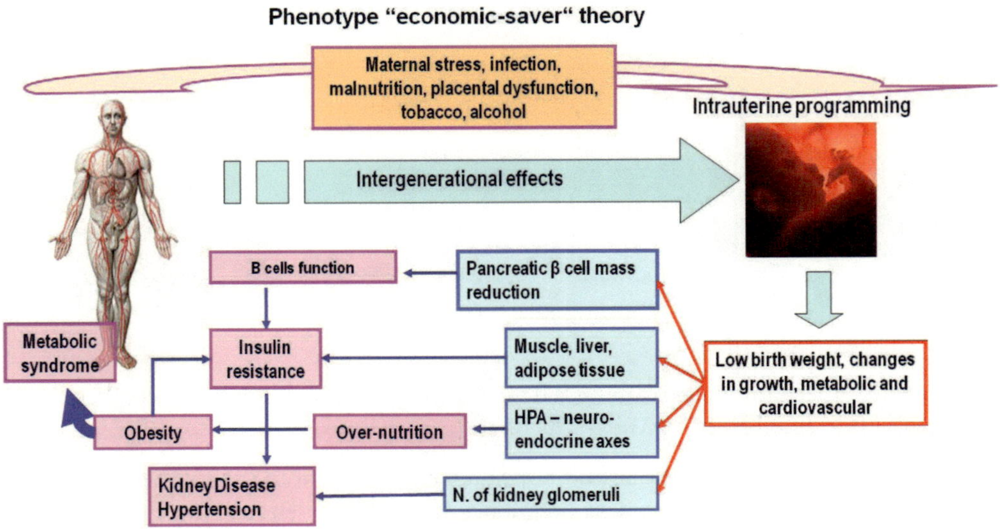

Fig. 5. Potential mechanisms explaining the relationship between low birth weight and obesity and metabolic syndrome in adults (Modified from McMillen, 2006).

The growth rate during early postnatal life may also influence the long-term health of an individual. The increase of the growth rate in the early postnatal period, also called "*catch-up growth*" is present in 30% of all children in any population well fed and occurs primarily in those who were underweight and had low length at birth. It has been suggested that the "*catch-up*" that occurs in the first 2 years is a mechanism that aims to restore the size that the child was supposed to have genetically. However, even though it presents short-term benefits, this situation is not positive in the long term because these children are going to exceed their genetic established target and will develop elevated body mass index and fat accumulation in the trunk. Levels of IGF-1 at 5 years of age are directly related to weight gain between 0 and 2 years (McMillen et al., 2006). Sayer, et al. have shown that infants suffering from intrauterine growth retardation and low birth weight develop alterations of body composition in adult life (Sayer et al., 2004). There is scientific evidence that nutrition in early postnatal life plays a role in the ability of leptin synthesis by adipocytes. It has been observed that the leptin / fat mass indices in teenagers is significantly higher in those who received enriched formula in comparison with those who received standard formula or human milk (from milk Banks) after a preterm birth. (Singhal et al., 2002). The protective effect of maternal milk on the development of obesity has also been widely tested (Koletzko et al., 2005; Li et al., 2003).

2.5 Programming of appetite

The action of the hypothalamus in controlling food intake is widely recognized, but only recently it has been shown to be an essential part in development programming associated with neonatal exposure to high-caloric diets (Cripps et al., 2005; McMillen et al., 2005;

Plagemann, 2005, 2006). In rodents, the hypothalamic nucleus continues to differentiate until day 20 of postnatal life (Grove et al., 2005); this period is therefore critical for studying the expression of key regulatory neuropeptides and receptors in the hypothalamus, the expression of which is permanently programmed through maternal-foetal dietary factors. The investigation of postnatal neuronal development in these animal models is directly relevant and applicable to other species, even for humans, since the extent of neuronal development also occurs in breast-feeding with hypothalamic maturation that begins at the uterus and continues in early postnatal life.

2.5.1 Central regulation of appetite

Neural circuits that mediate homeostatic functions such as eating patterns are distributed by various brain structures. Within these there are specific regions of the hypothalamus like the arcuate nucleus (ARC), ventromedial nucleus (VMN) and the lateral area. The solitary tract nucleus (STN) is also involved in food regulation. Neurons in this nucleus receive signals from vagus nerve with satiation stimulus. STN neurons have reciprocal connections with the forebrain areas such as the paraventricular nucleus (PVN) and the substrates have to respond to hormonal central effector peptides involved in energy homeostasis {(MC4 receptors, leptin receptors, and neurons containing propiomelanocortin (POMC)}. The hypothalamus is part of a system which integrates the regulation of body composition with food intake and energy expenditure. A series of stimuli in different systems related to the metabolic state are received in the hypothalamus, which modulate the release of hypothalamic peptides that regulate food intake and hypothalamic pituitary axis. The main hypothalamic areas involved in the regulation of eating behaviour are: 1) The VMN, where a possible lesion produces voracity and obesity. 2) The lateral hypothalamic area (LHA), whose injury produces decreased nutritional intake and anorexia. 3) The PVN, which receives information from other brain nuclei related to intake. 4) The ARC, whose neurons produce peptides that regulate food intake, stimulating it - as the neuropeptide Y, - or inhibiting such as POMC / *transcript regulated by cocaine and amphetamine* (CART). The two circuits send their signals primarily to PVN and also to other hypothalamic nuclei which directly modulate eating behaviour. Both circuits are influenced by peripheral hormones that can cross the hematoencephalic barrier. These cores are interconnected and the circuits generated in this brain area have a specialized role in energy homeostasis. The hypothalamus also receives different stimuli from the central nervous system (vagal and catecholaminergic), hormonal stimuli (insulin, leptin, cholecystokinin, and glucocorticoids) and gastrointestinal hormonal stimuli (ghrelin, peptide YY) (Schwartz & Brain, 2001).

The ARC is a critical component in the regulation of body weight located adjacent to the base of the 3rd ventricle in the mediobasal hypothalamus. Contains neurons that have axon terminals in direct contact with blood flow, although protected by the blood-brain barrier; these neurons are known as "the first-order neurons." They are able to sense and respond to hormonal ranges and nutrient signals such as insulin, leptin, ghrelin and glucose (Schwartz & Brain, 2001). There are 2 distinct groups of neurons in the ARC that will regulate energy balance. A group of them co-express neuropeptide Y (NPY) and related peptide agouti (AgRP), and another group of neurons co-expressing the POMC and CART (McMillen et al., 2005). The ARC is projected onto other second-order neurons, and these in turn project to other neurons of the solitary tract nucleus. Afferents related to satiety are transmitted to the STN in turn connected to ARC, via the vagus nerve and sympathetic fibres from the liver

and the gastrointestinal tract by peptides such as cholecystokinin (CCK). The connections between the ARC and other key sites in the central nervous system are known to regulate the dietary intake and energy balance in early postnatal life. Innervations between the ARC and PVN are present in the human foetus at 21 weeks gestation, although the density of these projections is greatly increased in the postnatal period (Grove et al., 2003).
Appetite and energy balance are regulated primarily by hypothalamic neuropeptides expressed in the adult. Neurons co-expressing NPY / AgRP are part of the energy balance anabolic pathway. Both NPY and AgRP are inhibited by leptin and insulin. The increase in NPY signals as a result of a decrease in energy balance not only determines hyperphagia and weight gain, but also contributes to systemic insulin resistance and glucose intolerance. By contrast, AgRP exerts an anabolic effect through antagonism of neuronal melanocortin receptors (MC3-R and MC4-R) that are involved in regulating appetite. Prolonged inhibition of melanocortin receptors determines weight gain and insulin resistance. The MC4-R mutations in humans are associated with obesity phenotypes (McMillen et al., 2005). In overfed newborn rats it has been observed an increase in adiposity (Davidowa & Plagemann, 2004). It has been shown that the overfeeding of rats with small amounts in the neonatal period, determines the development of hyperphagia, fat deposition and accelerates weight gain associated with hyperleptinemia and central leptin-resistance at the level of the arcuate nucleus (Velkoska et al., 2005). These studies suggest a bad programming of the hypothalamus that would take place during lactation. Kozak et al. (2000) have shown a direct involvement of the hypothalamus in the programming of obesity, having observed that adult offspring of rats fed a diet rich in fat (55% margarine) show an exaggerated response to food after injection of Neuropeptide Y (NPY) in the lateral ventricle, eating twice more than control animals (Kozak et al., 2000). Prenatal over nutrition in sheep also led to a change in appetite regulation in the early postnatal period (Muhlhausler et al., 2006).

2.5.2 Leptin

It has been suggested that high concentrations of circulating leptin determine a misalignment of the action of leptin and its receptors in the hypothalamus, thus there would be a disruption on the route of signal transduction that is required for suppression of appetite (Ahima & Flier, 2000). Leptin is synthesized in adipose tissue, with the size of adipocytes the determinant factor of this synthesis. Adipose tissue secretes the protein ob (leptin) that circulate in the blood reaches the ventromedial nucleus of the hypothalamus where it binds to its receptor, encoded by the gene db. This results in a decrease of NPY from the ARC, which suppresses appetite and increases the levels of norepinephrine from sympathetic terminals that innerve adipose tissue and affect other hormone actions, such as insulin secretion (Figure 6).
Sex is also important; there are higher levels of leptin in women compared to men, for an equivalent in mass (Martin-Gronert & Ozanne, 2005). The leptin receptor (ObRb) activates the Janus kinase (JAK), which phosphorylates some members of the pathway of signal transduction and transcription (STAT). Activation of the leptin receptor also induces the expression of suppressor of cytokine signalling--3 (SOCS-3), which in turn inhibits the subsequent signal transduction of leptin. The SOCS-3 can also potentially inhibit signals from Ins-Rb. In addition, sensitivity to insulin and leptin increases in the SOCS-3 of rats, giving them protection against the development of diet-induced obesity. Moreover, SOCS-3 is a key candidate for the regulator of diet-induced leptin as well as in the case of insulin

resistance. The presence of functional leptin receptors in pancreatic β cells and the observation that leptin directly inhibits insulin secretion, leads to the concept of "axis adipoinsular" (Kieffer & Habener, 2000) by which insulin stimulates adipogenesis and synthesis of leptin and leptin inhibits the production of insulin in the pancreas. It is proposed that the pancreatic resistance to leptin may be a mechanism that promotes obesity often associated with hyperinsulinemia and may contribute to later development of diabetes in obese individuals (Seufert et al., 1999).

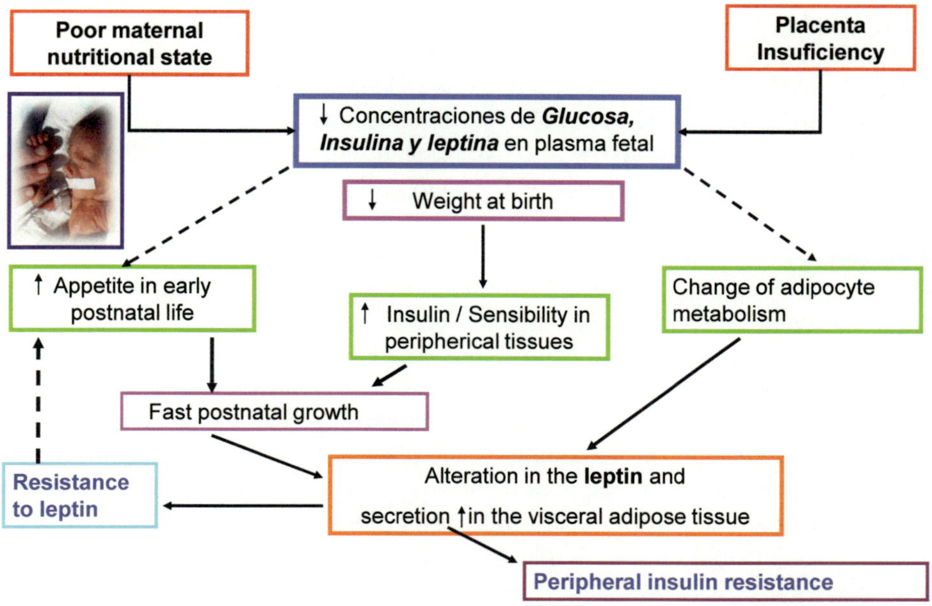

Fig. 6. Adipose tissue secretes the protein ob (leptin) that reaches the blood circulating through the hypothalamic ventromedial nucleus where it binds to its receptor, encoded by the gene db.

It has been shown a pivotal role of leptin in the programming of hypothalamic obesity after a study where leptin administered subcutaneously in the postnatal period (3-13 days) reversed the hyperphagia and obesity in adult rats born of rats with low dietary intake (malnutrition) (Vickers et al., 2005). A similar effect has been demonstrated by Yura et al. in normal rats observing that the early injection of leptin (8-10 days postnatal) determines an obese phenotype in the adult rat (Yura et al., 2005). A study in the developing hypothalamus in rats has shown that leptin promotes neuronal growth from the ARC to the paraventricular nucleus (PVN) during lactation, promoting a very close connection in neuronal hypothalamic regulatory system of appetite. Leptin appears to take part in the differentiation of 2 opposing pathways that control energy intake, promoting the development of the appetite stimulant NPY and agouti-related peptide projection (AgRP) from the ARC to the PVN by neural connections from melanocyte stimulating hormone-(α-MSH) - appetite suppressant derived from the POMC and present in all neurons (Bouret & Simerly, 2006; Horvath & Bruning, 2006).

Some programming models have shown evidence of impaired control of the sympathetic system (Khan et al., 2003), and a specific programming in neonatal hypothalamus by hyperleptinemia may also contribute to increased sympathetic tone that is intended for the development of hypertension-related obesity. In established obesity, there is a high level of circulating leptin, a selective resistance to leptin at the hypothalamic level that determines in part the attenuation of the anorectic leptin actions and of weight loss, and on the other hand, the preservation of vase-pressure actions of leptin at the central level that contribute to elevated blood pressure (Haynes, 2005). The selective leptin resistance causes a reduced availability of leptin to activate signalling mechanisms in the areas of appetite regulation of the ARC, keeping the sympathetic excitatory action of leptin in the cardiovascular system, related to the ventromedial nucleus (VMN) and dorsomedial (DMN) of the hypothalamus (Marsh et al., 2003). Given the neurotrophic role of leptin during the neonatal hypothalamic plasticity period, it seems that maternal hyperleptinemia and / or neonatal in the immediate postnatal period could program the selective resistance to leptin and thus the propensity for obesity and obesity-related hypertension (Howard et al., 2004).

2.5.3 Insulin: Glucose control and peripheral regulator of appetite

Insulin is secreted by pancreatic β cells in response to increased circulating glucose, amino acids or glucagon, as well as after stimulation of sympathetic nerve pathways (α) and parasympathetic (cholinergic). In adults, the β-cell mass is controlled by at least four independent mechanisms: a) β cell replication, b) β cell hypertrophy c) β cell neogenesis, d) β-cell apoptosis. The rate and type of response used depends on the adaptation of β cell mass to metabolic changes throughout adult life (Bonner-Weir, 2000). Insulin is the primary circulation factor involved in the control of body weight by the central nervous system (CNS). Insulin circulates in plasma at levels proportionate to the size of energy stores and enters the CNS in proportion to the plasma concentrations by a carrier linked to a specific receptor. Exogenous insulin administered directly into the brain, determines the reduction of food intake and body weight. The action of insulin in the brain is necessary for the upkeep of glucose homeostasis. The insulin receptor (Ins-Rb) is expressed in the ARC and the VMN and in the striatum and in the choroid plexus. Prolonged or chronic actions of insulin signalling will result in hyperphagia, increased plasma insulin and decreased sensitivity to insulin (Taylor & Poston, 2007).

3. Conclusions, public health messages and possible interventions

Recently, it has been reported that obesity during pregnancy clearly increases the risk of successful pregnancy after the study of 150000 Swedish women (Villamor et al., 2006), but also endangers the health of children, and in terms of public health, the health of future generations. The long term ultimate goal should be to reduce the incidence of obesity during pregnancy and increase public awareness of the importance of a balanced diet before and during pregnancy. The Obesity Committee of the American College of Obstetricians and Gynaecologists, have suggested that obstetricians should give pre-conception counselling and education about potential complications and should strongly recommend to obese patients to participate in a weight reduction program before pregnancy (American College of Obstetricians and Gynecologists [ACOG], 2005). So far, no similar recommendations have been made in Europe.

Recent research suggests that it should be avoided weight gain between pregnancies, and women should try to reach the initial weight before pregnancy before becoming pregnant again (Villamor et al., 2006). The Public Affairs Committee of the Teratology Society has also recommended counselling women about appropriate caloric intake, exercise and education about infant nutrition and the importance of breastfeeding (Scialli, 2006). However, although the benefits of breast-feeding are widely recognized, long term breastfeeding may promote obesity (Harder, 2005), and also, the milk of diabetic mothers and obese may be obesogenic to the developing baby (Rodekamp et al., 2005). To avoid rapid growth during the first year of life, infant formulas must be optimized. From a nutritional perspective, future research should focus on the identification of maternal nutritional insults that can be vectors of "health programming in your child," for example, the role of fat vs. carbohydrates and the saturated fat vs. unsaturated fats. Medically, the most effective treatment of maternal obesity and gestational diabetes, and specifically the control of hyperglycemia, hyperinsulinemia and hyperleptinemia, both before and during pregnancy can help to prevent programming of obesity.

In the future it is envisaged the use of pharmacological interventions with drugs that inhibit food intake but also peripheral acting drugs that modify the metabolism and energy balance as the antagonists of the 11β-HSD-1 (Wang et al., 2006). Agonists of PPAR-α and PPAR-γ, including the glitazones may improve insulin resistance (Guo & Tabrizchi, 2006) and enhance mitochondrial biogenesis in adipose tissue (Bogacka et al., 2005), offering a dual PPAR agonist therapy to treat risk factors of obesity (Gervois et al., 2004). There are also potentially effective new drugs acting on the cascade of signals related to adipocyte differentiation (Rodriguez et al., 2006). However, until the safety and efficacy of these drugs are proven, interventions on diet and lifestyle are the only resources available to fight obesity, especially during pregnancy. As for possible interventions in children, early identification of children at risk by measuring the rate of growth / BMI and early assessment of adiposity during the first years of life, and the identification of potential biomarkers of future obesity, could help to advise treatment with an early improvement of lifestyle and drug therapy in those at high risk. Research in this field offers a real chance to achieve strategies that can enable the effective prevention of obesity in future generations.

4. References

Ahima RS, Flier JS. (2000). Adipose tissue as an endocrine organ. *Trends in Endocrinology and Metabolism*, 11, 327-332

American College of Obstetricians and Gynecologists. ACOG Committee Opinion number 315, 2005. Obesity in pregnancy. *Obstet Gynecol*, 106, 671-675

Barker DJ. (1992). The foetal origins of diseases of old age. *Eur J Clin Nutr*, 46, Suppl 3:S3-9

Bayol SA, Simbi BH & Stickland NC. (2005). A maternal cafeteria diet during gestation and lactation promotes adiposity and impairs skeletal muscle development and metabolism in rat offspring at weaning. *J Physiol*, 567, 951-961

Bispham J, Budge H, Mostyn A, Dandrea J, Clarke L & Keisler D (2002). Ambient temperature, maternal dexamethasone, and postnatal ontogeny of leptin in the neonatal lamb. *Pediatric Research*, 52, 85-90

Bispham J, Gopalakrishnan GS, Dandrea J, Wilson V, Budge H, Keisler DH, Broughton Pipkin F, Stephenson T & Symonds ME. (2003). Maternal endocrine adaptation throughout pregnancy to nutritional manipulation: consequences for maternal plasma leptin and cortisol and the programming of fetal adipose tissue development. *Endocrinology*, 144, 3575-3585

Bjornsson H, Sigurdsson M, Fallin M, Irizarry R, Aspelund T Cui H, Yu W, Rongione M, Ekstrom T & Harris T. (2008) Intra-individual change over time in DNA methylation with familial clustering. *Jama*, 299, 2877–2883

Blewitt ME, Vickaryous NK, Paldi A, Koseki H &Whitelaw E. (2006). Dynamic reprogramming of DNA methylation at an epigenetically sensitive allele in mice. *PLoS Genet*, 2, e49

Bogacka I, Ukropcova B, McNeil M, Gimble JM & Smith SR. (2005). Structural and functional consequences of mitochondrial biogenesis in human adipocytes in vitro. *J Clin Endocrinol Metab*, 90, 6650–6656

Boney CM, Verma A, Tucker R & Vohr BR. (2005). Metabolic Syndrome in Childhood: Association With Birth Weight, Maternal Obesity, and Gestational Diabetes Mellitus, *Pediatrics*, 115, 3

Bonner-Weir S. (2000). Perspective: Postnatal pancreatic beta cell growth. *Endocrinology*, 141, 6, 1926-9

Bouret SG & Simerly RB. (2006). Developmental programming of hypothalamic feeding circuits. *Clin Genet*, 70, 295–301

Bouret SG, Draper SJ & Simerly RB. (2004). Trophic action of leptin on hypothalamic neurons that regulate feeding. *Science*, 304, 108–110

Breier BH, Vickers MH, Ikenasio BA, Chan KY & Wong WP. (2001). Fetal programming of appetite and obesity. *Mol Cell Endocrinol*, 185, 1, 73-9

Budge H, Gnanalingham MG, Gardner DS, Mostyn A, Stephenson T & Symonds ME. (2005). Maternal nutritional programming of fetal adipose tissue development: long-term consequences for later obesity. *Birth Defects Res C Embryo Today*, 75, 3, 193-9

Cetin I, Morpurgo PS, Radelli T, Taricco E, Cortelazzi D & Bellotti M. (2004). Fetal plasma leptin concentrations:relationship with different intrauterine growth patterns from 19weeks to term. *Pediatric Research*, 48, 646–651

Champagne F, Weaver I, Diorio J, Dymov S, Szyf, M & Meaney M. (2006). Maternal care associated with methylation of the estrogen receptor-alpha1b promoter and estrogen receptor-alpha expression in the medial preoptic area of female offspring. *Endocrinology*, 147, 2909–2915

Chinnery PF, Samuels DC, Elson J & Turnbull DM. (2002). Accumulation of mitochondrial DNA mutations in ageing, cancer, and mitochondrial disease: is there a common mechanism? *Lancet*, 360, 1323–1325

Christensen B, Houseman E, Marsit C, Zheng S, Wrensch M, Wiemels J, Nelson H, Karagas M, Padbury J &Bueno R. (2009). Aging and environmental exposures alter tissue-specific DNA methylation dependent uponCpGisland context. *PLoS Genet.*, 5

Clarke L, Bryant MJ, Lomax MA & Symonds ME. (1997). Maternal manipulation of brown adipose tissue and liver development in the ovine fetus during late gestation. *British Journal of Nutrition*, 77, 871–883

Clarke L, Heasman L, Juniper DT & Symonds ME. (1998). Maternal nutrition in early-mid gestation and placental size in sheep. *Br J Nutr*, 79, 359-364

Constantin A, Costache G, Sima A, Glavce C, Vladica M & Popov D. (2010). Leptin G-2548A and leptin receptor Q223R gene polymorphisms are not associated with obesity in Romanian subjects. *Biochem Biophys Res Commun*, 1, 391, 282-6

Corbett SW, Stern JS & Keesey RE. (1986). Energy expenditure in rats with diet-induced obesity. *Am J Clin Nutr,* 44, 173–180

Cottrell EC & Ozanne SE. (2008). Early life programming of obesity and metabolic disease. *Physiol Behav,* 22, 94, 17-28

Creemers JW, Lee YS, Oliver RL, Bahceci M, Tuzcu A, Gokalp D, Keogh J, Herber S, White A, O'Rahilly S & Farooqi IS. (2008). Mutations in the N-terminal region of pro-opiomelanocortin (POMC) in patients with early-onset obesity impair POMC sorting regulated secretory pathway. *J Clin Endocrinol Metab,* 93, 11, 4494-9

Cripps RL, Martin-Gronert MS & Ozanne SE. (2005). Fetal and perinatal programming of appetite. *Clin Sci,* 109, 1–11

Davidowa H & Plagemann A. (2004). Hypothalamic neurons of postnatally overfed, overweight rats respond differentially to corticotropin-releasing hormones. *Neurosci Lett,* 371, 64–68

Demmelmair H, von Rosen J & Koletzko B. (2006). Long-term consequences of early nutrition. *Early Hum Dev,* 82, 8, 567-574

Dunstan JA, Simmer K, Dixon G & Prescott SL. (2008). Cognitive assessment of children at age 2 ½ years after maternal fish oil supplementation in pregnancy: a randomised controlled trial. *Arch Dis Child Fetal Neonatal,* 93, F45-F50

Eriksson JG, Forsen T, Tuomilehto J, Jaddoe VW, Osmond C & Barker DJ. (2002). Effects of size at birth and childhood growth on the insulin resistance syndrome in elderly individuals. *Diabetologia,* 45, 342–348

Fajas L, Auboeuf D, Raspe E, Schoonjans K, Lefebvre AM & Saladin R. (1997). The organization, promoter analysis, and expression of the human PPAR_ gene. *J Biol Chem,* 272, 18779–89

Feldt K, Raikkonen K, Eriksson JG, Andersson S, Osmond C & Barker DJ. (2007). Cardiovascular reactivity to psychological stressors in late adulthood is predicted by gestational age at birth. *J Hum Hypertens,* 21, 5, 401-10

Fernández-Twinn DS & Ozanne SE. (2006). Mechanisms by which poor early growth programs type-2 diabetes, obesity and the metabolic syndrome. *Physiol Behav.* 88, 3, 234-43

Freinkel N. Of pregnancy and progeny. (1980). *Diabetes,* 29, 1023-1035

Gervois P, Fruchart JC & Staels B. (2004). Inflammation, dyslipidaemia, diabetes and PPars: pharmacological interest of dual PPARα and PPARγ agonists. *Int J Clin Pract Suppl,* 22–29

Gluckman PD & Hanson MA. (2004). Living with the past: evolution, development and patterns of disease. *Science,* 305, 1773—6

Gnanalingham MG, Mostyn A, Symonds ME & Stephenson T. (2005). Ontogeny and nutritional programming of adiposity in sheep: potential role of glucocorticoid action and uncoupling protein-2. *Am J Physiol Regul Integr Comp Physiol,* 289, R1407–R1415

Gnanalingham MG, Wilson V, Bispham J, Williams P, Pellicano A, Budge H, Stephenson T & Symonds ME. (2007). Nutritional manipulation between early to mid gestation: effects on uncoupling protein-2, glucocorticoid sensitivity, IGF-I receptor and cell proliferation but not apoptosis in the ovine placenta. *Reprod,* 134, 615-623

Godfrey KM. (2002). The role of the placenta in fetal programming. A review. *Placenta,* 23, Suppl A:S20-7

Graziewicz MA, Longley MJ & Copeland WC. (2006). DNA polymerase γ in mitochondrial DNA replication and repair. *Chem Rev,* 106, 383–405

Grove KL & Smith MS. (2003). Ontogeny of the hypothalamic neuropeptide Y system. *Physiological Behaviours,* 79, 47–63

Grove KL, Grayson BE, Glavas MM, Xiao XQ & Smith MS. (2005). Development of metabolic systems. *Physiol Behav,* 86, 646–660

Guo L & Tabrizchi R. (2006). Peroxisome proliferator-activated receptor γ as a drug target in the pathogenesis of insulin resistance. *Pharmacol Ther,* 111, 145–173

Hales CN & Barker DJ. (2001). The thrifty phenotype hypothesis. *Br Med Bull,* 60:5–20

Harder T, Bergmann R, Kallischnigg G & Plagemann A. (2005). Duration of breastfeeding and risk of overweight: a meta-analysis. *Am J Epidemiol,* 162, 397–403

Haynes WG. (2005). Role of leptin in obesity-related hypertension. *Exp Physiol,* 90, 683–688

Heijmans B, Tobi E, Stein A, Putter H, Blauw G, Susser E, Slagboom P & Lumey L. (2008). Persistent epigenetic differences associated with prenatal exposure to famine in humans. *Proc. Natl Acad. Sci. USA,* 105, 17046–17049

Helland IB, Smith L, Saarem K, Saugstad OD & Drevon CA. (2003). Maternal supplementation with very-long-chain n-3 fatty acids during pregnancy and lactation augments children's IQ at 4 years of age. *Pediatrics,* 111, e39-e44

Hibbeln JR, Davis JM, Steer C, Emmett P, Rogers I & Williams C. (2007). Maternal seafood consumption in pregnancy and neurodevelopmental outcomes in childhood (ALSPAC study): an observational cohort study. *Lancet,* 369, 9561, 578-85

Hiden U & Desoye G. (2010). Gestational Diabetes During and After Pregnancy. Part 4, 97-111, DOI: 10.1007/978-1-84882-120-0_7

Higgins L, Greenwood S, Wareing M & Mills T. (2011). Obesity & placenta: A consideration of nutrient exchange mechanisms in relation to aberrant fetal growth *Placenta,* 32, 1e7

Hinney A, Nguyen TT, Scherag A, Friedel S, Brönner G, Müller TD, Grallert H, Illig T, Wichmann HE, Rief W, Schäfer H & Hebebrand J. (2007). Genome wide association (GWA) study for early onset extreme obesity supports the role of fat mass and obesity associated gene (FTO) variants. *PLoS ONE,* 26, 2, 12

Horvath TL & Bruning JC. (2006). Developmental programming of the hypothalamus: a matter of fat. *Nat Med,* 12, 52–53

Howard JK, Cave BJ, Oksanen LJ, Tzameli I, Bjorbaek C & Flier JS. (2004). Enhanced leptin sensitivity and attenuation of diet-induced obesity in mice with haploinsufficiency of Socs3. *Nat Med,* 10, 734–738

Itoh E, Iida K, Kim DS, Del Rincon JP, Coschigano KT & Kopchick JJ. (2004). Lack of contribution of 11bHSD1 and glucocorticoid action to reduced muscle mass associated with reduced growth hormone action. *Growth Hormone & IGF Research,* 14, 462–66

Jaquet D, Leger J, Tabone MD, Czernicho P & Levy MC. (1999). High serum leptin concentrations during catch-up growth of children born with intrauterine growth retardation. *Journal of Clinical and Endocrinological Metabolism,* 84, 1949–1953

Jiang Y, Wilk JB, Borecki I, Williamson S, DeStefano AL, Xu G, Liu J, Ellison RC, Province M & Myers RH. (2004). Common Variants in the 5′ Region of the Leptin Gene Are Associated with Body Mass Index in Men from the National Heart, Lung, and Blood Institute Family Heart Study. *Am J Hum Genet,* 75, 220–230.

Jump DB. (2002). Dietary polyunsaturated fatty acids and regulation of gene transcription. *Curr Opin Lipidol*,13, 2, 155-6

Key YJ, Schatzkin A, Willett WC, Allen NE, Spencer EA & Travis RC. (2004). Diet, nutrition and the prevention of cancer. *Public Health Nutrition*, 7, 1A, 187–200

Khan IY, Taylor PD, Dekou V, Seed PT, Lakasing L & Graham D. (2003). Gender-linked hypertension in offspring of lard-fed pregnant rats. *Hypertension*, 41, 168–175

Kieffer TJ & Habener JF. (2000). The adipoinsular axis: effects of leptin on pancreatic beta-cells. *American Journal of Physiology, Endocrinology and Metabolism*, 278, E1–E14

King JC. Maternal obesity, metabolism, and pregnancy outcomes. (2006). *Annu Rev Nutr*, 26, 271-91

Kliewer SA, Xu HE, Lambert MH & Willson TM. (2001). Peroxisome proliferator-activated receptors: from genes to physiology. *Recent Prog Horm Res*, 56, 239–63

Koletzko B, Broekaert I, Demmelmair H, Franke J, Hannibal I & Oberle D. (2005). Protein intake in the first year of life: a risk factor for later obesity? The E.U. childhood obesity project. *Adv Exp Med Biol*, 5569, 69-79

Koletzko B. (2006). Long-term consequences of early feeding on later obesity risk. *Nestle Nutr Workshop Ser Pediatr Program*, 58, 1-18

Kozak R, Burlet A, Burlet C & Beck B. (2000). Dietary composition during fetal and neonatal life affects neuropeptide Y functioning in adult offspring. *Brain Res Dev Brain Res*, 125, 75–82

Krauss-Etschmann S, Shadid R, Campoy C, Hoster E, Demmelmair H, Jiménez M, Gil A, Rivero M, Veszprémi B, Decsi T & Koletzko BV (2007). Nutrition and Health Lifestyle (NUHEAL) Study Group. Effects of fish-oil and folate supplementation of pregnant women on maternal and fetal plasma concentrations of docosahexaenoic acid and eicosapentaenoic acid: a European randomized multicenter trial. *Am J Clin Nutr*, 85, 5, 1392-400

Lefebvre AM, Paulweber B & Fajas L. (1999). Peroxisome proliferator-activated receptor gamma is induced during differentiation of colon epithelium cells. *J Endocrinol*, 162, 331–40

Levy-Marchal C, Jaquet D &Czernichow P. (2004). Long term metabolic consequences of being born small for gestational age. *Seminars in Neonatology*, 9, 67–74

Li L, TJ Parsons & Power C. (2003). Breast feeding and obesity in childhood: cross Sectional study. *BMJ*, 327, 904-905

Lillycrop K, Phillips E, Torrens C., Hanson M, Jackson A & Burdge G. (2008). Feeding pregnant rats a protein-restricted diet persistently alters the methylation of specific cytosines in the hepatic PPAR alpha promoter of the offspring. *Br. J. Nutr*, 100, 278–282

Lillycrop KA, Phillips ES, Jackson AA, Hanson MA & Burdge GC. (2005). Dietary protein restriction of pregnant rats induces and folic acid supplementation prevents epigenetic modification of hepatic gene expression in the offspring. *J Nutr*, 135, 1382–1386

Lombardo YB & Chicco AG. (2006). Effects of dietary polyunsaturated n-3 fatty acids on dyslipidemia and insulin resistance in rodents and humans. A review. *J Nutr Biochem*, 17, 1, 1-13

Loos RJ, Beunen G, Fagard R, Derom C & Vlietinck R. (2001). Birth weight and body composition in young adult men - a prospective twin study. *International Journal of Obesity Related Metabolic Disorders*, 25, 1537–1545

Loos RJ, Beunen G, Fagard R, Derom C & Vlietinck R. Birth weight and body composition in young women: a prospective twin study. (2002). *Am J Clin Nutr*, 75, 4, 676-82

Loos RJ, Lindgren CM, Li S, Wheeler E, Zhao JH, Prokopenko I, Inouye M, Freathy RM, Attwood AP, Beckmann JS & Berndt SI; Prostate, Lung, Colorectal, and Ovarian (PLCO) Cancer Screening Trial. (2008). Common variants near MC4R are associated with fat mass, weight and risk of obesity. *Nat Genet*, 40, 6, 768-75

Lowell BB. (1999). PPARγ: an essential regulator of adipogenesis and modulator of fat cell function. *Cell*, 99, 239–42

Lucas A. (1994). Role of nutritional programming in determining adult morbidity. *Arch Dis Child*, 71, 4, 288-90

Lucas A. (2005). Long-term programming effects of early nutrition - implications for the preterm infant. *J Perinatol*, 25 Suppl 2, S2-6

Mammès O, Betoulle D, Aubert R, Herbeth B, Siest G, Fumeron F. (2000). Association of the G-2548A polymorphism in the 5' region of the LEP gene with overweight. *Ann Hum Genet*, 64, 5, 391-4

Marsh AJ, Fontes MA, Killinger S, Pawlak DB, Polson JW & Dampney RA. (2003). Cardiovascular responses evoked by leptin acting on neurons in the ventromedial and dorsomedial hypothalamus. *Hypertension*, 42, 488–493

Martin-Gronert MS & Ozanne SE. (2005). Programming of appetite and type 2 diabetes. *Early Hum Dev*, 81, 12, 981-8

McGowan P, Sasaki A, D'Alessio A, Dymov S, Labonte B, Szyf M, Turecki G & Meaney M. (2009). Epigenetic regulation of the glucocorticoid receptor in human brain associates with childhood abuse. *Nat. Neurosci*, 12, 342–348

McMillen IC, Adam CL & Mühlhäusler BS. (2005). Early origins of obesity: programming the appetite regulatory system. *J Physiol*, 15, 565, 9-17

McMillen, L J Edwards, J Duffield & BS Muhlhausler. (2006). Regulation of leptin synthesis and secretion before birth: implications for the early programming of adult obesity. *Reproduction*, 131, 415–27

Mostyn A, Litten JC, Perkins KS, Euden PJ, Corson AM, Symonds ME & Clarke L. (2005). Influence of size at birth on the endocrine profiles and expression of uncoupling proteins in subcutaneous adipose tissue, lung and muscle of neonatal pigs. *American Journal of Physiology*, 288, R1536 - R1542

Moulin K, Truel N, Andre M, Arnauld E, Nibbelink M & Cousin B. (2001). Emergence during development of the white-adipocyte cell phenotype is independent of the brown-adipocyte cell phenotype. *Biochemical Journal*, 356, 659–664

Muhlhausler BS, Adam CL, Findlay PA, Duffield JA & McMillen IC. (2006). Increased maternal nutrition alters development of the appetite-regulating network in the brain. *FASEB J*, 20, 1257–1259

Nuñez BS, Rogerson FM, Mune T, Igarashi Y, Nakagawa Y & Phillipov G. (1999). Mutants of 11ß-Hydroxysteroid Dehydrogenase (11-HSD2) With Partial Activity: Improved Correlations Between Genotype and Biochemical Phenotype in Apparent Mineralocorticoid Excess. *Hypertension*, 34, 638-42

Ollikainen M, Smith R, Joo E, Kiat N, Andronikos R, Novakovic B, Aziz K, Carlin J, Morley R, Saffery R & Craig J. (2010). DNA methylation analysis of multiple tissues from newborn twins reveals both genetic and intrauterine components to variation in the human neonatal epigenome. *Human Molecular Genetics*, 19, 21, 4176–4188

Oswal A, Yeo GS. (2007). The leptin melanocortin pathway and the control of body weight: lessons from human and murine genetics. *Obes Rev,* 8, 4, 293-306

Ozanne SE & Hales CN. (2002). Early programming of glucose-insulin metabolism. *Trends Endocrinol Metab*, 13, 368-373

Paracchini V, Pedotti P, Taioli E. (2005). Genetics of leptin and obesity: a HuGE review. *Am J Epidemiol*, 15, 162, 101-14

Parsons TJ, Power C & Manor O. (2001). Fetal and early life growth and body mass index from birth to early adulthood in 1958 British cohort: longitudinal study. *BMJ*, 8, 323, 1331-5

Plagemann A. (2005). Perinatal programming and functional teratogenesis: impact on body weight regulation and obesity. *Physiol Behav*, 86, 661–668

Plagemann A. (2006). Perinatal nutrition and hormone-dependent programming of food intake. *Horm Res,* 65, Suppl. 3, 83–89

Rae MT, Rhind SM, Kyle CE, Miller DW& Brooks AN. (2002). Maternal undernutrition alters triiodothyronine concentrations and pituitary response to GnRH in fetal sheep. *J Endocrinol,* 173, 449–455

Ravelli GP, Stein ZA & Susser MW. (1976). Obesity in young men after famine exposure in útero and early infancy. *New England Journal of Medicine,* 295, 349–353

Raygada M, Cho E & Hilakivi-Clarke L. (1998). High maternal intake of polyunsaturated fatty acids during pregnancy in mice alters offsprings' aggressive behavior, immobility in the swim test, locomotor activity and brain protein kinase C activity. *J Nutr,* ;128, 2505–2511

Reynolds RM,Walker BR, Syddall HE, Andrew R &Wood PJ. (2001). Altered control of cortisol secretion in adult men with low birth weight and cardiovascular risk factors. *J Clin Endocrinol Metab*, 86, 245–250

Ricote M, Li AC, Willson TM, Kelly CJ & Glass CK. (1998). The peroxisome proliferator-activated receptor-gamma is a negative regulator of macrophage activation. *Nature,* 1, 391, 79-82

Robitaille J, Brouillette C, Houde A, Lemieux S, Perusse L & Tchernof A. (2004). Association between the PPARa-L162V polymorphism and components of the metabolic syndrome. *J Hum Genet*, 49, 482–489

Rodekamp E, Harder T, Kohlhoff R, Franke K, Dudenhausen JW & Plagemann A. (2005). Long-term impact of breast-feeding on body weight and glucose tolerance in children of diabetic mothers: role of the late neonatal period and early infancy. *Diabetes Care,* 28, 1457–1462

Rodriguez WE, Joshua IG, Falcone JC & Tyagi SC. (2006). Pioglitazone prevents cardiac remodeling in high-fat, high-calorie-induced Type 2 diabetes mellitus. *Am J Physiol Heart Circ Physiol*, 291, H81–H87

Rosado EL, Bressan J, Hernández JA, Martins MF & Cecon PR. (2006). Effect of diet and PPARgamma2 and beta2-adrenergic receptor genes on energy metabolism and body composition in obese women. *Nutr Hosp,* 21, 3, 317-31

Ruiz-Pesini E, Mishmar D, Brandon M, ProcaccioV&Wallace DC. (2004). Effects of purifying and adaptive selection on regional variation in human mtDNA. *Science*, 303, 223–226

Sakai RR, Tamashiro KL, Yamazaki Y & Yanagimachi R. (2005). Cloning and assisted reproductive techniques: influence on early development and adult phenotype. *Birth Defects Res C Embryo Today*, 75, 151–162

Sayer AA & Cooper C. (2005). Fetal programming of body composition and musculoskeletal development. *Early Hum Dev*, 81, 9, 735-44

Sayer AA, Syddall HE, Dennison EM, Gilbody HJ, Duggleby SL & Cooper C. (2004). Birth weight, weight at 1 y of age, and body composition in older men: findings from the Hertfordshire Cohort Study. *Am J Clin Nutr*, 80, 199–203

Schwartz MW. (2001). Brain pathways controlling food intake and body weight. *Experimental Biology of Medicine*, 226, 978–981

Scialli A. (2006). Teratology public affairs committee position paper: maternal obesity in pregnancy. *Birth Defects Res A Clin Mol Teratol*, 76, 73–77

Sébert SP, Hyatt MA, Chan LL, Patel N, Bell RC, Keisler D, Stephenson T, Budge H, Symonds ME & Gardner DS. (2008). Maternal nutrient restriction between early-to-mid gestation and its impact upon appetite regulation following juvenile obesity. *Endocrinology*, 150, 2, 634-41

Seufert J, Kieffer TJ, Leech CA, Holz GG, Moritz W & Ricordi C. (1999). Leptin suppression of insulin secretion and gene expression in human pancreatic islets: implications for the development of adipogenic diabetes mellitus. *Journal of Clinical and Endocrinological Metabolism*, 84 670–676

Silverman BL, Metzger BE, Cho NH & Loeb CA. (1995). Impaired glucose tolerance in adolescent offspring of diabetic mothers. *Diabetes Care*, 18, 611-617

Simmons D & Breier BH. (2002). Fuel mediated teratogenesis driven by maternal obesity may be responsible for pandemic of obesity. *BMJ*, 324, 674

Simopoulos AP. (1999). Essential fatty acids in health and chronic disease. *Am J Clin Nutr*, ;70, 3 Suppl, 560S-569S

Singhal A, Farooqi IS, O'Rahilly S, Cole TJ, Fewtrell M & Lucas A. (2002). Early nutrition and leptin concentrations in later life. *Am J Clin Nutr*, 75, 6, 993-9

Stevens D, Alexander G & Bell AW. (1990). Effect of prolonged glucose infusion into fetal sheep on body growth, fat deposition and gestation length. *J Dev Physiol*, 13, 277–281

Stocker C, O'Dowd J, Morton NM,Wargent E, Sennitt MV & Hislop D. (2004). Modulation of susceptibility to weight gain and insulin resistance in low birthweight rats by treatment of their mothers with leptin during pregnancy and lactation. *Int J Obes Relat Metab Disord*, 28, 129–136.

Symonds ME, Budge H, Mostyn A, Stephenson T & Gardner DS. (2006). Nutritional programming of foetal development: endocrine mediators and long-term outcomes for cardiovascular health. *Curr Nutr Food Sci*, 2, 389-398.

Symonds ME, Mostyn A, Pearce S, Budge H & Stephenson T. (2003). Energy regulation in the fetus: endocrine control of adipose tissue development. *Journal of Endocrinology*, 179, 293–299

Symonds ME, Pearce S, Bispham J, Gardner DS & Stephenson T. (2004). Timing of nutrient restriction and programming of fetal adipose tissue development. *Proceedings of the Nutrition Society*, 63, 397–403

Symonds ME, Stephenson T, Gardner DS &Budge H. (2007). Long term effects of nutritional programming of the embryo and fetus: mechanisms and critical windows. *Rep Fertil Dev*, 19, 53-63

Symonds ME. (2007). Integration of physiological and molecular mechanisms of the developmental origins of adult disease: new concepts and insights. *Proc Nutr Soc*, 66, 442-450

Taylor PD & Poston L. (2007). Developmental programming of obesity in mammals. *Exp Physiol*, 92, 2, 287–298

Taylor PD, McConnell J, Khan IY, Holemans K, Lawrence KM & Asare-Anane H. (2005). Impaired glucose homeostasis and mitochondrial abnormalities in offspring of rats fed a fat-rich diet in pregnancy. *Am J Physiol Regul Integr CompPhysiol*, 288, R134–R139

Tobi E, Lumey L, Talens RP, Kremer D, Putter H, Stein A, Slagboom P & Heijmans B. (2009). DNA methylation differences after exposure to prenatal famine are common and timing- and sex-specific. *Hum. Mol. Genet*, 18, 4046–4053

Velkoska E, Cole TJ & Morris MJ. (2005). Early dietary intervention: long-term effects on blood pressure, brain neuropeptide Y, and diposity markers. *Am J Physiol Endocrinol Metab*, 288, E1236–E1243

Vickers MH, Breier BH, CutfieldWS, Hofman PL & Gluckman PD. (2000). Fetal origins of hyperphagia, obesity, and hypertension and postnatal amplification by hypercaloric nutrition. *Am J Physiol Endocrinol Metab*, 279, E83–E87

Vickers MH, Breier BH, McCarthy D & Gluckman PD. (2003). Sedentary behavior during postnatal life is determined by the prenatal environment and exacerbated by postnatal hypercaloric nutrition. *Am J Physiol Regul Integr Comp Physiol*, 285, R271–R273

Vickers MH, Gluckman PD, Coveny AH, Hofman PL, Cutfield WS & Gertler A. (2005). Neonatal leptin treatment reverses developmental programming. *Endocrinology*, 146, 4211–4216

Villamor E & Cnattingius S. (2006). Interpregnancy weight change and risk of adverse pregnancy outcomes: a population-based study. *Lancet*, 368, 1164–1170

Vottero A, Kino T, Combe H, Lecomte P & Chrousos GP. (2002). A Novel, C-Terminal Dominant Negative Mutation of the GR Causes Familial Glucocorticoid Resistance through Abnormal Interactions with p160 Steroid Receptor Coactivators. *The Journal of Clinical Endocrinology & Metabolism*, 87, 6, 2658–2667

Wake DJ &Walker BR. (2004). 11β-Hydroxysteroid dehydrogenase type 1 in obesity and the metabolic syndrome. *Mol Cell Endocrinol*, 215, 45–54

Wang SJ, Birtles S, de Schoolmeester J, Swales J, Moody G & Hislop D. (2006). Inhibition of 11β-hydroxysteroid dehydrogenase type 1 reduces food intake and weight gain but maintains energy expenditure in diet-induced obese mice. *Diabetologia*, 49, 1333–1337

Waterland RA. (2006). Assessing the effects of high methionine intake on DNA methylation. *J Nutr*, 136, 1706S–1710S

Wells JC. (2007). The thrifty phenotype as an adaptative maternal effect. *Biol Rev Camb Philos Soc*, 82, 1, 143-72

Whorwood CB, Firth KM, Budge H & Symonds ME. (2001). Maternal undernutrition during early- to mid-gestation programmes tissue-specific alterations in the expression of the glucocorticoid receptor, 11b-hydroxysteroid dehydrogenase isoforms and type 1 angiotensin II receptor in neonatal sheep. *Endocrinology*, 142, 2854-2864

Widdowson EM, McCance RA. (1963). The effect of finite periods of undernutrition at different ages on the composition and subsequent development of the rat. *Proc R Soc Lond Biol Sci*, 158, 329–42

Williams P, Kurlak LO, Perkins A, Budge H, Stephenson T, Keisler DH, Symonds ME & Gardner DS. (2007). Impaired renal function and hypertension accompany juvenile obesity: effect of prenatal diet. *Kidney Int*, 772, 279-289

Wilson FH, Hariri A, Farhi A, Zhao H, Petersen KF & Toka HR. (2004). A cluster of metabolic defects caused by mutation in a mitochondrial tRNA. *Science*, 306, 1190–1194

Wisloff U, Najjar SM, Ellingsen O, Haram PM, Swoap S & Al-Share Q. (2005). Cardiovascular risk factors emerge after artificial selection for low aerobic capacity. *Science*, 307, 418–420

Yuen BS, Owens PC, Muhlhausler BS, Roberts CT, Symonds ME & Keisler DH. (2003). Leptin alters the structural and functional characteristics of adipose tissue before birth. *FASEB Journal*, 17, 1102–1104

Yura S, Itoh H, Sagawa N, Yamamoto H, Masuzaki H &Nakao K. (2005). Role of premature leptin surge in obesity resulting from intrauterine undernutrition. *Cell Metab*, 1, 371–378

6

Childhood Inmigration and Obesity – An Emerging Problem

I. Díez López[1] and M. Carranza Ferrer[2]
[1]*Pediatric Endocrinology Unit, Txagorritxu Hospital, HUA,*
[2]*Pediatric Endocrinology Unit, Nuestra Señora de Meritxell Hospital,*
[1]*Spain*
[2]*Andorra*

1. Introduction

Overweight and obesity are rapidly increasing among children and adults. In 1998, the World Health Organisation recognized obesity as a major worldwide public health epidemic [1].

In the World Health conference at Geneva called for specific action to halt this epidemic [2]. Overweight and obesity can lead to a wide array of health and social consequences. Childhood overweight appears to be associated with cardiovascular risk factors such a high blood pressure; hyperlipidemia, elevated insulin levels [3] and non-insulin-dependent diabetes mellitus (type 2 diabetes). Other comorbidities include asthma and orthopedic problems as well as a varity of more rare disorders [3,4]. Ultimately overweight in childhood is associated with premature mortality especially if combined with intrauterine growth retardation (small for gestacional age SGA). The psychological well-being and the quality of life can also be affected [3,5,6].

Furthermore overweight and obesity in childhood, particularly in adolescence tends to persist into adulthood. The risk of adult overweight is about twofold increased for individuals who were overweight as children compared with individuals who were not overweight [7,8]. Adulthood overweight are at increased risk of dyslipidaemia, hypertension and type 2 diabetes even if the extra weight was lost during adulthood [6]. Psychological consequences include social and psychological stress, with increased risk of negative self- esteem, social isolation and negative influence on the career and family incomes [7].

There are wide geographical variations of overweight. Comparing reported prevalences of childhood overweight in Europe, Lobstein et al. [9] point out that children residing in central and Eastern Europe have a lower level of overweight than children from other parts of Europe, especially from Southern Europe. Average prevalences in Eastern Europe range from 10% to 18% among children aged 7 to 11 years, whereas values around 20% to 35 % have been reported from countries like Greece and Spain [9,10]. It is suggested that the low obesity prevalence in Eastern Europe is a consequence of the huge economic burden and the associated poverty following the political transition in the 1990s.

2. A new reality, a new global illness: Obesity in children

Studies in industrialized countries show that children from families with lower socio-economic status particularly suffer from excess weight [11,12]. In less industrialized societies excess weight is found predominantly among children from families with higher socio-economic status [9].

The process of migration, with its economic, social and environmental consequences may also affect health and body weight among migrants. Several US studies show differences in body mass index (BMI) among ethnic minorities [13,14] but empirical data on BMI in children among different ethnic groups in Europe are scarce. In Europe children from non-Europe ethnic groups nowadays make up a large percentage of children overall, more in countries such us Spain, Italy…. In some cities up to 50% of all children entering school may be first, second or third generation migrants [15]. There are several studies or health reports on overweight and obesity among migrant children at school entry [16-19]. Migrant children were consistently found to be more frequently overweight. Obesity was noted as a particular problem among children of Turkish origin [20].

However, since the assessment of migration status is not uniform, comparisons between studies are difficult. In addition, family socioeconomic status and duration of migration are not routinely evaluated. It will be important investigated the prevalence of overweight and obesity among migrant and not migrant children at school entry and to assess the influence of duration of migration and socioeconomic status on overweight and obesity in childhood.

We can found in papers same examples about this fact: among boys in Bavaria, Kalies [21] found that the frequency of overweight and obesity in non-German compared to German children was 1.9 times higher for overweight and 2.4 times higher for obesity.

Results of one study that our city demonstrated in our city in Spain the obesity was more important and prevalence in children from Latino-America and East-Europe than not migrant [22]. We conclude that immigrant's children have a higher rate of obesity; their obesity was more severe, leave to assists to the consult with more frequency and get poor results losing BMI than Spanish children. Difficulties with language, different culture and the lack of perception of illness in the problem of obesity make this collective more vulnerable for obesity.

But the choice of reference and the definition of migrant status (see below) may also contribute to the slightly different results. In Europe, only a few studies on Body Mass Index (BMI) examined the potential impact of ethnicity or migration status on overweight and obesity. In a UK survey [23] showed that Indian and Pakistani boys had a higher prevalence of overweight compared with boys in the general.

UK population while Bangladeshi and Chinese boys had a lower overweight prevalence. Among girls, Afro-Caribbean and Pakistani girls more frequently were overweight while Indian and Chinese girls had a lower overweight prevalence compared to girls from the general population.

In our study the obesity was more prevalence in children from Latino-america and East-Europe than not migrant [22]. In France, the children of Maghrebian immigrants were more obese than French children in cross-sectional surveys conducted in the 1970ies and the 1990ies [30]. The overall prevalence of obesity increased from 8% to 13% over this period. Data from health surveys in 1992/93 and 1993/94 among children in the Netherlands showed that the average body mass index was higher among Turkish and Moroccan children than among Dutch children [24].

Geographical differences in overweight in Europe were demonstrated by Lobstein et al. [9]. Children from countries in Central and East Europe generally showed a low prevalence of overweight. On the other hand, a higher prevalence of overweight was found in children in Southern European countries. Recent data from Edirne in Turkey demonstrate comparatively low prevalences of overweight and obesity among adolescents [25,26].

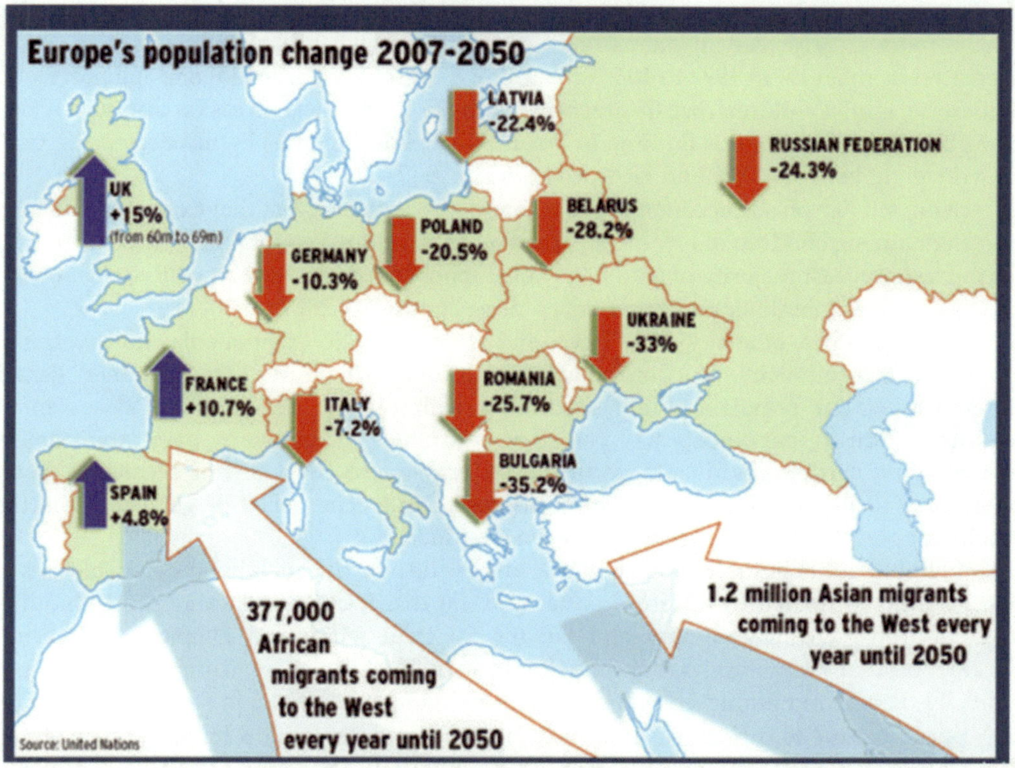

3. Other considerations

The international variability of definitions concerning paediatric overweight and obesity implies methodological difficulties when comparing prevalences internationally. In adults, the BMI cut-points of 25 and 30 are widely used to define overweight and obesity. Unlike in adults, BMI in children varies substantially by age and gender during childhood and adolescence. Unfortunately no commonly accepted standard has yet emerged. Different reference systems have been proposed, so it is very difficult compare different studies of obesity in children.

It appears disputable whether the use of national reference data is preferable when assessing overweight and obesity among migrant children. The comparison to reference curves from the country of origin would disregard the environmental changes associated with migration in many instances. An international standard appeared the most suitable option in this situation (migrant children).

Additional indexes of social class, social capital, or social context are rarely obtained in research surveys on diets and health. Undoubtedly, the arbitrary choice of cut-points and other problems associated with BMI-based classification systems in childhood will require further debate [27-28].

An association of overweight among migrant children with a long duration stay in Europe has not been reported previously. Social and political circumstances as potential explanation needs to be considered. The possible impact of such changes, however in opposite direction, can be more clearly seen in data from Russia. The prevalence of overweight in Russia decreased from 26.4% in 1992 to 10.2% in 1998 in 6–9 y-old children [35] and the prevalence of underweight in children rose during same time [9]. Economical recession during this time plausible explanation of this finding. In Poland, Koziel al. found a slightly decreasing trend in overweight between 1987 and 1997 in 14y-old boys [27].

In general, studies on socioeconomic status and overweight suggest that overweight is more prevalent among children of low income families in developed countries.

In contrast, the vast majority of studies in developing countries show a positive relationship between socioeconomic status and obesity among children [9,28].

In other fact, Race/ethnicity may have underlying genetic components; however, self-identified race/ethnicity is complicated by genetic admixture [29]. Whether genetic differences across populations are associated with obesity development also remains unclear. A "thrifty genotype" may confer an advantage in an energy-poor environment, which would become disadvantageous in an energy-dense environment because it would predispose to increased accumulation of adipose tissue. The genes or gene variants that would support this hypothesis have not been identified.

One possible contributor to racial/ethnic disparities in the metabolic comorbidities of obesity may be related to different patterns of fat distribution. African American adults and children have less visceral and hepatic fat than white and Hispanic individuals (22,28). Another possibility is that there are fundamental metabolic differences by race or ethnicity. Racial and ethnic differences in resting metabolic rate have been found (28) but may partly be due to differences in fat-free mass or organ mass and have not been shown to account for weight gain over time within populations (28) Some differences in insulin secretion and response among racial/ethnic groups have been found. African American and Hispanic children have lower insulin sensitivity than white children. African Americans have higher circulating insulin levels than whites, due to not only a more robust β-cell response to glucose but also decreased clearance of insulin in the liver. Hispanics also have lower insulin sensitivity than whites, after controlling for BMI and body composition, and have higher insulin levels in compensation for their relative insulin resistance (29).

There are differences in lipids and lipoproteins related to race/ethnicity (30). African Americans have lower rates of basal lipolysis than whites (30). This could be a metabolic risk factor for both the development of obesity and the risk of obesity-related comorbidities. African Americans also have lower levels of adiponectin than white subjects during childhood and adolescence, which may help explain their increased risk of diabetes and cardiovascular disease despite having less visceral adiposity (30). In summary, there is circumstantial evidence for biological differences in obesity development and the occurrence of comorbidities by race/ethnicity; however, the relationships are far from definitive (22).

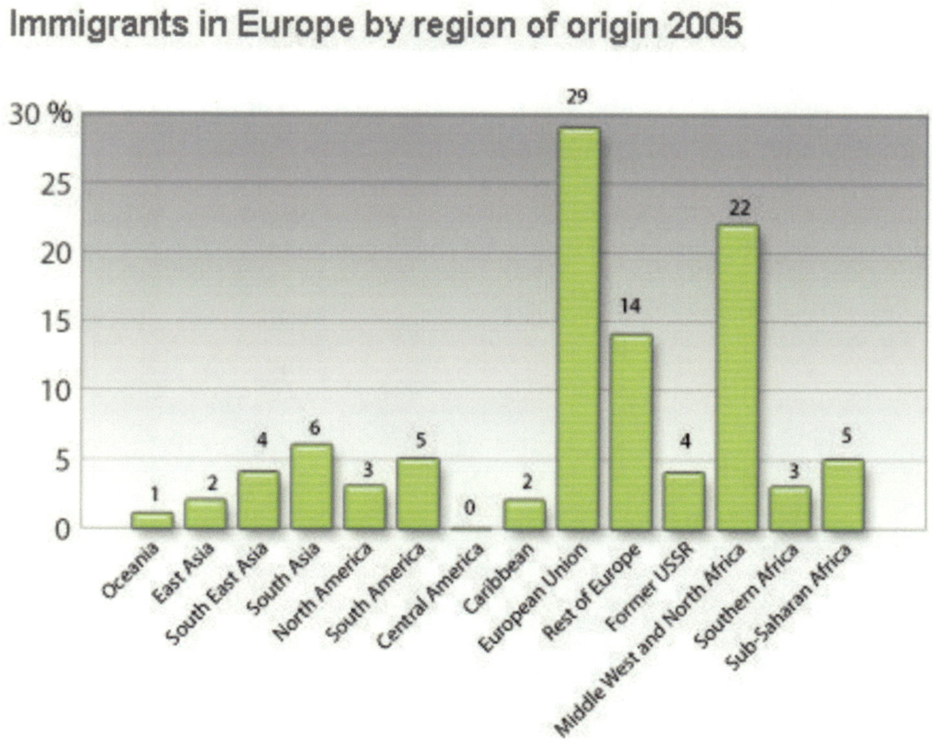

4. A new social reality, new challenges

The prevalence of obesity among immigrants depending on education level and the origin of their countries. While immigrants with Hispanic ethnicity appear to exhibit increase in obesity as their stay in the Europe (12-16) becomes longer, Asian and white immigrants do not experience any statistically significant increase.

Another point that is important is the more time has passed since the time of arrival in the new host country, the incidence of obesity is higher (18-22)

Same keys of this fact could be, Counseling on diet and physical activity in the early phase of their arrival may therefore help arrest the growing prevalence of obesity among immigrants. Such counseling is likely to be more effective if directed at low-educated immigrants and on those who arrived at a relatively young age since these two groups are most likely to experience increases in obesity after arrival in Europe.

From another point of view, immigrants from low socioeconomic backgrounds are less likely to have access to quality healthcare (22). They also have limited or no counseling for diet and physical exercise. This research therefore suggests that resources for counseling on diet and physical exercise should be committed to help the most vulnerable populations, e.g. the low educated, those who immigrate when young and among ethnic groups, resources should be channeled toward providing counseling to Latino immigrants (26-30).

A key of Europe healthy will be control the BMI of our children, in special the immigrant children. The number of born of immigrant's families and the rate of immigrant in same countries of Europe will be a great role influence in our more nearest future.

5. Summary

The increase of population in Europe in recent years at the expense of increased immigration is a fact.

These new populations tend to maintain their eating habits but ill adapted to the new reality in which they live: easy and cheap access to food, many high-calorie, reduced physical activity, increased sedentary ...... is called the "syndrome of the new rich."

There is also a human feeling to give the children what the parents have lacked, which often leads to overeating phenomenon of immigrant child population.

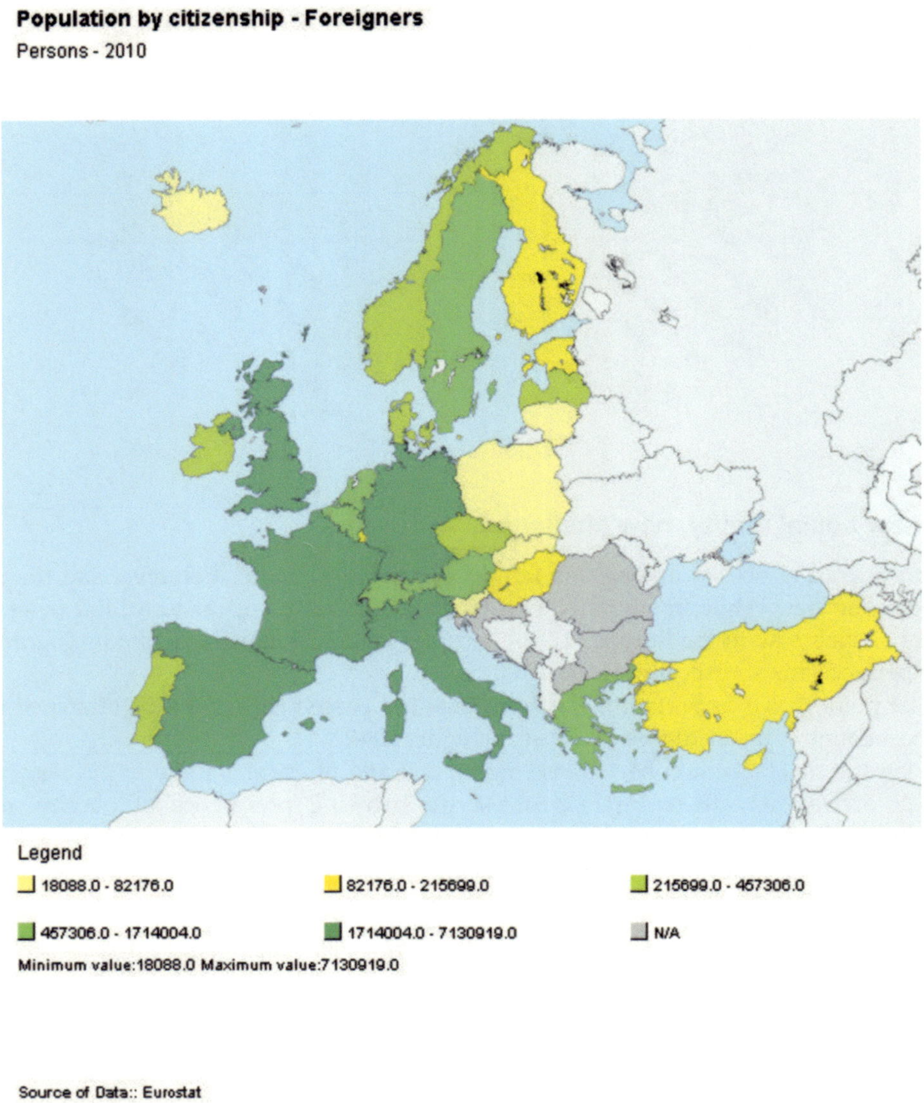

On the other hand is the fact of the possibility that part of the immigrant population has a higher rate of "energy-saving genes," a fact that has led to a survival advantage in their countries of origin but a clear disadvantage in the "rich Europe".

These fact combined with a possible increased susceptibility to the development of metabolic disease is causing an increase in the prevalence of obesity and obesity-related diseases in child and adolescent population of immigrants.

This is a major challenge for the future of European health systems. Coping with new social, economic and adjusting the existing health resources against a disease increasingly pressing, which, to do nothing, will lead to an unprecedented increase in health spending due to metabolic and cardiovascular diseases.

Of the health conscious this problem depends on the current reality obese children, does not become a majority of young adults sick.

6. List of abbreviations

BMI: Body mass index

7. Competing interests

The author(s) declare that they have no competing interest

8. References

[1] World Health Organization: Obesity: Preventing and managing the global epidemic. WHO technical report series. *Volume 894*. Geneva, WHO; 2000.

[2] World Health Organization: Fifty-seventh world health assembly. Global strategy on diet, physical activity and health. Geneva, 17-22 May. 2004.

[3] Deckelbaum RJ, Williams CL: Childhood obesity: the health issue. *Obes Res* 2001, 9 Suppl 4:239S-243S.

[4] Reilly JJ, Methven E, McDowell ZC, Hacking B, Alexander D, Stewart L, Kelnar CJ: Health consequences of obesity. *Arch Dis Child* 2003, 88:748-752.

[5] Must A, Anderson SE: Effects of obesity on morbidity in children and adolescents. *Nutr Clin Care* 2003, 6:4-12.

[6] Dietz WH: Health consequences of obesity in youth: childhood predictors of adult disease. *Pediatrics* 1998, 101:518-525.

[7] 7 Dietz WH: Childhood weight affects adult morbidity and mortality. *J Nutr* 1998, 128:411S-414S.

[8] Must A: Morbidity and mortality associated with elevated body weight in children and adolescents. *Am J Clin Nutr* 1996, 63:445S-447S.

[9] Lobstein T, Frelut ML: Prevalence of overweight among children in Europe. *Obes Rev* 2003, 4:195-200.

[10] Krassas GE, Tzotzas T, Tsametis C, Konstantinidis T: Prevalence and trends in overweight and obesity among children and adolescents in Thessaloniki, Greece. *J Pediatr Endocrinol Metab* 2001, 14 Suppl 5:1319-1326.

[11] Kromeyer-Hauschild K, Zellner K, Jaeger U, Hoyer H: Prevalence of overweight and obesity among school children in Jena (Germany). *Int J Obes Relat Metab Disord* 1999, 23:1143-1150.

[12] Langnäse K, Mast M, Muller MJ: Social class differences in overweight of prepubertal children in northwest Germany. *Int J Obes Relat Metab Disord* 2002, 26:566-572.

[13] Haas JS, Lee LB, Kaplan CP, Sonneborn D, Phillips KA, Liang SY: The association of race, socioeconomic status, and health insurance status with the prevalence of overweight among children and adolescents. *Am J Public Health* 2003, 93:2105-2110.
[14] Nelson JA, Chiasson MA, Ford V: Childhood overweight in a New York City WIC population. *Am J Public Health* 2004, 94:458-462.
[15] Ministerium für Schule Jugend und Kinder des Landes Nordrhein- Westfalen: Ausländische und ausgesiedelte Schülerinnen und Schüler, Ausländische Lehrerinnen und Lehrer im Schuljahr 2003/04. 2004, 344:.
[16] Gawrich S: Wie gesund sind unsere Schulanfänger?- Zur Interpretation epidemiologischer Auswertungen der Schuleingangsuntersuchung. *Hessisches Ärzteblatt* 2004, 2:73-76.
[17] Erb J, Winkler G: Role of nationality in overweight and obesity in preschool children in Germany. *Monatsschrift Kinderheilkunde* 2004, 152:291-298.
[18] Bauer C, Rosemeier A: A handicap for life - Overweight and obesity in pre-school children in Karlsruhe. *Gesundheitswesen* 2004, 66:246-250.
[19] Gesundheitsamt der Stadt Dortmund: Die Gesundheit der Schulanfängerinnen und Schulanfänger in Dortmund- Ergebnisse der schulärztlichen Untersuchungen von 1985-1996. 1997, 5:.
[20] Delekat D: Zur Gesundheitlichen Lage von Kindern in Berlin- Ergebnisse und Handlungsempfehlungen auf Basis der Einschulungsuntersuchungen 2001.Spezialbericht 2003-2. Berlin, Senatsverwaltung für Gesundheit, Soziales und Verbraucherschutz; 2003.
[21] Kalies H, Lenz J, von Kries R: Prevalence of overweight and obesity and trends in body mass index in German pre-school children, 1982-1997. *Int J Obes Relat Metab Disord* 2002, 26:1211-1217.
[22] Díez López I, Rodríguez Estévez A Revista Española de Obesidad Vol. 6 2008 6:280-285
[23] Saxena S, Ambler G, Cole TJ, Majeed A: Ethnic group differences in overweight and obese children and young people in England: cross sectional survey. *Arch Dis Child* 2004, 89:30-36.
[24] Roville-Sausse F: [Increase during the last 20 years of body mass of children 0 to 4 years of age born to Maghrebian immigrants]. *Rev Epidemiol Sante Publique* 1999, 47:37-44.
[25] Brussaard JH, Erp-Baart MA, Brants HA, Hulshof KF, Lowik MR: Nutrition and health among migrants in The Netherlands. *Public Health Nutr* 2001, 4:659-664.
[26] Oner N, Vatansever U, Sari A, Ekuklu E, Guzel A, Karasalihoglu S, Boris NW: Prevalence of underweight, overweight and obesity in Turkish adolescents. *Swiss Med Wkly* 2004, 134:529-533.
[27] Neovius M, Linne Y, Barkeling B, Rossner S: Discrepancies between classification systems of childhood obesity. *Obes Rev* 2004, 5:105-114.
[28] Wang Y, Wang JQ: A comparison of international references for the assessment of child and adolescent overweight and obesity in different populations. *Eur J Clin Nutr* 2002, 56:973-982.
[29] Wang Y, Monteiro C, Popkin BM: Trends of obesity and underweight in older children and adolescents in the United States, Brazil, China, and Russia. *Am J Clin Nutr* 2002, 75:971-977.
[30] Koziel S, Kolodziej H, Ulijaszek SJ: Parental education, body mass index and prevalence of obesity among 14-year-old boys between 1987 and 1997 in Wroclaw, Poland. *Eur J Epidemiol* 2000, 16:1163-1167.
[31] Wang Y: Cross-national comparison of childhood obesity: the epidemic and the relationship between obesity and socioeconomic status. *Int J Epidemiol* 2001, 30:1129-1136.

Part 2

Childhood Obesity – Prevention and Future Life

7

Comorbidities of Childhood Obesity

Ambar Banerjee[1] and Dara P. Schuster[2]
[1]*Center for Minimally Invasive Surgery, Division of General and Gastrointestinal Surgery, The Ohio State University, Columbus, Ohio*
[2]*Department of Internal Medicine, Division of Endocrinology, Diabetes and Metabolism, The Ohio State University, Columbus, Ohio*
USA

1. Introduction

The epidemic of obesity is known to contribute annually to 2.6 million deaths worldwide. [1] Excessive adiposity is the primary etiology of major metabolic diseases and related mortality. These deaths are attributed mainly to the comorbidities associated with obesity, including hypertension (HTN), cardiovascular disease (CVD), and diabetes mellitus (DM). The global escalation of childhood obesity is a matter of grave concern. Recent data have demonstrated a nearly fourfold rise in the prevalence of childhood obesity, making the pediatric age group the fastest growing subpopulation of obese individuals in this country. [1] Corresponding data examining global obesity trends demonstrate similar patterns worldwide with rates of overweight—defined as having a body mass index (BMI) greater that 25 kg/m^2—occurring in 40% of men and 30% of women and rates of obesity (BMI≥30 kg/m^2) at approximately 25%. [2] This condition can have far-reaching consequences on the physical and mental health of the young obese patients with many of these chronic diseases surging in childhood rather than adulthood.

The normal BMI values used for defining overweight and obesity in adults cannot be extrapolated to the pediatric population as BMI is known to change with age and gender during childhood and adolescence. Center for Disease Control (CDC) BMI-for-age growth charts for girls and boys provide standard translation of a BMI number into a percentile with age and gender specific normograms. [3] Children with BMI equal to or exceeding the age-gender-specific 95th percentile are defined obese. Those with BMI equal to or exceeding the 85th but are below 95th percentiles are defined overweight. [4]

2. Risk factors

An inter-relationship of genetics and the environment is central to the regulation of energy balance, and thus body weight. Hence risk factors of the pandemic of obesity can be stratified on the basis of genetic and environmental sources.

Genetic influence of obesity is related to two primary processes: (1) susceptibility to overeating despite normal energy requirements, and (2) presence of a normal drive to eat despite low energy requirements. Appetite and the drive to eat may be impacted by several genetically programmed metabolic pathways, and this is demonstrated in the specific but rare syndromes such as Prader–Willi and Bardet–Biedl. [5] Obesity caused by single-gene mutations has been well documented in mice and other rodents but is relatively rare and ill-defined in humans. [6] These include the agouti, leptin, and leptin receptor gene mutations. These mutations produce phenotypes of severe hyperphagia, obesity, DM, defective thermogenesis, and infertility. The polygenic mouse models of obesity more closely resemble the human obesity phenotypes than single gene models and have mutations that influence obesity, plasma cholesterol levels, body fat distribution, and propensity toward development of obesity on a high-fat diet. [4]

The impact of the environment on the regulation of energy balance, and thus body weight is paramount. The changes in the macronutrient content of the diet (i.e., carbohydrate, protein and fat), energy density, sugar-sweetened beverages, and portion size have been associated with the soaring trend of obesity over the last couple of decades. In addition, the global trend of increasing technology, automation, motorized transportation and sedentary occupations contributes to a lifestyle that requires minimal physical activity. While once essential for survival, regular physical activity is optional in our modern, low energy-demanding environment, thereby making its contribution to the escalation of the pandemic. Poor socioeconomic status with less consumption of more expensive fruits and vegetables and suboptimal cognitive stimulation at home mediate development of obesity in children. [7-9] The dietary habits of the parents significantly modify child food preferences and the degree of parental adiposity is a relatively direct measure of the child's dietary preferences. [10-12]

3. Pathophysiology

A breakdown in the complex interplay of the central nervous system, the gastrointestinal system and the adipose tissue of the body culminates in obesity. The central nervous system provides the feedback control system for integration of energy expenditure and for digestion, absorption, transport, and storage of nutrients and mobilization and use of fuels. Signals regarding alterations in fuel usage are tightly regulated and come primarily from adipocytes and from the gastrointestinal tract. This interaction of the different systems is responsible for the weight and fat balance of the human body.

Adipose tissue is now known to play a significant role in metabolic and immune function, possibly through the production of pro-inflammatory cytokines and other hormones secreted by adipocytes. [13-14] In the past decade, pro-inflammatory adipocytokines, including TNF-α, IL-6, and leptin, resistin, and many others, have received tremendous attention for their potential role in fuel metabolism, glucose homeostasis, insulin resistance, and perhaps atherosclerosis. [13-15] In contrast to the proinflammatory hormones, adiponectin, a 244-amino-acid peptide solely produced and secreted by adipose tissue, has been reported to improve insulin sensitivity and indeed could prevent diabetes mellitus and atherosclerosis. [16] Leptin, also produced by the adipocytes, circulates at levels proportionate to levels of body fat. It binds to receptors in the hypothalamus, activating signals to inhibit food intake and increase energy expenditure. In addition, leptin affects other hormones, both anorectic and orexigenic. [17-18]

Previous research has implicated gut hormones or incretins in appetite regulation, gastrointestinal motility, satiety, and changes in glucose, and in this regard may possibly play a role in the occurrence of obesity. [19] In the foregut, ghrelin, produced in the stomach and duodenum, increases before meals and decreases after meals. [20] Ghrelin is elevated in the setting of obesity and increased after diet-induced weight loss, suggesting a role in the compensatory changes in appetite and energy expenditure that make maintenance of diet-induced weight loss difficult. [21] In the hind-gut, where the suppression of gastrointestinal motility is modulated by hormones, such as peptide YY (PYY), neurotensin, glucagon-like peptide −1 (GLP-1), and oxyntomodulin, perturbations in hormone release have been demonstrated with weight loss secondary to Roux-en-Y gastric bypass. Peptide YY is a hormone released after meals whose function is to reduce appetite. [22] Its postprandial levels have been found to remain markedly elevated after bariatric surgery. [23] Better understanding of the interactions of the gut hormones on appetite and fuel metabolism will hopefully provide important information on the development of future obesity management strategies.

4. Co-morbidities related to obesity

Obesity in children and adolescents appears to be identical to obesity in adults, in both pathophysiology and consequences of obesity-related co-morbidities. These can be categorized broadly into medical and psychosocial. The medical consequences can result in metabolic effects, involving the cardiovascular, endocrine, gastrointestinal and renal systems, and mechanical effects involving the pulmonary, skeletal and central nervous systems.

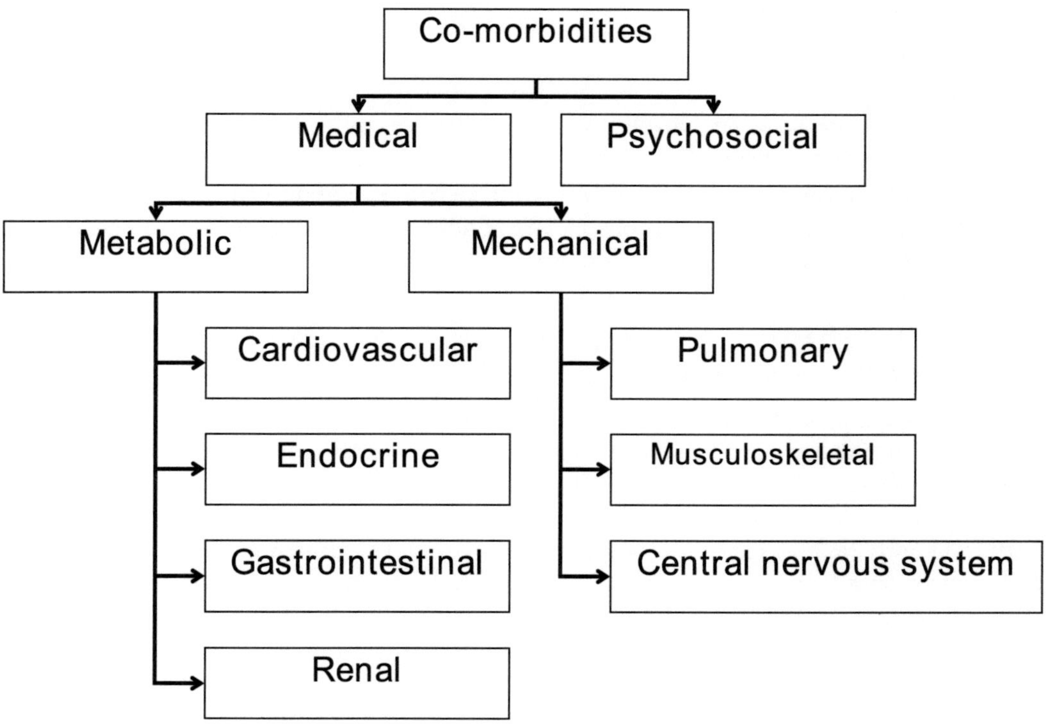

Fig. 1. Categories of co-morbidities

4.1 Metabolic consequences
4.1.1 Endocrine system
4.1.1.1 Insulin resistance

Obesity has a negative impact on multiple associated alterations in the glucose/insulin axis and on lipid metabolism. In particular, obese adults demonstrate reduced glucose disposal, primarily at the level of skeletal muscle (peripheral insulin resistance) [24] as well as impairment in insulin action on non-esterified fatty acid oxidation, [25] leading to insulin resistance and abnormal lipolysis. Yet it is unclear when these abnormalities occur in the setting of acute versus chronic obesity. Polonsky and coworkers [26] found that insulin secretory rates were significantly higher in the obese group when compared with the normal weight group. Furthermore, there was no difference in insulin clearance or hepatic insulin extraction between the groups. There was a diminished hepatic insulin extraction noted in a subset of the obese group that demonstrated a greater degree of hyperinsulinemia. To characterize this further, Monti and coworkers [27] examined obese children with normo-insulinemia to characterize early metabolic derangement and found peripheral insulin resistance in the obese children when compared with normal weight children but no significant differences in non-esterified fatty acids response to insulin infusion. Le Stunff and coworkers [28] found that the earliest abnormality in glucose metabolism in obese children (those with short duration of obesity) was an abnormal insulin response to a meal stimuli and that maximal glucose uptake decreased with age and obesity duration. Thus, it appears that one of the earliest negative effects of obesity is the development of insulin resistance.

4.1.1.2 Metabolic syndrome

The metabolic syndrome complex is comprised of hyperglycemia, HTN, dyslipidemia and obesity where truncal fat and insulin resistance are thought to be the primary problems. There is no consensus in the definition of this syndrome in children and its role in future cardiovascular events can only be extrapolated from corresponding adult studies. Goodman et al. [29] identified four groups of risk factors in adolescents and inferred that obesity had maximal influence on cumulative cardio-metabolic risk. Each of the components of this syndrome complex is found to aggravate with increasing obesity independent of age, sex and pubertal status. [30]

4.1.1.3 Type 2 diabetes mellitus

The prevalence of pediatric DM has increased significantly over the last decade with significant variability based on race and ethnicity. Obesity and DM have been tightly linked in both animal models and adult humans. Recently, data on increasing incidence and prevalence of DM in adolescents demonstrate that insulin resistance and increases in both total body fat and visceral fat play a role in DM development in adolescents, similar to that seen in adults. [31-32] Obesity is associated with increased TNF-α levels which lead to increased release of free fatty acids in adipocytes, blockade of the synthesis of adiponectin and activation of the insulin receptor. [33] Moreover, IL-6, released mainly by macrophages and adipocytes, influences glucose tolerance through antagonizing the secretion of adiponectin and by enhancing gluconeogenesis, glycogenolysis and inhibiting glycogenesis. [34] There are numerous other adipokines like resistin, adipsin and others which are believed to be the missing link between obesity and target tissue resistance to insulin resulting in Type DM. [35-37] With early onset of obesity, the population is believed to be more susceptible to the disease and its inadvertent complications.

4.1.1.4 Gynecological disorders

4.1.1.4.1 Polycystic ovarian syndrome (PCOS)

Polycystic ovarian disease is one of the most common endocrine abnormalities and typically begins in adolescence. It is often accompanied by hyperandrogenism and hyperinsulinemia. Although the exact mechanism for this relationship is unclear, it is postulated that high circulating levels of insulin play a role in ovarian cyst development due to the anabolic effect of insulin at the IGF receptors on the ovaries. Up to 30% of women with polycystic ovarian disease are overweight/obese. Obesity can worsen the picture of polycystic ovary syndrome (PCOS) by increasing insulin resistance, diabetes, and metabolic syndrome, thereby commencing a vicious cycle. This cycle may culminate in infertility . The prevalence of impaired glucose tolerance in obese young women with PCOS has been estimated to be as high as 30-40%, with an additional 5-10% having frank DM. [38] Yet, there remains debate in the literature about the nature of the relationship between obesity and PCOS.

4.1.1.4.2 Menstrual abnormalities

Body weight and body fat are considered to be significant physiological triggers of menarche. [39] Hence, obese girls often present with menarche before the age of 10 years. [40] Obesity can also lead to oligomenorrhea or amenorrhea at the other end of the spectrum, all leading to an increased risk of complicated pregnancies.

4.1.2 Cardiovascular system

4.1.2.1 Hypertension

Multiple studies showed childhood obesity to be a major determinant of the cardiovascular risk factors in adulthood. [41-42] In addition to overall increased adiposity, truncal obesity is associated with increased atherothrombotic events and increased inflammatory markers. [43-44] Hypertension, especially systolic, in children and adolescents is closely associated with adiposity. [45-46] Intima media thickness (IMT), a noninvasive marker for early atherosclerotic changes, was found to be significantly increased in the obese children as compared with non-obese children of similar age, sex, and pubertal stage. [47-50] Reinehr et al. further demonstrated a significant association between these atherogenic changes and CVD risk factors, HTN, impaired glucose metabolism, and chronic inflammation. [51]

4.1.2.2 Left ventricular hypertrophy and coronary artery disease

The onset of left ventricular hypertrophy (LVH) was believed to date back to the adolescent years and developed into a formidable CVD risk factor by young adulthood in this sub-population. [52] Maggio et al. showed the onset of this relationship between obesity and LVH in the pre-pubertal age group and proposed the initiation of prevention and treatment of obesity to prevent end-stage organ damage. [53] A prospective follow-up over 57 years of the landmark Harvard Growth Study of 1922-1935 revealed that being overweight in adolescence was associated with a greater than two-fold increase in the relative risk of coronary artery disease mortality, independent of adult weight.[54] Hence, these patients with an advanced vascular age may need intensive management, including pharmacotherapy for risk factor modification, with the final goal of halting the progression of atherosclerosis and altering the lifetime risk of excess morbidity and mortality.

4.1.3 Gastrointestinal system

4.1.3.1 Non-alcoholic steatohepatitis (NASH)

The incidence of hepatic steatosis is 38% in obese children. The underlying cause is unknown, but the condition is associated with DM, obesity, rapid weight loss, and hyperlipidemia—all of which are characterized by impaired fat metabolism. Non-alcoholic fatty liver disease (NAFLD) is the primary hepatic complication of obesity and insulin resistance, and may be considered the early hepatic manifestation of metabolic syndrome. [55] One study demonstrated that non-alcoholic fatty liver disease is associated with insulin resistance even in patients with normal glucose tolerance. In the pediatric population, results demonstrate increased adipose tissue lipolytic activity with resulting increased rates of fatty acid release into plasma throughout the day. This continual excess in fatty acid flux supports the hypothesis that adipose insulin resistance is implicated in the pathogenesis of steatosis and contributes to the metabolic complications associated with NASH. [56] The fats accumulate largely in adipose tissue and, inappropriately, in muscle and liver. The sequence of events leading to the ectopic accumulation of triglycerides which cause development of insulin resistance has been referred to as the "overflow hypothesis". [57] The severe cases of this disease are notorious to progress to hepatic fibrosis and cirrhosis.

4.1.3.2 Gallstones

The dyslipidemia induced by obesity is responsible for increased biliary excretion of cholesterol, thereby increasing the likelihood of gallstone formation. Unlike the majority of children, this subgroup of the population complains of gallstones without any underlying diseases like hemolytic disorders. Obesity is incriminated to cause 8% to 33% of gallstones in children, with insulin resistance and metabolic syndrome being other potential risk factors.[58-59]

4.1.4 Renal system

Obesity plays a major role in the development of chronic kidney disease (CKD). It predisposes the individual to diabetic nephropathy, hypertensive nephrosclerosis, focal and segmental glomerular sclerosis and urolithiasis. Even in the absence of other comorbidities, obesity has been found to cause structural changes such as glomerulomegaly and glomerular basement membrane (GBM) thickening resulting in obesity-related nephropathy. [60-61] The physiological modification in renal hemodynamics in the setting of obesity is comprised of hyperfiltration associated with hyperperfusion, which together play a role in renal injury. An increased glomerular filtration rate (GFR) was observed in overweight compared with lean subjects, being significantly positively related to BMI [62-63] and insulin resistance. [64] However, pathologic changes within the nephron can be seen before overt proteinuria and renal disease. A recent study conducted in our institution revealed that bariatric surgery induced weight loss is associated with an improvement in the overall long term renal function in the morbidly obese adult. [65] Such data are lacking for the pediatric population. Recent European studies concluded that renal impairment may not be an early manifestation of adiposity in childhood but may contribute to the development of the disease in the long term. [66]

4.2 Mechanical consequences

4.2.1 Pulmonary system

4.2.1.1 Obstructive sleep apnea

Although there is limited data on obstructive sleep apnea (OSA) in children, the published estimate of prevalence is 7% in obese children. Obese children are six times more likely than lean, age-matched children to have OSA. This condition is known to cause daytime somnolence and neurocognitive deficits like concentration and memory lapses secondary to poor quality of sleep. [67-68] Sleep disturbance is linked to higher inflammatory biomarkers, such as CRP and IL-6. [69] Other hormone changes seen in OSA include a drop in leptin, an increase in ghrelin, increased insulin levels, and a decrease in insulin sensitivity. The etiology for these changes is unclear but felt to be related to the intermittent hypoxemia that may potentiate the inflammatory cascade which triggers systemic inflammation. [70-71]

4.2.1.2 Bronchial hyperactivity and exacerbation of asthma

Obesity is demonstrated to be significantly related to current asthma among children and adolescents with the association being stronger in non-atopic children than in atopic children. [72-73] The state of systemic inflammation, induced by adiposity, is hypothesized to result in this morbid condition. Overweight & obese children show a decreased response to inhaled steroids in the setting of asthma. [74] Childhood and adolescent adiposity is reported to be associated with significantly increased risk of asthma in the long term as well, thereby increasing the dependence on chronic medication. [75] Inability to exercise leads to the progression of obesity and the cycle continues.

4.2.2 Musculoskeletal system

Childhood obesity has been linked to increase frequency and severity of orthopedic problems in children. It appears that the orthopedic issues occur due to increased stress and strain on bone and cartilage that was not designed to carry excess weight. The more common orthopedic problems include bowing of the tibia and femurs that result in overgrowth of the medial aspect of the proximal tibial metaphysis or Blount syndrome and slipped capital femoral epiphysis due to increased weight on the growth plate of the hip. [76] Obesity during the growth spurt may increase the likelihood of fractures during falls as bone development does not adequately cope with excess weight. This weight/bone mass imbalance also places high levels of stress on growing bones and joints that may result in joint damage and may contribute to osteoarthritis in later years. [77] The occurrence of more severe fractures and bone disorders lead to the increased requirement of complex surgeries and joint replacements, especially in the setting of pediatric trauma, thus amplifying the physical and financial load of the disease in this population. [78]

4.2.3 Central nervous system

Corbett et al reported increased incidence of idiopathic intracranial hypertension at a relatively young age of less than 20 years in 90% of patients who had childhood obesity. [79] Moreover, about 30%-50% of children with pseudotumor cerebri are obese and probably this subgroup accounts for the majority of cases that are not associated with infection or medication. [80] It is thought that the increased intra-abdominal pressure due to obesity causes rise in intra-thoracic pressure which is transmitted to the head as increased resistance to venous return from the brain. [81]

4.3 Psychosocial consequences

Childhood obesity represents a dynamic process, in which behavior, cognition and emotional regulation interact mutually with each other. The interconnection between obesity and psychological problems seems to be cyclical, in that clinically meaningful psychological distress might precipitate weight gain and obesity may lead to further psychosocial problems. [82] Depression in adulthood has been found to be related to obesity in adolescence. [83] Females appear to have a stronger association than males. These patients are found to have obsessive concern due to social stigma about body image, low esteem and poor self-perception of physical appearance. The expectation of rejection leads to further progression of depression. Overweight adolescents frequently reported reduced health-related quality of life in physical, emotional and social aspects. [84-86] These factors tend to have a negative influence on these individuals. A vicious cycle ensues and some of these obese adolescents may consequently have less education, lower incomes and higher poverty rates. [87-88]

5. Conclusion

Despite the lack of full understanding of the pathophysiology of obesity, it is clear that there are consistent findings of insulin resistance and inflammation seen in both obese adults and children. These metabolic abnormalities play a role in the development of obesity-related comorbidities that are manifested early in the disease process. Inflammation in the adipose tissue is the result of increased oxidative stress, possibly secondary to hypoxia. Hypoxia is precipitated by the overgrowth of adipose tissue during obesity. Adipose tissue is responsible for the production of a significant proportion of systemic interleukin-6 (IL-6) which may induce a degree of systemic inflammation in this population. Along with this, it is also believed to activate CD8+ T cells which promote the recruitment and activation of macrophages in the tissue. [89] The inflammatory markers secreted by the cells and oxygen free radicals resulting from oxidative stress increase vascular endothelial permeability and cause endothelial dysfunction. [90-91] These abnormalities lay the foundation for all the derangements associated with obesity. Unfortunately, there is very limited data on the progress of the various comorbidities from childhood and adolescence to their culmination in adulthood. A study reported that 43% of obese children persisted to be obese adults and another 29% were overweight as adults. [92] Early onset obesity is a risk factor for significant morbidity and mortality later in life, where the rates of DM, CAD, atherosclerosis, metabolic syndrome are increased. A heightened degree of suspicion is warranted when confronted with adult and pediatric obese patients to avoid underdiagnosing of the various diseases. Given the negative short- and long-term impact of obesity on children, careful attention should be paid to the unique health issues of this "at-risk" population with both prevention and aggressive early intervention strategies.

6. References

[1] Kimm, S.Y. and E. Obarzanek, *Childhood obesity: a new pandemic of the new millennium.* Pediatrics, 2002. 110(5): p. 1003-7.

[2] Kirn, T. (2007) *Worldwide survey finds adult obesity rate of around 25%*. Circulation, DOI: *epub doi:10.1161/ circulationaha.106.676379*. Available from: http://www.cdc.gov/growthcharts/.
[3] Donohoue, P., *Obesity*. Nelson Textbook of Pediatrics 17th Ed, ed. R.M.K. R E Behrman, H B Jenson. 2004, Philadelphia: WB Saunders; pp. 173-7.
[4] Woods, S.C., et al., *Signals that regulate food intake and energy homeostasis*. Science, 1998. 280(5368): p. 1378-83.
[5] Bray GA, Fisler J, York DA. *Neuroendocrine control of the development of obesity: Understanding gained from studies of experimental animal models. Front Neuroendocrinol 1990;11:128.*
[6] Strauss, R.S. and J. Knight, *Influence of the home environment on the development of obesity in children*. Pediatrics, 1999. 103(6): p. e85.
[7] Neumark-Sztainer, D., et al., *Correlates of inadequate fruit and vegetable consumption among adolescents*. Prev Med, 1996. 25(5): p. 497-505.
[8] Kennedy, E. and R. Powell, *Changing eating patterns of American children: a view from 1996*. J Am Coll Nutr, 1997. 16(6): p. 524-9.
[9] Fisher, J.O. and L.L. Birch, *Fat preferences and fat consumption of 3- to 5-year-old children are related to parental adiposity*. J Am Diet Assoc, 1995. 95(7): p. 759-64.
[10] Ray, J.W. and R.C. Klesges, *Influences on the eating behavior of children*. Ann N Y Acad Sci, 1993. 699: p. 57-69.
[11] *Donohoue PA. Obesity. In: Behrman RE, Kleigman RM, Jenson HB, editors. Nelson textbook of pediatrics. 17th ed. Philadelphia: WB Saunders; 2004. pp. 173–7.*
[12] Engeli, S., et al., *Association between adiponectin and mediators of inflammation in obese women*. Diabetes, 2003. 52(4): p. 942-7.
[13] Straczkowski, M., et al., *Increased plasma-soluble tumor necrosis factor-alpha receptor 2 level in lean nondiabetic offspring of type 2 diabetic subjects*. Diabetes Care, 2002. 25(10): p. 1824-8.
[14] Deiuliis, J., et al., *Visceral adipose inflammation in obesity is associated with critical alterations in tregulatory cell numbers*. PLoS One. 6(1): p. e16376.
[15] Foster, G.D., et al., *Resting energy expenditure, body composition, and excess weight in the obese*. Metabolism, 1988. 37(5): p. 467-72.
[16] Considine, R.V., et al., *Serum immunoreactive-leptin concentrations in normal-weight and obese humans*. N Engl J Med, 1996. 334(5): p. 292-5.
[17] Bray, G.A. and D.A. York, *Clinical review 90: Leptin and clinical medicine: a new piece in the puzzle of obesity*. J Clin Endocrinol Metab, 1997. 82(9): p. 2771-6.
[18] Griffen, W.O., Jr., et al., *Gastric bypass for morbid obesity*. World J Surg, 1981. 5(6): p. 817-22.
[19] Hickey, M.S., et al., *A new paradigm for type 2 diabetes mellitus: could it be a disease of the foregut?* Ann Surg, 1998. 227(5): p. 637-43; discussion 643-4.
[20] Cummings, D.E., et al., *Plasma ghrelin levels after diet-induced weight loss or gastric bypass surgery*. N Engl J Med, 2002. 346(21): p. 1623-30.
[21] Taylor, I.L., *Role of peptide YY in the endocrine control of digestion*. J Dairy Sci, 1993. 76(7): p. 2094-101.
[22] Korner, J., et al., *Effects of Roux-en-Y gastric bypass surgery on fasting and postprandial concentrations of plasma ghrelin, peptide YY, and insulin*. J Clin Endocrinol Metab, 2005. 90(1): p. 359-65.
[23] Del Prato, S., et al., *Insulin regulation of glucose and lipid metabolism in massive obesity*. Diabetologia, 1990. 33(4): p. 228-36.

[24] Lillioja, S., et al., *Free fatty acid metabolism and obesity in man: in vivo in vitro comparisons.* Metabolism, 1986. 35(6): p. 505-14.

[25] Polonsky, K.S., et al., *Quantitative study of insulin secretion and clearance in normal and obese subjects.* J Clin Invest, 1988. 81(2): p. 435-41.

[26] Monti, L.D., et al., *Insulin regulation of glucose turnover and lipid levels in obese children with fasting normoinsulinaemia.* Diabetologia, 1995. 38(6): p. 739-47.

[27] Le Stunff, C. and P. Bougneres, *Early changes in postprandial insulin secretion, not in insulin sensitivity, characterize juvenile obesity.* Diabetes, 1994. 43(5): p. 696-702.

[28] Goodman, E., et al., *Factor analysis of clustered cardiovascular risks in adolescence: obesity is the predominant correlate of risk among youth.* Circulation, 2005. 111(15): p. 1970-7.

[29] Weiss, R., et al., *Obesity and the metabolic syndrome in children and adolescents.* N Engl J Med, 2004. 350(23): p. 2362-74.

[30] Pinhas-Hamiel, O., et al., *Increased incidence of non-insulin-dependent diabetes mellitus among adolescents.* J Pediatr, 1996. 128(5 Pt 1): p. 608-15.

[31] Richards, G.E., et al., *Obesity, acanthosis nigricans, insulin resistance, and hyperandrogenemia: pediatric perspective and natural history.* J Pediatr, 1985. 107(6): p. 893-7.

[32] Lastra, G., C.M. Manrique, and M.R. Hayden, *The role of beta-cell dysfunction in the cardiometabolic syndrome.* J Cardiometab Syndr, 2006. 1(1): p. 41-6.

[33] Fonseca-Alaniz, M.H., et al., *Adipose tissue as an endocrine organ: from theory to practice.* J Pediatr (Rio J), 2007. 83(5 Suppl): p. S192-203.

[34] Steppan, C.M., et al., *The hormone resistin links obesity to diabetes.* Nature, 2001. 409(6818): p. 307-12.

[35] Steppan, C.M. and M.A. Lazar, *The current biology of resistin.* J Intern Med, 2004. 255(4): p. 439-47.

[36] Pyrzak, B., et al., *Adiponectin as a biomarker of the metabolic syndrome in children and adolescents.* Eur J Med Res, 2010. 15 Suppl 2: p. 147-51.

[37] Ehrmann, D.A., et al., *Prevalence of impaired glucose tolerance and diabetes in women with polycystic ovary syndrome.* Diabetes Care, 1999. 22(1): p. 141-6.

[38] Frisch, R.E., *Body fat, puberty and fertility.* Biol Rev Camb Philos Soc, 1984. 59(2): p. 161-88.

[39] Crawford, J.D. and D.C. Osler, *Body composition at menarche: The Frisch-Revelle hypothesis revisited.* Pediatrics, 1975. 56(3): p. 449-58.

[40] Berenson, G.S., et al., *Association between multiple cardiovascular risk factors and atherosclerosis in children and young adults. The Bogalusa Heart Study.* N Engl J Med, 1998. 338(23): p. 1650-6.

[41] Raitakari, O.T., M. Juonala, and J.S. Viikari, *Obesity in childhood and vascular changes in adulthood: insights into the Cardiovascular Risk in Young Finns Study.* Int J Obes (Lond), 2005. 29 Suppl 2: p. S101-4.

[42] Eriksson, P., et al., *Adipose tissue secretion of plasminogen activator inhibitor-1 in non-obese and obese individuals.* Diabetologia, 1998. 41(1): p. 65-71.

[43] Shimomura, I., et al., *Enhanced expression of PAI-1 in visceral fat: possible contributor to vascular disease in obesity.* Nat Med, 1996. 2(7): p. 800-3.

[44] Raj, M., et al., *Obesity in Indian children: time trends and relationship with hypertension.* Natl Med J India, 2007. 20(6): p. 288-93.

[45] Sorof, J.M., et al., *Overweight, ethnicity, and the prevalence of hypertension in school-aged children.* Pediatrics, 2004. 113(3 Pt 1): p. 475-82.

[46] Wunsch, R., G. de Sousa, and T. Reinehr, *Intima-media thickness in obesity: relation to hypertension and dyslipidaemia.* Arch Dis Child, 2005. 90(10): p. 1097.

[47] Woo, K.S., et al., *Overweight in children is associated with arterial endothelial dysfunction and intima-media thickening.* Int J Obes Relat Metab Disord, 2004. 28(7): p. 852-7.
[48] Mangge, H., et al., *Low grade inflammation in juvenile obesity and type 1 diabetes associated with early signs of atherosclerosis.* Exp Clin Endocrinol Diabetes, 2004. 112(7): p. 378-82.
[49] Zhu, W., et al., *Arterial intima-media thickening and endothelial dysfunction in obese Chinese children.* Eur J Pediatr, 2005. 164(6): p. 337-44.
[50] Reinehr, T., et al., *Intima media thickness in childhood obesity: relations to inflammatory marker, glucose metabolism, and blood pressure.* Metabolism, 2006. 55(1): p. 113-8.
[51] Sivanandam, S., et al., *Relation of increase in adiposity to increase in left ventricular mass from childhood to young adulthood.* Am J Cardiol, 2006. 98(3): p. 411-5.
[52] Maggio, A.B., et al., *Associations among obesity, blood pressure, and left ventricular mass.* J Pediatr, 2008. 152(4): p. 489-93.
[53] Must, A., et al., *Long-term morbidity and mortality of overweight adolescents. A follow-up of the Harvard Growth Study of 1922 to 1935.* N Engl J Med, 1992. 327(19): p. 1350-5.
[54] Fu, J.F., et al., *Non-alcoholic fatty liver disease: An early mediator predicting metabolic syndrome in obese children?* World J Gastroenterol. 17(6): p. 735-42.
[55] E. Fabbrini, D.d.a.D.D., *Alterations in fatty acid kinetics in obese adolescents with increased intrahepatic triglyceride content, Obesity 17 (2008),* pp. 25-29.
[56] Pagano, G., et al., *Nonalcoholic steatohepatitis, insulin resistance, and metabolic syndrome: further evidence for an etiologic association.* Hepatology, 2002. 35(2): p. 367-72.
[57] Friesen, C.A. and C.C. Roberts, *Cholelithiasis. Clinical characteristics in children. Case analysis and literature review.* Clin Pediatr (Phila), 1989. 28(7): p. 294-8.
[58] Holcomb, G.W., Jr., J.A. O'Neill, Jr., and G.W. Holcomb, 3rd, *Cholecystitis, cholelithiasis and common duct stenosis in children and adolescents.* Ann Surg, 1980. 191(5): p. 626-35.
[59] Kato, S., et al., *Pathological influence of obesity on renal structural changes in chronic kidney disease.* Clin Exp Nephrol, 2009. 13(4): p. 332-40.
[60] Kopple, J.D., *Obesity and chronic kidney disease.* J Ren Nutr, 2010. 20(5 Suppl): p. S29-30.
[61] Serra, A., et al., *Renal injury in the extremely obese patients with normal renal function.* Kidney Int, 2008. 73(8): p. 947-55.
[62] Cindik, N., et al., *Effect of obesity on inflammatory markers and renal functions.* Acta Paediatr, 2005. 94(12): p. 1732-7.
[63] Chagnac, A., et al., *Glomerular hemodynamics in severe obesity.* Am J Physiol Renal Physiol, 2000. 278(5): p. F817-22.
[64] Schuster, D.P., et al., *Effect of bariatric surgery on normal and abnormal renal function.* Surg Obes Relat Dis.
[65] Savino, A., et al., *Implications for kidney disease in obese children and adolescents.* Pediatr Nephrol. 26(5): p. 749-58.
[66] Redline, S. and K.P. Strohl, *Recognition and consequences of obstructive sleep apnea hypopnea syndrome.* Otolaryngol Clin North Am, 1999. 32(2): p. 303-31.
[67] Rhodes, S.K., et al., *Neurocognitive deficits in morbidly obese children with obstructive sleep apnea.* J Pediatr, 1995. 127(5): p. 741-4.
[68] Suarez, E.C., *Self-reported symptoms of sleep disturbance and inflammation, coagulation, insulin resistance and psychosocial distress: evidence for gender disparity.* Brain Behav Immun, 2008. 22(6): p. 960-8.
[69] Meslier, N., et al., *Impaired glucose-insulin metabolism in males with obstructive sleep apnoea syndrome.* Eur Respir J, 2003. 22(1): p. 156-60.
[70] Somers, V.K., et al., *Sympathetic neural mechanisms in obstructive sleep apnea.* J Clin Invest, 1995. 96(4): p. 1897-904.

[71] Visness, C.M., et al., *Association of childhood obesity with atopic and nonatopic asthma: results from the National Health and Nutrition Examination Survey 1999-2006.* J Asthma, 2010. 47(7): p. 822-9.
[72] Noal, R.B., et al., *Childhood body mass index and risk of asthma in adolescence: a systematic review.* Obes Rev, 2011. 12(2): p. 93-104.
[73] Forno, E., et al., *Decreased response to inhaled steroids in overweight and obese asthmatic children.* J Allergy Clin Immunol, 2011. 127(3): p. 741-9.
[74] Reilly, J.J. and J. Kelly, *Long-term impact of overweight and obesity in childhood and adolescence on morbidity and premature mortality in adulthood: systematic review.* Int J Obes (Lond), 2010.
[75] Kelsey, J.L., K.J. Keggi, and W.O. Southwick, *The incidence and distrubition of slipped capital femoral epiphysis in Connecticut and Southwestern United States.* J Bone Joint Surg Am, 1970. 52(6): p. 1203-16.
[76] Goulding, A., et al., *Overweight and obese children have low bone mass and area for their weight.* Int J Obes Relat Metab Disord, 2000. 24(5): p. 627-32.
[77] Rana, A.R., et al., *Childhood obesity: a risk factor for injuries observed at a level-1 trauma center.* J Pediatr Surg, 2009. 44(8): p. 1601-5.
[78] Corbett, J.J., et al., *Visual loss in pseudotumor cerebri. Follow-up of 57 patients from five to 41 years and a profile of 14 patients with permanent severe visual loss.* Arch Neurol, 1982. 39(8): p. 461-74.
[79] Scott, I.U., et al., *Idiopathic intracranial hypertension in children and adolescents.* Am J Ophthalmol, 1997. 124(2): p. 253-5.
[80] Sugerman, H.J., et al., *Increased intra-abdominal pressure and cardiac filling pressures in obesity-associated pseudotumor cerebri.* Neurology, 1997. 49(2): p. 507-11.
[81] Puder, J.J. and S. Munsch, *Psychological correlates of childhood obesity.* Int J Obes (Lond). 34 Suppl 2: p. S37-43.
[82] Herva, A., et al., *Obesity and depression: results from the longitudinal Northern Finland 1966 Birth Cohort Study.* Int J Obes (Lond), 2006. 30(3): p. 520-7.
[83] Zeller, M.H., et al., *Health-related quality of life and depressive symptoms in adolescents with extreme obesity presenting for bariatric surgery.* Pediatrics, 2006. 117(4): p. 1155-61.
[84] Schwimmer, J.B., T.M. Burwinkle, and J.W. Varni, *Health-related quality of life of severely obese children and adolescents.* JAMA, 2003. 289(14): p. 1813-9.
[85] Williams, J., et al., *Health-related quality of life of overweight and obese children.* JAMA, 2005. 293(1): p. 70-6.
[86] Gortmaker, S.L., et al., *Social and economic consequences of overweight in adolescence and young adulthood.* N Engl J Med, 1993. 329(14): p. 1008-12.
[87] Sargent, J.D. and D.G. Blanchflower, *Obesity and stature in adolescence and earnings in young adulthood. Analysis of a British birth cohort.* Arch Pediatr Adolesc Med, 1994. 148(7): p. 681-7.
[88] Nishimura, S., et al., *CD8+ effector T cells contribute to macrophage recruitment and adipose tissue inflammation in obesity.* Nat Med, 2009. 15(8): p. 914-20.
[89] Hadi, H.A., C.S. Carr, and J. Al Suwaidi, *Endothelial dysfunction: cardiovascular risk factors, therapy, and outcome.* Vasc Health Risk Manag, 2005. 1(3): p. 183-98.
[90] Esposito, K., et al., *Oxidative stress in the metabolic syndrome.* J Endocrinol Invest, 2006. 29(9): p. 791-5.
[91] Maffeis, C., et al., *Insulin resistance and the persistence of obesity from childhood into adulthood.* J Clin Endocrinol Metab, 2002. 87(1): p. 71-6.

8

Behavioral and Psychosocial Factors in Childhood Obesity

Fernando L. Vazquez[1] and Angela Torres[2]
[1]Department of Clinical Psychology, Faculty of Psychology
[2]Department of Psychiatry, Faculty of Medicine and Odontology
University of Santiago de Compostela
Spain

1. Introduction

Obesity has been recognized as a major public health problem and one of the most important causes of the burden of disease worldwide (Ezzati et al, 2002). Its prevalence has escalated over the last two decades, reaching pandemic levels in the developed countries and also increasing in the developing world (Wang & Lobstein, 2006). In fact, in the newsletter of the World Health Organization/Europe, called *The Bridge*, published in 2010, it's stated that "Paradoxically coexisting with under-nutrition, an escalating global epidemic of overweight and obesity - *globesity* - is spreading over many parts of the world" (p. 11). The pandemic of obesity originated in the United States of America and crossed to Europe and the world's poorest countries (Prentice, 2006).

The obesity phenomenon is observed not only in adults. Despite large differences among countries and regions, a global childhood obesity epidemic has also emerged worldwide. In many countries, including the United Kingdom, the United States, Australia, Brazil and China, child overweight is increasing at a faster rate than is adult obesity (Popkin et al, 2006). Of particular concern is the upward trend in countries that have traditionally experienced low rates of overweight (Lissau et al, 2004). In fact, obesity in children and adolescents is well recognized as a major public health concern (Institute of Medicine, 2005) because of alarming trends in the prevalence, severity, and occurrence of adverse health and psychosocial consequences over the life cycle. Compared with the past two decades, the rates of children who are obese has doubled, while the number of adolescents who are obese has tripled. So, in the United States, according to the National Health and Nutrition Examination Survey [NHANES] (Odgen et al, 2010), almost 32% of children and adolescents aged 2-19 years were overweight (Body Mass Index [BMI] at or above 85th percentile), while almost 17% were obese (BMI at or above 95th percentile). NHANES data indicated disparities among racial/ethnic groups, with Hispanic boys and non-Hispanic black girls disproportionately affected by obesity.

Childhood obesity also poses a serious problem in Europe. Studies conducted in Scotland (Craig et al, 2010) and England (Stamatakis et al, 2010) showed that in the United Kingdom there is a clear socioeconomic gradient with high prevalence of being overweight and obese in low socioeconomic strata. Mediterranean countries also present high levels of childhood overweight in Europe. In Spain the nationwide enKid study reported prevalences of 12.4% for overweight and 13.9% for obesity among 2-24-year-olds, with the highest values observed between 6 and 13 years of age (Serra Majem et al, 2006). Spanish preadolescents (10-12 years) appear to be at particularly high risk, reaching prevalences of overweight and obesity of 29.9% and 8.9% respectively (Vázquez et al, 2010). Greece presents childhood obesity statistics as high as Spain (Lagiou & Parava, 2008). In Eastern Europe, rates are climbing substantially. Hungary has reported that 20% of children between the ages of 11 and 14 years are obese; in Poland rates have increased from 8% to 18% from 1994 to 2000 (World Health Organization, 2005).

Childhood obesity also extends to other areas of the world besides the United States and Europe. In the Middle East, the situation is critical: Eighteen percent of all children are overweight and 7% obese (Lobstein & Frelut, 2003). In Israel, the rate of 13.9% is on the rise (Keinan-Boker et al, 2005). In the Oceania region, Australia's current rates in children are among the highest in the developed world, with 20% of children overweight and 10% obese (Barnett, 2006). In New Zealand, 20% of children between the ages of 5 and 14 years are overweight, with another 10% obese. Approximately, 31% of Maori and Pacific Islander children are affected (Baur, 2006).

Estimates of the prevalence of overweight and obesity in school-aged youth from 34 countries (Janssen et al, 2005) showed a similar picture in prevalence rates to those noted above. The three countries with the highest prevalence of overweight youth were Malta (25.4%), the United States (25.1%), and Wales (21.2%). The countries with the highest prevalence of obesity were Malta (7.9%), the United States (6.8%), and England (5.1%). The three countries with the lowest prevalence of overweight and obese youth were Lithuania (5.1% and 0.4%), Russia (5.9% and 0.6%), and Latvia (5.9% and 0.5%).

Given de current prevalence of childhood obesity and the wide geographic distribution throughout the world, the term *pandemic* is appropriated to describe the picture of the new millennium (Kimm & Obarzanek, 2002). The Healthy People 2010 Program in the United States sets the goals of reducing obesity prevalence to 5% in children (U.S. Department of Health and Human Services, 2006), which is unlikely to be met.

It must also be noted that obesity is related to health problems in children, adolescents and adults. High BMI in children and adolescents may have immediate consequences on health, with particular impact on high cholesterol and high blood pressure, which are risk factors for cardiovascular disease (CVD). In one study (Freedman et al, 2007), 70% of obese children had at least one CVD risk factor, and 39% had two or more. Also, children with obesity are more likely to have increased risk of impaired glucose tolerance, insulin resistance and type 2 diabetes (Whitlock et al, 2005). Psychological problems such as depression and worsening quality of life are also correlates of serious obesity (Daniels et al, 2005). In addition, obese children are more likely to become obese adults (Biro & Wien, 2010). In the analysis of three nationally representative cohorts of children (Van Cleave et al, 2010), it was reported that for all cohorts, 37% of children with obesity at the beginning of the study were so classified six years later. Both overweight and obesity also are major risk factors for a number of chronic diseases in adults, including diabetes, cardiovascular disease and certain cancers (National Institutes of Health, 1998).

The high prevalence of overweight and obesity, and the many adverse impacts associated with them, provide evidence of the need for a clear understanding of its causes to guide effective prevention and treatment. Obesity is believed to be of multifactorial etiology, but the mechanisms involved in its development are not well understood. This chapter will review the relevant literature concerning both behavioral and psychosocial factors involved in childhood obesity, and the impact of childhood obesity on mental health.

2. The contribution of psychosocial and cultural factors to understanding childhood obesity

Although the mechanism of development of childhood obesity is not fully understood, it is clear that obesity occurs when energy intake exceeds energy expenditure. There are multiple factors for this imbalance; hence the rising prevalence of childhood obesity cannot be attributed to a single etiology. The causes of childhood obesity are complex and multifaceted because it is a condition with many genetic, biological, environmental and psychosocial influences. Genetic factors influence susceptibility to obesity (Franks & Ling, 2010; Lyon & Hirschhorn, 2005; Seal, 2011). However, behavioral and social factors seem to play significant roles in the rising prevalence of childhood obesity worldwide, rather than changes in biological or genetic factors (Dunton et al, 2009; Ferreira et al, 2006). These include, among others, dietary factors and eating habits, physical activity and social factors (Ben-Sefer et al, 2009).

2.1 Dietary and eating behavior patterns

Weight gain occurs as a result of energy imbalance, particularly when energy intake through food intake exceeds energy expenditure for body functions and physical activity. Recent research and reviews indicate that so-called *energy balance related behaviors* can contribute to the development of overweight and obesity, particularly a combination of increased fat intake, decreased physical activity and increased *screen time* (Ekelund et al, 2004). Screen time is the amount of time that a child spends watching television, playing on the computer and with videogames.

Factors that are named frequently as contributors to excess energy intake include restaurant food, sweetened beverages, large portion sizes, and the frequency of meals and snacks. Diverse eating patterns confound the understanding of the relationship between nutrient intake and chronic diseases, including obesity. These eating patterns seem to be related more consistently to increased total energy intake than to actual weight status (Krebs et al, 2007). Some studies showed that children (Bowman et al, 2004; Paeratakul et al, 2003) and adolescents (French et al, 2001) who consumed fast food more frequently had higher energy intakes and poorer diet quality, compared with those who did not. Overweight adolescents are less likely than their leaner counterparts to compensate for the increased energy in the food by adjusting energy intake throughout the day (Ebbeling et al, 2004). It has also been reported that energy intake has been related positively to consumption of sweetened beverages by children and adolescents (Nielsen & Popkin, 2004). Research studies have consistently found that when adults and children eat out instead of eating at home, they consume more fat and calories, more fried foods, more soft drinks, fewer fruits and vegetables, and less fiber (French et al, 2000; Zoumas-Morse et al, 2001).

The environment we live in has been described as *obesogenic*. The concept of an obesogenic environment has been defined as "the sum of influences that the surroundings, opportunities or conditions of life have on promoting obesity in individuals or populations" (Swinburn et al, 1999, p. 564). Many cultural and environmental factors are considered obesogenic by having negatively influenced eating behaviors and the physical activity levels of children and adolescents. Time and economic pressures force many parents to minimize food costs and meal preparation time, resulting in an increase in availability and consumption of high-calorie and high-fat convenience foods and beverages, fewer family meals, more meals eaten away from home, and greater portion sizes (Johnson et al, 2008; Newby, 2007).

A school food policy to promote healthy eating behavior can also impact the food intake of children, reducing the intake of sugar and fat in food (Neumark-Sztainer et al, 2005). But other food policies and initiatives such us the presence of vending machines in schools (Belderson et al, 2003), the consumption of packed lunches at school (Whincup et al, 2005), or the use of breakfast clubs (New & Livingstone, 2003) can increase overweight/obesity.

All of the factors described above are contributing to create a "toxic environment" that promotes in the population the consumption of unhealthy foods because they are better tasting, are highly accessible and are less expensive, as compared with healthy foods (Schwartz & Brownell, 2007). So, the increasing prevalence of obesity, particularly in the developed world, is partially explained by societal changes that promote both consumption of energy-dense foods and unhealthy eating patterns (Centers for Disease Control and Prevention, 2011).

2.2 Physical activity and sedentary behavior

Physical activity is an important factor of health and well-being for people of all ages. There is evidence supporting the link between physical inactivity and obesity in children (Tremblay & Willms, 2003) and adolescents (Janssen et al, 2006). Children who are physically active may gain immediate and long-term positive effects (Hartmann et al, 2010). However, low levels of fitness (Tomkinson et al, 2003) and recent declines in active transportation, such as walking and cycling to school (Carlin et al, 1997), have been reported among children in many developed countries.

Physical activity patterns established during childhood may continue into adulthood (Friedman et al, 2008), but longitudinal studies show a decline in physical activity with increasing age (Telama et al, 2005), with physical activity tracking at low to moderate levels across the life span (Malina, 2001). Studies reveal a decrease in physical activity participation during adolescence (Kimm et al, 2002; Van Mechelen et al, 2000) and differences in patterns of physical activity participation for males and females (Sallis et al, 2000). Moreover, perceived sports competency (females), and cardio-respiratory fitness, playing sports outside school and having active fathers (males) in childhood and adolescence were positively associated with being persistently active during the transition from adolescence to adulthood (Jose et al, 2011).

There is evidence that decreased opportunities and participation in physical activity contributes to overweight. Opportunities for children's physical activity include participation in structured activities, such as physical education at school and in organized sports teams, as well as less structured activities such as walking and cycling to school and active free-play (Pangrazi, 2000). School physical education programs have decreased because of the pressure to increase test scores, so children's opportunities to participate in recess and physical education activities during school time are decreasing. And it seems that children are not compensating for the lost physical activity time by increasing their physical activity level after school or on holiday (Andersen & van Mechelen, 2005). In fact, contemporary children may also engage in sedentary activities after school, and spend less time walking to school and playing outside. Moreover, sedentary behaviors, such as watching television, playing on the computer and with videogames have increased (American Academy of Pediatrics, 2006; Barlow & the Expert Committee, 2007). It has been reported that preschool children spend around 80% of their time in activities classified as sedentary (Reilly et al, 2004). However, the relationship between sedentary behavior and obesity is not explained solely by reduced physical activity. In a population of adolescent females, correlation between percentage of body fat and Internet viewing time persisted even after controlling for physical activity (Schneider et al, 2007).

The Centers for Disease Control and Prevention (2003) recommended that children be active daily at least 60 minutes. In addition, the American Academy of Pediatrics (2003) recommended that children accumulate no more than two hours per day of screen time. Despite these recommendations, it seems that the real situation is quite different. In the U.S., in a nationally representative cross-sectional study of 2,964 children aged 4 to 11 years (Anderson et al, 2008), it was found that 37.3% had low levels of activity play, 65% had high screen time, and 26.3% had both those behaviors.

Children spend more time with media than in any other activity except for sleeping—an average of more than seven hours/day (Rideout, 2010). Children and teenagers who use a lot of media may tend to be more sedentary in general (Jordan, 2007; Vandewater et al, 2004). Children and teenagers who watch more TV tend to consume more calories or eat higher-fat diets, and to have poor eating behaviors (Barr-Anderson et al, 2009; Pearson et al, 2011; Zimmerman & Bell, 2010). In a prospective study of 3-year-old children, TV viewing and physical activity measures at age 3 were better predictors of BMI at age 6 than eating habits (Jago et al, 2005). Moreover, TV viewing has been identified as the strongest connection between a specific behavior and childhood obesity (Whitaker, 2003).

Undoubtedly media play an important role in the current epidemic of childhood and adolescent obesity. Screen time may displace more active pursuits, advertising of junk food and fast food increases children's requests for those particular foods and products, snacking increases while watching TV or movies (Council on Communications and Media, 2011). Late-night screen time is known to displace or disturb children's and teens' sleep patterns, and there is evidence that later bedtimes and less sleep may be associated with a greater risk of obesity (Bell & Zimmerman, 2010; Taheri, 2006).

Recently, a new generation of video games that requires interactive physical activity, known as *exergaming*, has become popular. These new video games have the potential to attract children to become more physically active and could have particular value for extremely sedentary individuals or those who may shun traditional forms of exercise. For example, a study of preteens playing *Dance Revolution* and *Nintendo's Wii Sports* found that energy expenditure was equivalent to moderate-intensity walking (Graf et al, 2009).

However, despite protective effects of physical activity on adiposity of childhood obesity (particularly in adolescents), significant methodological limitations related to the validity of the measurements of both physical activity and body fatness must be considered (Reichert et al, 2009).

2.3 Socioeconomic and cultural factors

One consistent epidemiological finding is the fact that, in highly developed countries at least, the prevalence of obesity is inversely associated with both socioeconomic status and educational status (Mustillo et al, 2003; Prentice, 2006). Economic poverty and/or lack of education impair a person's ability to resist the current obesogenic environment, so in highly developed societies, obesity may be a cause of economic disadvantage rather than simply a consequence (O'Rahilly & Farooqi, 2008). Data have suggested that in industrialized countries, excess weight gain in children was more prevalent among lower-income families (Veugelers & Fitgerald, 2005; Wang et al, 2002). Low-income families face numerous barriers including food insecurity, lack of safe places for physical activity, and lack of consistent access to healthful food choices, especially fruits and vegetables (American Academy of Pediatrics, 2003).

There are large disparities in obesity between socio-demographic groups. Findings from nationally representative surveys conducted by the Centers for Disease Control and Prevention, the National Health and Nutrition Examination Survey, and the Youth Risk Behavior Surveillance System in the United Sates (Wang, 2011) indicated that some population groups are affected more seriously than others. For example, Native American, Black and Mexican-American children have the highest prevalence of obesity, whereas Asians have the lowest rate among all ethnic groups; preschool age children have a lower obesity prevalence than older children; young people in some states and cities are twice as likely to be overweight or obese than those living in other regions; low socioeconomic status is associated with obesity only among some population groups.

Beliefs about what foods are desirable or appropriate, what is an attractive or healthy weight, how families should share meals, and the authority parents have over children at different ages, as well as many other attitudes that affect lifestyle habits are influenced by cultural values and beliefs. For example, some studies have examined differences between identified racial, ethnic, or cultural groups; it has been pointed out that black girls are more satisfied with heavier bodies than are white girls (Kimm et al, 1997). A study of low-income minority parents of preschool-aged children showed that Hispanic parents had indulgent feeding styles more often than did low-income black parents (Hughes et al, 2005).

Sociocultural factors in the household are the most investigated environmental factors for all *energy balance related behaviors*. It must be noted first that a systematic review of environmental factors of obesity-related eating behaviors in children and adolescents (Van der Horst et al, 2007) showed consistent evidence for relationships between parental and children's fat, fruit and vegetable intake; for parental and siblings' intakes with adolescents' energy and fat intake; and for parental educational level with adolescents' fruit and vegetable intake. In addition, a systematic review of studies on factors influencing physical activity level (Ferreira et al, 2006) identified fathers' physical activity habits, school physical activity-related policies and time spent outdoors as potential determinants of physical activity in children. As we noted previously, the emergence of the technology revolution with handheld videogames and cell phones may also promote sedentary lifestyles and reduced children's physical activity levels (McMurray et al, 2000).

3. Behavioral and emotional problems associated with childhood obesity

Overweight and obesity have received a great deal of attention in psychological and psychiatric research. It was postulated that obese people suffer from their weight situation given the fact that obesity is a highly visible condition meaning that everybody can evaluate the weight status of others and make commentaries about it (Warschburge, 2005). Consequently there are a wide range of behavioral and emotional outcomes that have been studied in association with obesity in children and adolescents, particularly those related to stigma, psychological well-being, and mental health problems.

3.1 Stigma

It is generally agreed that being obese or even being overweight is one of the most stigmatizing and least socially acceptable conditions in childhood (Schwimmer et al, 2003). Modern societal prejudice against obesity and overweight is widespread, even toward children and adolescents.

A stigma is defined as a mark or attributes that link a person to undesirable characteristics or negative stereotypes (Goffman, 1963). Stigma is part of a cultural system of shared meanings or schemas that allow people to control behavior, interpret the world, respond to differences, express disapproval or explain danger or inferiority (Jones et al, 1984; Page, 1984). It can be seen as a relationship between an attribute and a stereotype (Jones et al, 1984). There are three related concepts which comprise a set of issues to be considered in any stigmatized situation: Associative stigma, internalized stigma, and stigma management. *Associative stigma*, which Goffman (1963) called *courtesy stigma*, is ascribed to people who are voluntarily attached as caregivers or acquaintances to people who are stigmatized, such as dying or mentally ill patients. *Internalized stigma*, or accepting the discrediting of one's worth conveyed by society, can occur without the experience of overt mistreatment and can lower a person's sense of self-esteem and prestige because he or she is aware of the threat of censure and rejection (Jones et al, 1984). *Stigma management* is central to coping with carrying a stigma; that is, being aware of the real or potential negative reactions of others and attempting to minimize their effects (Jones et al, 1984; Page, 1984). The stigmatized person who strives to manage the stigma must consider the problems of concealment, disclosure, and "passing" as normal, secrecy, information management, and social visibility (Goffman, 1963; Page, 1984).

There are weight-related beliefs and attitudes that are expressed as stereotypes, prejudice and rejection toward children and adolescents because they are overweight or obese. In a society where slimness is valued and self-determination is emphasized, obese people are often viewed as undesirable, lazy and responsible for their condition. As a result, obese children are often subject to negative stereotyping, discrimination and social rejection. Often they encounter physical bullying by peers (such us pushing, hitting, or kicking), verbal teasing (name calling, being made fun of), and social exclusion (such us being excluded from peer activities, being avoided or ignored). Research on Canadian children aged 11–16 years reported that overweight and obese boys and girls were more likely to be the victims of physical, verbal and relational bullying than their normal weight peers (Janssen et al, 2004). A study in the United States, found that, compared with average weight children, obese children reported being teased at least three times more often (Neumark-Sztainer et al, 2002). It was found that between a quarter and a third of those teenagers report being teased by peers for reasons of weight, with obese girls and thin boys showing the highest levels of teasing (Eisenberg et al, 2003). A review of gender differences found that overweight girls were stigmatized significantly more often than boys and they typically faced more teasing, bullying and social marginalization in both friendships and romantic relationships (Tang-Peronard & Heitmann, 2008).

In addition, it appears that obese children and adolescents have difficulties with peer relationships. As many as one-third of obese children have no reciprocated friendships

(Zeller et al, 2008). Peers rank obese children among the least desirable playmates (Zametkin et al, 2004). Obese youngsters themselves report being less socially accepted (McCullough et al, 2009).

Obese and overweight children are also susceptible to negative attitudes from teachers, parents, and even health professionals. The term *civilized oppression* was used to describe the pervasive pattern of ongoing, daily denigration and condemnation that constitutes living as an obese person (Rogge et al, 2004). Adults have been found to stigmatize obese children citing that they are untidy and lack self-control (Zametkin et al, 2004). Children as well as adults stereotype the obese as "lazy," "ugly" and "stupid" (Latner & Stunkard, 2003). There are also current prejudicial beliefs well documented among health professionals that obese people are "gluttonous," "lazy," "bad," "weak," "stupid," "worthless" and "lacking in self control" (Schwartz et al, 2003). Even obesity prevention initiatives for children often inappropriately label large numbers of children as "overweight" or "fat" (Szwarc, 2004–2005).

3.2 Psychological well-being

Psychological well-being is a relatively complex notion with a variety of components that may contribute to it. The elements of psychological well-being believed to be most seriously compromised in obesity are self-esteem, body image and emotional well-being (focused primarily on quality of life and social functioning).

Studies on self-esteem in obese children and adolescents report inconsistent results. Martyn-Nemeth et al (2009) found that low self-esteem is clearly associated with overeating and weight gain in adolescents. Many other studies indicate that overweight and obese children and adolescents have moderately lower self-esteem than non-obese peers (French et al, 1996; Friedlander et al, 2003; Hesketh et al, 2004). Other studies reveal no differences in self-esteem between population-based groups of obese children and adolescents and non-obese controls (Renman et al, 1999; Strauss, 2000). Furthermore, studies report that self-esteem is not significantly lower in obese populations once body image is controlled for (French et al, 1995; Pesa et al, 2000).

Clinical samples of obese children also report higher levels of psychosocial maladjustment and lower self-esteem than population-based samples of either obese or normal-weight children (Hill, 2005; Sjoberg, 2005). Obesity in children seeking clinical treatment is often more severe than in children in the general population (Flodmark, 2005). This may reflect the different characteristics of those who are seeking treatment because they are more negatively affected psychologically by their obesity or they feel unable to control it (Wardle & Cook, 2005).

Self-esteem in obese children varies with gender, age and ethnicity (Walker & Hill, 2009; Wardl & Cooke, 2005). Obese females seem to be at greater risk for self-esteem problems because body image is an important component of their self-esteem; adolescents appear more at risk than younger children, and whites are more susceptible than Hispanics or African-Americans. But in a recent systematic review the differences between children and adolescents were not so clear (Griffiths et al, 2010).

As for body image, the most consistently replicated finding is that obese children and adolescents have a more negative body image than their peers and often believe that they have been responsible for their obesity (Ben-Sefer et al, 2009). Overweight children as young as age 5 can also develop a negative body image (Pallan et al, 2011). A relationship between increasing weight status and body dissatisfaction in older children has been observed in many different cultural communities (Crow et al, 2006; Duncan et al, 2006; Fonseca et al, 2009; Mirza et al, 2005). However, it does not appear to be inevitable, and many obese children are not aware that they are overweight (Wardle & Cooke, 2005). Moreover, researchers of both American and Australian adolescents suggested that the perception of being obese appears to be more predictive of mental disorders than actual obesity status (Ali et al, 2010; Allen et al, 2006).

Obesity in children also may correlate with poorer quality of life (Flodmark, 2005). A cross-sectional study of children and adolescents between ages 5 and 18 years demonstrated that severely obese children and adolescents have lower health-related quality of life than children and adolescents who are healthy, and similar quality of life as those diagnosed as having cancer (Schwimmer et al, 2003). In addition, given the importance placed on body shape and size in occidental culture, overweight children may experience elevated peer problems and peer rejection compared to non-overweight children. The psychosocial burden of excess weight appears to be significant even in young children. A cross-sectional survey conducted in 100 primary schools of a large French region, with 2,341 children aged 6–11 randomly selected (Pitrou et al, 2010) found that overweight was strongly associated with poor social functioning and with higher rates of peer difficulties.

Other studies, however, have different findings to those already mentioned in relation to childhood obesity and psychological well-being. In an extensive review of the empirical evidence on the relationship between childhood obesity and psychological well-being (Wardle & Cooke, 2005), the authors concluded that obese children seem to have psychological resilience to the adverse consequences of obesity. In fact, after examining the most relevant studies in this area, they find that while levels of body dissatisfaction are higher in community samples of overweight and obese children and adolescents than in their normal-weight counterparts, few are significantly depressed or have low self-esteem. A number of potential moderators and mediators of the association between obesity and psychological well-being have been proposed. Emerging most strongly are gender, age and ethnicity, but future research has some way to go before the risk and protective factors are fully established.

3.3 Mental health problems

Bruch and Touraine (1940) were the first authors to show a particular interest in the emotional functioning of obese children and adolescents. Since earliest publication, the psychopathological features of children with overweight and obesity have been studied extensively. The understanding of the relationship between obesity and common mental health disorders in children and adolescents is less advanced, and results are inconsistent (Gatineau & Dent, 2011). In addition, it must be noted that research in this area is subjected to many limitations (Costello et al, 2005; Pitrou et al, 2010, Vila et al, 2004; Wardle et al, 2005) such as the use of clinical samples that may not reflect the general population, the infrequent inclusion of structured clinical interviews based on diagnostic criteria, the lack of use of control groups in the study design, etc.

Despite these limitations, there are a number of interesting findings about childhood obesity in relation to mental health problems. Several studies have found mental health problems in young people with obesity. Higher rates of depression, anxiety, eating disorders, social withdrawal and behavioral problems have been found among obese children and youth

(Bosch et al, 2004; Zametkin et al, 2004). For example, a study carried out in 155 French children and adolescents referred and followed for obesity (Vila et al, 2004) reported that when administered diagnostic interviews with the Kiddie Schedule for Affective Disorders and Schizophrenia (K-SADS-R), 58% of obese children had at least one DSM-IV psychiatric diagnosis, and between 50% and 64% scored positive on questionnaire screening techniques. The most frequent disorder was anxiety disorder (32%), followed distantly by disruptive behavior disorder (16%), and affective disorder (12%). Psychopathology was particularly prominent in those children whose parents scored high on the General Health Questionnaire (GHQ-28; a screening questionnaire of psychiatric and non-psychotic morbidity). Compared with diabetic children, they displayed significantly higher internalized and externalized questionnaire scores and poorer social skills. Another study reported that a substantial number of referred obese youngsters suffered from mental disorders (Van Vlierberghe et al, 2009). In this research there were also differences in the prevalence of psychiatric disorders, and in the psychological symptoms between referred and non-referred overweight youngsters: Referred youth displayed significantly more eating disorders and binge-eating disorders than non-referred youngsters and exhibited a significantly greater severity of internalized symptoms.

Related to eating disturbances, Stice et al (2002) found that emotional eating was positively associated with binge-eating disorder (BED), and BED was predictive of obesity (but negative affect alone was not related to BMI). However, BED has been rarely found in samples of obese children seeking inpatient or outpatient treatment (Decaluwé & Braet, 2003). In fact, eating disturbances such as binge eating, episodic overeating and the use of inappropriate compensatory behaviors are more common in adolescents and young adults (Britz et al, 2000; Decaluwé et al, 2003).

In contrast, some population-based studies did not report significant associations between overweight and psychopathology (Drukker et al, 2009; Erermis et al, 2004; Lamertz et al, 2002; Wardle et al, 2006). This contrasts with those studies using clinical samples that generally show a clear positive association between overweight and levels of depressive symptoms and anxiety disorders (Pine et al, 2001; Van Vlierberghe et al, 2009; Vila et al, 2004), and oppositional defiant disorders (Mustillo et al, 2003). One possible explanation is that people who suffer mentally from their elevated weight status, significantly more often seek professional help than those who do not, and thereby bias the clinical samples toward higher levels of psychopathology (Pitrou et al, 2010).

Prospective studies in the literature also found an association between obesity and psychopathology. For example, in a community-based cohort of 820 youths, studied longitudinally at four occasions spanning childhood and early adulthood (Anderson et al, 2006), it was found that DSM disorders of anxiety and depression were associated with higher BMIs in females but not in males.

Moreover, childhood obesity has been associated with emotional and behavioral problems from a very young age, but findings are inconsistent. Results from the UK's Millennium Cohort Study (Griffiths et al, 2011) indicated that at age 5, obese boys are at particular risk of hyperactivity and inattention problems, conduct problems, and peer relationship problems when the Strengths and Difficulties Questionnaire (SDQ) is used to screen psychopathology outcomes. But in a cross-sectional study of a national representative sample of 4- to 5-year-old Australian children (Sawyer et al, 2006) it was found that differences in rates of SDQ mental health problems experienced by young children of different weight status appear relatively small. It seems that higher rates of mental health problems experienced by many obese boys may reflect differences in their socio-demographic characteristics rather than their weight status per se.

Related to hyperactivity and inattention problems, it has been suggested that the impulsivity and poor behavioral regulation often found in youth with Attention-Deficit/Hyperactivity Disorder (ADHD) may lead to the development of eating patterns that put youth at increased risk for obesity. Research conducted in clinical samples (Holtkamp et al, 2004; Hubel et al, 2006; Lam & Yang, 2007) linked overweight and ADHD in children. And even a large cross-sectional study of children and adolescents aged 5 to 17 years (Waring & Lapane, 2008) reported that unmedicated children with ADHD are more likely to be overweight.

It was also reported that disordered sleep may be one of the many contributors to excessive weight during childhood (Beebe et al, 2007). Longitudinal studies have documented that shorter sleep times predict the later emergence of overweight (Agras et al, 2004). A cross-sectional study of 383 youths ages 11–16 years (Gupta, 2002) indicated that overweight youths experienced less total sleep time than non-obese youths, although there were no significant differences between the groups in measures of sleep disturbance. Some studies also suggest that children and adolescents with major depression disorders and a high BMI have more fragmented sleep than healthy controls (Wojnar et al, 2010).

The relationship of obesity and common mental health disorders is complex and multi-factorial, especially with depression. Depression itself is often associated with abnormal patterns of eating and physical activity that could result in future obesity; however, obesity may also result in psychosocial problems that can produce depression. Evidence supports both hypotheses. Pine et al (2001) found that youths with depression are at greater risk to develop an increased BMI. Anderson et al (2006) found that depression in childhood predicted higher weight over time among female youths but not male youths. Results from longitudinal studies also suggest that depression precedes obesity in adolescents—girls, but not boys—and that obesity precedes depression in adults. In one study (Richardson et al, 2003) 1,037 New Zealanders were assessed to determine the presence of obesity and major depression in early adolescence (ages 11, 13, and 15), late adolescence (ages 18 and 21), and adulthood (age 26). After controlling for sex, socioeconomic status, maternal obesity and depression, and baseline obesity, it was reported that depression in early adolescence was associated with a slightly lower risk of adulthood obesity in both boys and girls; but the relationship between late-adolescent depression and adulthood obesity differed across the sexes: Boys who were depressed at age 18 or 21 were less likely to be obese at age 26 than were boys without depression in late adolescence; girls with late-adolescent depression, however, were twice as likely to be obese at age 26 than were girls who were not depressed at 18 or 21. Furthermore, the prevalence of obesity among girls increased linearly with the number of assessment periods at which they were depressed.

Results from the longitudinal Northern Finland 1966 Birth Cohort Study (Herva et al, 2006) indicated that obesity in adolescence may be associated with later depression in young adulthood, and being overweight/obese both in adolescence and adulthood may be a risk factor for depression among female subjects. Examining longitudinally by meta-analysis whether overweight and obesity increase the risk of developing depression, and whether depression increases the risk of developing overweight and obesity, bidirectional associations were found between depression and obesity, particularly in adults (Luppino et al, 2010): Obese persons had a 55% increased risk of developing depression over time, whereas depressed persons had a 58% increased risk of becoming obese. In this study, the association between depression and obesity was stronger than the association between depression and overweight, which reflects a dose-response gradient.

Several mediating and moderating factors must be considered in understanding the direction and strength of the relationship between obesity and psychopathology (Markowitz et al, 2008; Napolitano & Foster, 2008). The mediating factors are those that help to explain the relationship of the two conditions, while the moderating variables might influence the strength of such relationship. The main mediating factors for obesity causing mental disorders in children and adolescents include low self-esteem, body dissatisfaction, lack of physical activity, weight-based teasing and eating disorders (Gatineau & Dent, 2011). As for moderating factors, gender and age could affect the direction and/or strength of the relationship between obesity and common psychiatric disorders in children and adolescents. Girls may be particularly vulnerable to the emotional costs of obesity (Cornette, 2008; Israel & Ivanova, 2002; Stradmeijer et al, 2000). A review of gender differences found that overweight girls were stigmatized significantly more often than boys and they typically faced more teasing, bullying and social marginalization in both friendships and romantic relationships (Tang-Peronard & Heitmann, 2008). The negative impact of obesity on mental health in children appears to increase as they get older, although research results in this area are contradictory. Some findings suggest that obese adolescents had a particular risk of emotional and psychosocial problems, while in younger children the emotional impact of overweight would be limited (Hill, 2005; Walker & Hill, 2009). However, recent findings of The Millennium Cohort Study (Griffiths et al, 2011) indicate that childhood obesity may be associated with emotional and behavioral problems from a very young age, with obese boys at particularly high risk.

4. Conclusions

This chapter reviewed the relevant literature concerning both behavioral and psychosocial factors involved in childhood obesity, and the impact of childhood obesity on mental health. The main conclusions of this review and some recommendations are summarized below:

1. Epidemiologic trends in the prevalence and worldwide distribution of overweight and obesity in children and adolescents suggest the existence of a real new pandemic in the new millennium.
2. Childhood obesity represents a dynamic process rather than a stable condition, in which genetic, psychosocial and environmental factors mutually interact as children grow and develop in different contexts.
3. Weight gain occurs from an imbalance between energy consumed and energy expended. The impact of energy balance related behaviors, particularly the combination of increased fat intake, decreased physical activity and increased screen time, on the development of childhood overweight and obesity is mediated and moderated by socioeconomic and cultural factors.
4. The disparities in obesity between different socio-demographic groups of children and adolescents indicate that obesogenic environmental changes may affect some groups more than others, which is also why different groups may have responded differently to the environmental conditions.

5. Obesity is well recognized as a major public health concern that can create tremendous social and emotional adversity both in children and in their families.
6. Stigma related to overweight and obesity is pervasive, even in children. Although environmental approaches to prevent obesity are promising because they move away from the individual as the source of the problem, they are not without stigmatized risks.
7. The relationship between obesity and psychological well-being (self-esteem, body image and emotional well-being) show inconsistent results.
8. The most frequently implicated mental health conditions in obese children are internalized problems (depression and anxiety), behavioral problems, uncontrolled eating behavior, and attention-deficit/hyperactivity disorder.
9. The relationship between obesity and mental health problems is complex and seems to be bi-directional in that clinically meaningful psychological distress might foster weight gain, and obesity may lead to emotional problems.
10. Girls may be particularly vulnerable to the emotional costs of overweight and obesity.
11. Despite the extensive current literature about the implications of childhood globesity, further research is needed, particularly long-term follow-up studies, for a better understanding of the developmental trajectories that may improve prevention and treatment efforts.
12. The holistic treatment of childhood obesity should encompass psychosocial and emotional consequences as well as physical effects.

5. References

Agras, WS, Hammer, LD, McNicholas, F, & Kraemer, HC (2004). Risk factors for childhood overweight: A prospective study from birth to 9.5 years. *Journal of Pediatrics*, Vol. 145, pp. (20–25)

Ali, MM, Fang, H, & Rizzo, JA (2010). Body weight, self-perception and mental Elath outcomes among adolescents. *Journal of Mental Health & Policy Economics*, Vol. 13, pp. (53-63)

Allen, KL, Byrne, SM, Blair, EM, & Davis, EA (2006). Why do some overweight children experience psychological problems? The role of weight and shape concern. *International Journal of Pediatric Obesity*, Vo. 1, pp. (239-47)

American Academy of Pediatrics (2003). Prevention of pediatric overweight and obesity. *Pediatrics*, Vol. 112, pp. (424-430)

American Academy of Pediatrics (2006). Active healthy living: Prevention of childhood obesity through increased physical activity. *Pediatrics*, Vol. 117, pp. (1834-1842)

Andersen, LB, & van Mechelen, W (2005). Are children of today less active than before and is their health in danger? What can we do? *Scandinavian Journal of Med & Science in Sports*, Vol. 15, pp. (268-270)

Anderson, SE, Cohen, P, Naumova, EN, & Must, A (2006). Association of depression and anxiety disorders with weight change in a prospective community-based study of children followed up into adulthood. *Archives of Pediatrics & Adolescence Medicine*, Vol. 160, pp. (285-291)

Anderson, SE, Economos, CD, & Must, A (2008). Active play and screen time in US children aged 4 to 11 years in relation to sociodemographic and weight status characteristics:

a nationally representative cross-sectional analysis. *BioMed Central Public Health*, Vol. 8, No. 366. Avaliable from http://www.biomedcentral.com/1471-2458/8/366

Barlow, SE & the Expert Committee (2007). Expert committee recommendations regarding the prevention, assessment, and treatment of child and adolescent overweight and obesity: Summary report. *Pediatrics*, Vol. 120, pp. (164-192)

Barnett, AH (2006) How well do rapid-acting insulins work in obese individuals? *Diabetes, Obesity and Metabolism*, Vol. 8, pp. (388–395)

Barr-Anderson, DJ, Larson, NI, Nelson, MC, Neumark-Sztainer, D, & Story, M (2009). Does televisión viewing predict dietary intake five years later in high school students and young adults? *International Journal of Behavioral Nutrition and Physical Activity*, Vol. 6, No. 7. Available from: http://www.ijbnpa.org/content/6/1/7

Baur, L (2006). The millennium disease. In: *The Millenium Disease*, Barnett G, (ed.), pp. (4-6). Australian Parliament House, Launceston

Beebe, DW, Lewin, D, Zeller, M, McCabe, M, MacLeod, K, Daniels, SR, & Amin, R (2007). Sleep in overweight adolescents: Shorter sleep, poorer sleep quality, sleepiness, and sleep-disordered breathing. *Journal of Pediatic Psychology*, Vol. 32, pp. (69–79)

Belderson, P, Harvey, I, Kimbell, R, O'Neill, J, Russell, J, & Barker, ME (2003). Does breakfast-club attendance affect schoolchildren's nutrient intake? A study of dietary intake at three schools. *British Journal of Nutrition*, Vol. 90, pp. (1003–1006)

Bell, JF & Zimmerman ,FJ (2010). Shortened nighttime sleep duration in early life and subsequent childhood obesity. *Archives of Pediatrics & Adolescence Medicine*, Vol. 164, pp. (840–845)

Ben-Sefer, E, Ben-Natan, M, & Ehrenfeld, M (2009). Childhood obesity: Current literature, policy and implications for practice. *International Nursing Review*, Vol. 56, pp. (166–173)

Biro, FM & Wien, M (2010). Childhood obesity and adult morbidities. *American Journal of Clinical Nutrition*, Vol. 91, pp. (1499-1505)

Bosch, J, Stradmeijer, M, & Seidell, J (2004). Psychosocial characteristics of obese children/youngsters and their families: Implications for preventive and curative interventions. *Patient Education and Counselling*, Vol. 55, pp. (353–362)

Bowman, SA, Gortmaker, SL, Ebbeling, CB, Pereira, MA, & Ludwig, DS (2004). Effects of fast-food consumption on energy intake and diet quality among children in a national household survey. *Pediatrics*, Vo. 113, pp. (112–118)

Britz, B, Siegfried, W, Ziegler, A, Lamertz, C, Herpertz-Dahlmann, BM, Remschmidt, H, Wittchen, H-U, & Hebebrand, J (2000). Rates of psychiatric disorders in a clinical study group of adolescents with extreme obesity and in obese adolescents ascertained via population based study. *International Journal of Obesity*, Vol. 24, pp. (1707-1714)

Bruch, H & Touraine, G (1940). Obesity in childhood. *Psychosomatic Medicine*, Vol. 2, pp. (141–206)

Carlin, J, Stevenson, M, Roberts, I, Bennett, C, Gelman, A, & Nolan, T (1997). Walking to school and traffic exposure in Australian children. *Australian and New Zealand Journal of Public Health*, Vol. 21, pp. (286–292)

Centers for Disease Control and Prevention (2003). *Physical activity levels among children aged 9-13 years. United States 2002*. MMWR, Vol. 52, pp. (785-788)

Centers for Disease Control and Prevention (2011). CDC Grand Rounds: Childhood obesity in the United States. *Journal of the American Medical Association*, Vol. 305, pp. (988-991)

Cornette, R (2008). The emotional impact of obesity on children. *Worldviews on Evidence-based Nursing*, Vo. 5, pp. (136–141)

Costello, EJ, Egge, RH, & Angold, A (2005). 10-year research update review: The epidemiology of child and adolescent psychiatric disorders: I. Methods and public health burden. *Journal of the American Academy of Child & Adolescence Psychiatry*, Vol. 44, pp. (972-986)

Council on Communications and Media (2011). Children, adolescents, obesity, and the media. *Pediatrics*, Vol. 128, pp. (201-208)

Craig, LC, McNeill, G, Macdiarmid, JI, Masson, LF & Holmes, BA (2010). Dietary patterns of school-age children in Scotland: Association with socio-economic indicators, physical activity and obesity. *British Journal of Nutrition*, Vol. 103, pp. (319–34)

Crow, S, Eisenberg, ME, Story, M, & Neumark-Sztainer, D (2006). Psychosocial and behavioural correlates of dieting among overweight and non-overweight adolescents. *Journal of Adolescent Health*, Vol. 38, pp. (569–574)

Decaluwé, V, & Braet, C (2003). Prevalence of binge-eating disorder in obese children and adolescents seeking weight-loss treatment. *International Journal of Obesity*, Vol. 27, pp. (404–409)

Decaluwé, V, Braet, C, & Fairburn CG (2003). Binge eating in obese children and adolescents. *The International Journal of Eating Disorders*, Vol. 33, pp. (78-84)

Daniels SR, Arnett DK, Eckel RH, Gidding SS, Hayman LL, Kumanyika S, Robinson TN, Scott BJ, St Jeor S & Williams CL (2005). Overweight in children and adolescents: Pathophysiology, consequences, prevention, and treatment. *Circulation*, Vol. 111, pp. (1999-2012)

Drukker, M, Wojciechowski, F, Feron, FJM, Mengelers, R, & van Os J (2009). A community study of psychosocial functioning and weight in young children and adolescents. *International Journal of Pediatric Obesity*, Vol. 4, pp. (91-97)

Duncan, MJ, Al-Nakeeb, Y, Nevill, AM, & Jones, MV (2006). Body dissatisfaction, body fat and physical activity in British children. *International Journal of Pediatric Obesity*, Vol. 1, pp. (89–95)

Dunton, GF, Kaplan, J, Wolch, J, Jerrett, M & Reynolds, KD (2009). Physical environmental correlates of childhood obesity: A systematic review. *Obesity Reviews*, Vol.10, pp. (393–402)

Ebbeling, CB, Sinclair, KB, Pereira, MA, Garcia-Lago, E, Feldman, HA, & Ludwig ,DS (2004). Compensation for energy intake from fast food among overweight and lean adolescents. *Journal of the American Medical Association*, Vol. 291, pp. (2828–2833)

Eisenberg, ME, Neumark-Sztainer, D, & Story, M (2003). Associations of weight-based teasing and emotional well-being among adolescents. *Archives of Pediatrics & Adolescent Medicine*, Vol. 157, pp. (733-738)

Ekelund, U, Sardinha, LB, Anderssen, SA, Harro, M, Franks, PW, Brage, S, Cooper, AR, Andersen, LB, Riddoch, C, & Froberg, K (2004). Associations between objectively assessed physical activity and indicators of body fatness in 9- to 10-y-old European children: A population-based study from 4 distinct regions in Europe (the European Youth Heart Study). *American Journal of Clinical Nutrition*, Vol. 80, pp. (584-590)

Erermis, S, Cetin, N, Tamar, M., Bukusoglu, N, Akdeniz, F, & Goksen, D (2004). Is obesity a risk factor for psychopathology among adolescents? *Pediatrics International*, Vol. 46, pp. (296–301)

Ezzati, M, Lopez, AD, Rodgers, A, Vander Hoorn, S & Murray, CJL (2002) Selected major risk factors and global and regional burden of disease. *Lancet*, Vol. 360, pp. (1347–1360)

Ferreira, I, van der Horst, K, Wendel-Vos, W, Kremers , S, van Lenthe, FJ & Brug, J (2006). Environmental correlates of physical activity in youth: A review and update. *Obesity Reviews*, Vol. 8, pp. (129-154)

Flodmark, CE (2005). The happy obese child. *International Journal of Obesity*, Vol. 29, pp. (331–339)

Fonseca, H, Matos, MG, Guerra, A, & Pedro, JG (2009). Are overweight and obese adolescents different from their peers? *International Journal of Pediatric Obesity*, Vol. 4, pp. (166-174)

Franks, PW & Ling, Ch (2010). Epigenetics and obesity: The devil is in details. *BMC Medicine*, Vol. 8, No. 88. Available from: <http://www.biomedcentral.com/1741-7015/8/88>

Freedman, DS, Mei, Z, Srinivasan, SR, Berenson, GS, & Dietz ,WH (2007). Cardiovascular risk factors and excess adiposity among overweight children and adolescents: The Bogalusa Heart Study. *Journal of Pediatrics*, Vol. 150, pp. (12-17)

French, SA, Harnack, I, & Jeffery, RW (2000). Fast food restaurant use among young women in the Pound of Prevention study: Dietary, behavioral, and demographic correlates. *International Journal of Obesity and Related Metabolic Disorders*, Vol. 24, pp. (1353-1359)

French, SA, Perry, CL, Leon, GR, & Fulkerson, JA (1996). Self-esteem and change in body mass index over 3 years in a cohort of adolescents. *Obesity Research*, Vol. 4, pp. (27-33)

French, SA, Story, M, & Perry, CL (1995). Self-esteem and obesity in children and adolescents: A literature review. *Obesity Research*, Vol. 3, pp. (479–490)

French, SA, Story, M, Neumark-Sztainer, D, Fulkerson, JA, & Hannan, P (2001). Fast food restaurant use among adolescents: Associations with nutrient intake, food choices and behavioral and psychosocial variables. *International Journal of Obesity and Related Metabolic Disorders*, Vol. 25, pp. (1823–1833)

Friedlander, SL, Larkin, EK, Rosen, CL, Palermo, TM, & Redline, S (2003). Decreased quality of life associated with obesity in school-aged children. *Archives of Pediatrics and Adolescent Medicine*, Vol. 157, pp. (1206–1211)

Friedman, HS, Martin, L R, Tucker, J S, Criqui, MH, Kern, ML, & Reynolds, CA (2008). Stability of physical activity across the lifespan. *Journal of Health Psychology*, Vol. 13, pp. (1092-1104)

Gatineau, M, & Dent, M (2011). *Obesity and Mental Health.* National Obesity Observatory, Oxford.

Goffman, E (1963). *Stigma: Notes on the management of spoiled identity*. Englewood Cliffs, NJ, Prentice Hall.

Graf, DL, Pratt, LV, Hester, CN, & Short, KR (2009). Playing active video games increases energy expenditure in children. *Pediatrics* , Vol. 124, pp. (534 -540)

Griffiths, LJ, Dezateux, C, & Hill, A (2011). Is obesity associated with emotional and behavioural problems in children? Findings from the Millennium Cohort Study. *International Journal of Pediatric Obesity*, Vol. 6, pp. (423-432)

Griffiths, LJ, Parsons, TJ, & Hill, AJ (2010). Self-esteem and quality of life in obese children and adolescents: A systematic review. *International Journal of Pediatric Obesity*, Vol. 5, pp. (282-304)

Gupta, NK, Mueller, WH, Chan, W, & Meininger, JC (2002). Is obesity associated with poor sleep quality in adolescents? *American Journal of Human Biology*, Vol. 14, pp. (762–768)

Hartmann, T, Zahner, L, Pühse, U, Puder, JJ, & Kriemler, S (2010). Effects of a school-based physical activity program on physical and psychosocial quality of life in elementary school children: A cluster-randomized trial. *Pediatric Exercise Science*, Vol. 22, pp. (511-522)

Herva, A, Laitinen, J, Miettunen, J, Veijola, J, Karvonen, JT, Läksy, K, & Joukamaa, M (2006). Obesity and depression: Results from the longitudinal Northern Finland 1966 Birth Cohort Study. *International Journal of Obesity*, Vol. 30, pp. (520-527)

Hesketh, K, Wake, M, & Waters, E (2004). Body mass index and parent-reported self-esteem in elementary school children: Evidence for a causal relationship. *International Journal of Obesity Related Metabolic Disorders*, Vol. 28, pp. (1233–1237)

Hill, AJ (2005). Fed up and friendless? *The Psychologist*, Vol. 1, pp. (280-283)

Institute of Medicine (2005). *Preventing childhood obesity: Health in the balance*. Institute of Medicine, Washington DC.

Holtkamp, K, Konrad, K, Muller, B, Heussen, N, Herpertz, S, Herpertz-Dahlmann, B, & Hebebrand, J (2004). Overweight and obesity in children with attention-deficit/hyperactivity disorder. *International Journal of Obesity and Related Metabolic Disorders*, Vol. 28, pp. (685–689)

Hubel, R, Jass, J, Marcus, A, & Laessle, RG (2006). Overweight and basal metabolic rate in boys with attention-deficit/hyperactivity disorder. *Eating & Weight Disorders*, Vol. 11, pp. (139–146)

Institute of Medicine (2005). *Overview of the IOM report on food marketing to children and youth: Threat or opportunity?*. Institute of Medicine. Academies Press, Washington DC.

Hughes, SO, Anderson, CB, Power, TG, Micheli, NE, Jaramillo, SJ, & Nicklas, TA (2006). Measuring feeding in low-income African-American and Hispanic parents. Appetite, Vol. 46, pp. (215-223)

Israel, A, & Ivanova, M (2002). Global and dimensional selfesteem in preadolescent children who are overweight: Age and gender differences. *International Journal of Eating Disorders*, Vol. *31*, pp. (424–429)

Jago, R, Baranowski, T, Baranowski, JC, Thompson, D, & Greaves, KA (2005). BMI from 3-6 years of age is predicted by TV viewing and physical activity, not diet. *International Journal of Obesity*, Vol. 29, pp. (557–564)

Janssen, I, Boyce, WF, Simpson, K, & Pickett, W (2006). Influence of individual- and area-level measures of socioeconomic status on obesity, unhealthy eating, and physical inactivity in Canadian adolescents. *American Journal of Clinical Nutrition*, Vol. 83, pp. (139-145)

Janssen, I, Craig, WM, Boyce, WF, & Pickett, W (2004). Associations between overweight and obesity with bullying behaviors in school-aged children. *Pediatrics*, Vol. 113, pp. (1187-1194)

Janssen, I, Katzmarzyk, PT, Boyce, WF, Vereecken, C, Mulvihill, C, Roberts, C, Currie, C, Pickett, W & The Health Behaviour in School-Aged Children Obesity Working Group (2005). Comparison of overweight and obesity prevalence in school-aged youth from 34 countries and their relationships with physical activity and dietary patterns. *Obesity Reviews*, Vol. 6, pp. (123–132)

Johnson, L, Mander, AP, Jones, LR, Emmett, PM, & Jebb, SA (2008) Energy-dense, low-fibre, high-fat dietary pattern is associated with increased fatness in childhood. *American Journal of Clinical Nutrition*, Vol. 87, pp. (846-54)

Jones, EE, Farina, A, Hastarf, HH, Markus, H, Miller, DT, & Scott, RA (1984). *Social stigma: The psychology of marked relationships*. W. H. Freeman, New York

Jordan, AB (2007). Heavy television viewing and childhood obesity. *Journal of Children and Media*, Vol. 1, pp. (45–54)

Jose, KA, Blizzard, L, Dwyer, T, McKercher, C, & Venn, AJ (2011). Childhood and adolescent predictors of leisure time physical activity during the transition from adolescence to adulthood: A population based cohort study. *International Journal of Behavioral Nutrition and Physical Activity*, Vol. 8, No. 54. Avaliable from: <http://www.ijbnpa.org/content/8/1/54>

Keinan-Boker, L, Noyman, N, Chinich, A, Green, MS, & Nitzan-Kaluski, D (2005) Overweight and obesity prevalence in Israel: Findings of the First National Health and Nutrition Survey (MABAR). *Israel Medical Association Journal*, Vol. 7, pp. (219-223)

Kimm, SY, Barton, BA, Berhane, K, Ross, JW, Payne, GH, & Schreiber, GB (1997). Self-esteem and adiposity in black and white girls: The NHLBI Growth and Health Study. *Annals of Epidemiology*, Vol. 7, pp. (550–560)

Kimm, SY, Glynn, N, Kriska, AM, & Barton, B (2002). Decline in physical activity in black and white girls during adolescence. *New England Journal of Medicine*, Vol. 347, pp. (709-806)

Kimm, SYS & Obarzanek, E (2002). Childhood obesity: A new pandemic of the new millennium. *Pediatrics*, Vol. 110, pp. (1003-1007)

Krebs, NF, Himes, HM, Jacobson, D, Nicklas, Th A, Guilday, & P, Styne, D(2007). Assessment of child and adolescent overweight and obesity. *Pediatrics*, Vol. 120, Suppl. 4, pp. (193-228)

Lagiou, A & Parava, M (2008). Correlates of childhood obesity in Athens, Greece. *Public Health Nutrition*, Vol. 11, pp. (940–945)

Lam, LT & Yang, L (2007). Overweight/obesity and attention deficit and hyperactivity disorder tendency among adolescents in China. *International Journal of Obesity*, Vol. 31, pp. (584–590)

Lamertz, CM, Jacobi, C, Yassouridis, A, Arnold, K, & Henkel A (2002). Are obese adolescents and young adults at higher risk for mental disorders? A community survey. *Obesity Research*, Vol. 10, pp. (1152-1160)

Latner, JD, & Stunkard, AJ (2003). Getting worse: The stigmatization of obese children. *Obesity Research*, Vol. 11, pp. (452–456)

Lissau, I, Overpeck, MD, Ruan, WJ, Due, P, Holstein, BE, Hedige, ML, & the Health Behaviour in School-aged Children Obesity Working Group (2004). Body mass index and overweight in adolescents in 13 European countries, Israel and USA. *Archives of Pediatric and Adolescent Medicine*, Vol. 158, pp. (29–40)

Lobstein, T & Frelut, M (2003) Prevalence of overweight among children in Europe. *Obesity Review*, Vol. 4, pp. (195–200)

Luppino, FS, de Wit, LM, Bouvy, PF, Stijnen, Th, Cuijpers, P, Penninx, BWJH, & Zitman, FG (2010). Overweight, obesity, and depression. *Archives of General Psychiatry*, Vol. 67, pp. (220-222)

Lyon, HN & Hirschhorn, JN (2005). Genetics of common forms of obesity: A brief overview. *American Journal of Clinical Nutrition*, Vol. 82 (suppl.), pp. (215–217)

Malina, R (2001). Physical activity and fitness: Pathways from childhood to adulthood. *American Journal of Human Biology*, Vol. 13, pp. (162-172)

Markowitz, S, Friedman, MA, & Arent, SM (2008). Understanding the relation between obesity and depression: Causal mechanisms and implications for treatment. *Clinical Psychology: Science and Practice*, Vol. 15, pp. (1-20)

Martyn-Nemeth, P, Penckofer, S, Gulanick, M, Velsor-Friedrich, B, & Bryant, FB (2009). The relationships among self-esteem, stress, coping, eating behavior, and depressive mood in adolescents. *Research in Nursing & Health*, Vol. 32, pp. (96-109)

McCullough, N, Muldoon, O, & Dempster, M (2009). Self-perception in overweight and obese children: A cross-sectional study. *Child: Care, Health and Development*, Vol. 35, pp. (357–364)

McMurray, R, Hurrell, J, & Deng, S (2000). The influence of physical activity, socioeconomic status, and ethnicity on the weight status of adolescents. *Obesity Research*, Vol. 8, pp. (130–139)

Mirza, NM, Davis, D, & Yanovski, JA (2005). Body dissatisfaction, self-esteem, and overweight among inner-city Hispanic children and adolescents. *Journal of Adolescent Health*, Vo. 36, pp. (267.e16 -267.e20).

Mustillo, S, Worthman, C, Erkanli, A, Keeler, G, Angold, A, & Costello, EJ (2003). Obesity and psychiatric disorder: Developmental trajectories. *Pedatrics*, Vol. 111, pp. (851–859)

Napolitano, MA, & Foster, GD (2008). Depression and obesity: Implications for assessment treatment, and research. *Clinical Psychology: Science and Practice*, Vol. 15, pp. (21-27)

National Institute of Health (1998). *Clinical Guidelines on the Identification, Evaluation, and Treatment of Overweight and Obesity in Adults: The Evidence Report*. National Institute of Health, US Department of Health and Human Services, Bethesda, MD

Neumark-Sztainer, D, Falkner, N, Story, M, Perry, C, Hannan, PJ, & Mulert, S (2002). Weight-teasing among adolescents: Correlations with weight status and disordered eating behaviors. *International Journal of Obesity*, Vol. 26, pp. (123–131)

Neumark-Sztainer, D, French, SA, Hannan, PJ, Story, M, & Fulkerson, JA (2005). School lunch and snacking patterns among high school students: Associations with school food environment and policies. *Internacional Journal of Behavioral Nutrition and Physical Activity*, Vol. 2, pp. 14. Available from http://www.ncbi.nlm.nih.gov/pmc/articles/PMC1266392/?tool=pubmed

New, SA, & Livingstone, MB (2003). An investigation of the association between vending machine confectionery purchase frequency by schoolchildren in the UK and other dietary and lifestyle factors. *Public Health Nutrition*, Vol. 6, pp. (497-504)

Newby, PK (2007). Are dietary intakes and eating behaviors related to childhood obesity? A comprehensive review of the evidence. *Journal of Law, Medicine & Ethics*, Vol. 35, pp. (35–60)

Nielsen, SJ & Popkin, BM (2004). Changes in beverage intake between 1977 and 2001. *American Journal of Preventive Medicine*, Vol. 27, pp. (205–210)

O'Rahilly, S & Farooqi, IS (2008). Human obesity: A heritable neurobehavioral disorder that is highly sensitive to environmental conditions. *Diabetes*, Vol. 57, pp. (2905-2910)

Ogden, CL, Carroll, MD, Curtin, LR, Lamb, MM, & Flegal, KM (2010). Prevalence of high body mass index in U.S. children and adolescents, 2007–2008. *Journal of the American Medical Association*, Vol. 303, pp. (242–249)

Paeratakul, S, Ferdinand, DP, Champagne, CM, Ryan, DH, & Bray, GA (2003). Fast-food consumption among US adults and children: Dietary and nutrient intake profile. *Journal of the American Dietetic Association*, Vol. 103, pp. (1332–1338)

Page, R (1984). *Stigma*. Routledge & Kegan Paul, London.

Pallan, MJ, Hiam, LC, Duda, JL, & Adab, P (2011). Body image, body dissatisfaction and weight status in South Asian children: A cross-sectional study. *BMC Public Health*, Vol. 9, pp. (11-21). Avaliable from: < http://www.biomedcentral.com/1471-2458/11/21>

Pangrazi, R (2000). Promoting physical activity for youth. *Journal of Science and Medicine in Sport*, Vol. 3, pp. (280–286)

Pearson, N, Ball, K, & Crawford, D (2011). Mediators of longitudinal associations between television viewing and eating behaviours in adolescents. *International Journal of Behavioral Nutrition and Physical Activity*, Vol. 8, No. 23. Available from: http:// www.ijbnpa.org/content/6/1/23

Pesa, JA, Syre, TR, & Jones, E (2000). Psychosocial differences associated with body weight among female adolescents: The importance of body image. *Journal of Adolescent Health*, Vol. 26, pp. (330–337)

Pine, DS, Goldstein, RB, Wolk, S, & Weissman, MM (2001). The association between childhood depression and adulthood body mass index. *Pediatrics,* Vol. 107, pp. (1049-1056)

Pitrou, I, Shojaei, T, Wazana, A, Gilbert, F, & Kovess-Masféty, V (2010). Child overweight, associated psychopathology, and social functioning: A French school-based survey in 6- to 11-year-old children. *Obesity,* Vol. 18, pp. (809–817)

Popkin, BM, Conde, W, Hou, N, & Monteiro C (2006). Is there a lag globally in overweight trends for children compared with adults? Obesity, Vol. 14, pp. (1846–1853)

Prentice, AM (2006). The emerging epidemic of obesity in developing countries. *International Journal of Epidemiology,* Vol. 35, pp. (93-99)

Reichert, FF, Baptista Menezes, AM, Wells, JC, Carvalho Dumith, S, & Hallal, PC (2009). Psysical activity as a predictor of adolescente body fatness: A systematic review. *Sports Medicine,* Vol. 39, (279-294)

Reilly, JJ, Jackson, DM, Montgomery, C, Kelly, LA, Slater, C, Grant, S, & Paton, JY (2004). Total energy expenditure and physical activity in young Scottish children: Mixed longitudinal study. *Lancet,* Vol. 363, pp. (211-212)

Renman, C, Engstrom, I, Silfverdal, SA, & Aman, J (1999). Mental health and psychosocial characteristics in adolescent obesity: A population-based case-control study. *Acta Paediatrica,* Vol. 88, pp. (998–1003)

Richardson, LP, Davis, R, Poulton R, McCauley, E, Moffitt, TE, Caspi, A, & Connell, F (2003). A longitudinal evaluation of adolescent depression and adult obesity. *Archives of Pediatrics & Adolescent Medicine,* Vol. 157, pp. (739–745)

Rideout, V (2010). *Generation M2: Media in the Lives of 8- to 18-Year-Olds.* Kaiser Family Foundation. Menlo Park, CA

Rogge, MM, Greenwald, M, & Golden, A (2004). Obesity, stigma, and civilized oppression. *Advances in Nursing Science,* Vo. 27, pp. (301–315)

Sallis, J, Prochaska, J, & Taylor, W (2000). A review of correlates of physical activity of children and adolescents. *Medicine & Science in Sports & Exercise* , Vol. 32, pp. (963-975)

Sawyer, MG, Miller-Lewis, L, Guy, S, Wake, M, Canterford, L, & Carlin, JB (2006). Obesity and mental health problems in 4- to 5-year-old australian children. *Ambulatory Pediatrics,* Vol. 6, pp. (306–311)

Schneider, M, Dunton, GF, & Cooper, DM (2007). Media use and obesity in adolescent females. *Obesity,* Vo. 15, pp. (2328–2335)

Schwartz, M, & Brownell, K (2007). Actions necessary to prevent childhood obesity: Creating the climate for change. *Journal of Law Medicine & Ethics,* Vol. 35, pp. (78–89)

Schwartz, MB, Chambliss, HO, Brownell, KD, Blair, SN, & Billington, C (2003). Weight bias among health professionals specializing in obesity. *Obesity Research,* Vol. 11, pp. (1033-1039)

Schwimmer, JB, Burwinkle, TM, & Varni, JW (2003). Health-related quality of life of severely obese children and adolescents. *Journal of the American Medical Association,* Vol. 289, pp. (1813-1819)

Seal, N (2011). Introduction to genetics and childhood obesity: Relevance to nursing practice. *Biological Research for Nursing,* Vol. 13, pp. (61-69)

Serra-Majem, Ll, Aranceta Bartrina, J, Perez-Rodrigo, C, Ribas-Barba, L & Delgado-Rubio, A (2006). Prevalence and deteminants of obesity in Spanish children and young people. *British Journal of Nutrition*, Vol. 96, Suppl. 1, pp. (67–72)

Sjoberg, RL (2005). Obesity, shame, and depression in school-aged children: A population-based study. *Pediatrics*, Vol. 116, pp. (389-392)

Stamatakis, E, Wardle, J & Cole, TJ (2010). Childhood obesity and overweight prevalence trends in England: Evidence for growing socioeconomic disparities. *International Journal of Obesity* , Vol. 34, pp. (41–47)

Stice, E, Presnell, K, & Spangler, D (2002). Risk factors for binge eating onset in adolescent girls: A 2-year prospective investigation. *Health Psychology*, Vol. 21, pp. (131–138)

Stradmeijer, M, Bosch, J, Koops, W, & Seidell, J (2000). Family functioning and psychosocial adjustment in overweight youngsters. *International Journal of Eating Disorders*, Vol 27, pp. (110–114)

Strauss, RS (2000). Childhood obesity and self-esteem. *Pediatrics*, Vol. 105, pp. (e15-e19)

Swinburn, B, Egger, G, & Raza, F (1999). Dissecting obesogenic environments: The development and application of a framework for identifyingand prioritizing environmental interventions for obesity. *Preventive Medicine*, Vol. 29, pp. (563–570)

Szwarc, S (2004–2005). Putting facts over fears: examining childhood anti-obesity initiatives. *International Quarterly of Community Health Education*, Vol. 23, pp. (97–116)

Taheri, S (2006). The link between short sleep duration and obesity: We should recommend more sleep to prevent obesity. *Archives of Disease in Childhood*, Vol. 91, pp. (881– 884)

Tang-Peronard, JL, & Heitmann, BL (2008). Stigmatization of obese children and adolescents, the importance of gender. *Obesity Reviews*, Vol. 9, pp. (522–534)

The Bridge (2010). *Newsletter of WHO/Europe*. World Health Organization. Regional Office for Europe, Issue No. 29, autumn-winter.

Telama, R, Yang, XL, Viikari, J, Valimaki, I, Wanne, O, & Raitakari, O (2005). Physical activity from childhood to adulthood - A 21-year tracking study. *American Journal of Preventive Medicine*, Vol. 28, pp. (267-273)

Tomkinson, G, Leger, A, Olds, T, & Cazorla, G (2003). Secular trends in the performance of children and adolescents (1980–2000): An analysis of 55 studies of the 20m shuttle run test in 11 countries. *Sports Medicine*, Vol. 33, pp. (285–300)

Tremblay, MS, & Willms, JD (2003). Is the Canadian childhood obesity epidemic related to physical inactivity? *International Journal of Obesity and Related Metabolic Disorders*, Vol. 27, pp. (1100-1105)

U.S. Department of Health and Human Services (2006). *Healthy People 2010*. Available from: http://www.healthypeople.gov/

Van Cleave, J, Gortmaker, SL & Perrin, JM (2010). Dynamics of obesity and chronic health conditions among children and young. *Journal of the American Medical Association*, Vol. 303, No. 7, pp. (623-630)

Van der Horst, K, Oenema, A, Ferreira, I, Wendel-Vos, W, Giskes, K, Van Lenthe, F, & Brug, J (2007). A systematic review of environmental correlates of obesity-related dietary behaviors in youth. *Health Education Research*, Vol. 22, pp (203-226)

Van Mechelen, W, Twisk, JW, Post, GB, Snel, J, & Kemper, HC (2000). Physical activity of young people: The Amsterdam Longitudinal Growth and Health Study. *Medicine & Science in Sports & Exercise*, Vol. 32, pp. (1610-1616)

Van Vlierberghe, L, Braet, C, Goossens, L, & Mels, S (2009). Psychiatric disorders and symptom severity in referred versus non-referred overweight children and adolescents. *European Child and Adolescent Psychiatry*, Vol. 18, pp. (164-173)

Vandewater, E, Shim, M, & Caplovitz, A (2004). Linking obesity and activity level with children's television and video game use. *Journal of Adolescence*, Vol. 27, pp. (71-85)

Vázquez, FL, Díaz, O, & Pomar, C (2010). Prevalence of overweight and obesity among preadolescent schoolchildren in Galicia, Spain. *Child: Care, Health and Development*, Vol. 36, pp. (392-395)

Veugelers, PJ, & Fitzgerald, AL (2005). Prevalence of and risk factors for childhood overweight and obesity. *Canadian Medical Association Journal*, Vol. 173, pp. (607-613)

Vila, G, Zipper, E, Dabbas, M, Bertrand, C, Robert, JJ, Ricour, C, & Mouren-Simeoni, MCh (2004). Mental Disorders in obese children and adolescents. *Psychosomatic Medicine*, Vol. 66, pp. (387–394)

Walker, L, & Hill, AJ (2009). Obesity: The role of child mental health services. *Child and Adolescent Mental Health*, Vol. 14, pp. (114-120)

Wang, Y (2011). Disparities in pediatric obesity in the United States. *Advances in Nutrition*, Vol. 2, pp. (23-31)

Wang, Y, & Lobstein, T (2006). Worldwide trends in childhood overweight and obesity. *International Journal of Pediatric Obesity*, Vol. 1, pp. (11-25)

Wang, Y, Monteiro, C, & Popkin, BM (2002). Trends of obesity and underweight in older children and adolescents in the United States, Brazil, China, and Russia. *American Journal of Clinical Nutrition*, Vol. 75, pp. (971–977)

Wardle, J, & Cooke, L (2005). The impact of obesity on psychological well-being. *Best Practice & Research Clinical Endocrinology & Metabolism*, Vol. 19, pp. (421-440)

Wardle, J, Williamson, S, Johnson, F, & Edwards, C (2006). Depression in adolescent obesity: Cultural moderators of the association between obesity and depressive symptoms. *International Journal of Obesity*, Vol. 30, pp. (634–643)

Warschburger, P (2005). The unhappy obese child. *International Journal of Obesity*, Vol. 29, pp. (127-129).

Waring, ME, & Lapane, KL (2008). Overweight in children and adolescents in relation to attention-deficit/hyperactivity disorder: Results from a national sample. *Pediatrics*, Vol. 122, pp. (e1-6)

Whincup, PH, Owen, CG,, Sattar, N, & Cook, DG (2005). School dinners and markers of cardiovascular health and type 2 diabetes in 13–16 year olds: A cross-sectional study. *British Medical Journal*, Vol. 331, pp. (1060–1061)

Whitaker, RC (2003). Obesity prevention in pediatric primary care: Four behaviors to target. *Archives of Pediatrics and Adolescence Medicine*, Vol. 157, pp. (725–727)

Whitlock, EP, Williams, SB, Smith, PR & Shipman, SA (2005). Screening and intervention for childhood overweight: A summary of evidence for the US Preventive Service Task Force. *Pediatrics*, Vol. 116, pp. (125-144)

Wojnar,J, Brower, KJ, Dopp, R, Wojnar, M, Emslie, G, Rintelmann, J, Hoffmann, RF, & Armitage, R (2010). Sleep and body mass index in depressed children and healthy controls. *Sleep Medicine*, Vol. 11, pp. (295-301)

World Health Organization (2005). Fact sheet Copenhagen 2005, the challenge of obesity in the WHO European Region. 3. Available from http://www.euro.who.int/__data/assets/pdf_file/0018/102384/fs1305e.pdf

Zametkin, AJ, Zoon, CK, Klein, HW, & Munson, S (2004). Psychiatric aspects of child and adolescent obesity: A review of the past 10 years. *Journal of the American Academy of Child and Adolescent Psychiatry*, Vol. 43, pp. (134–150)

Zeller, MH, Reiter-Purtill, J, & Ramey, C (2008). Negative peer perceptions of obese children in the classroom environment. *Obesity*, Vol. 16, pp. (755–762)

Zimmerman, FJ & Bell, JF (2010). Associations of television content type and obesity in children. *American Journal of Public Health*, Vol. 100, pp. (334 –340)

Zoumas-Morse, C, Rock, CL, Sobo, EJ, & Neuhouser, ML (2001). Children's patterns of macronutrient intake and associations with restaurant and home eating. *Journal of the American Dietetic Association*, Vol. 101, pp. (923-5)

9

Obesity and Quality of Life in Communities of Diverse Ethnicity and Low Socioeconomics

Joan Griffith
University of Toledo Health Science Campus
USA

1. Introduction

The prevalence of childhood overweight and obesity is increasing throughout the world, in both developed and developing countries (Wang & Lobstein, 2006). Based on available data, the prevalence of childhood overweight and obesity has increased in almost all countries with exceptions in Russia and Poland where the prevalence rates for overweight among school-age children decreased during the 1990s (Wang & Lobstein, 2006). Globally, obesity and overweight have risen more in economically developed countries and in urbanized populations (Wang & Lobstein, 2006). North America, Europe, and parts of the Western Pacific have the highest prevalence of overweight children while parts of South East Asia and much of sub-Saharan Africa have the lowest prevalence (Wang & Lobstein, 2006).

Socioeconomic status and ethnicity can affect overweight and obesity prevalence for adults and children, and may be modified by the economics of the country. Among middle-income countries, members of better-off households are more likely to be at risk than members of poorer households, and urban residents may be more at risk than rural ones (Wang & Lobstein, 2006). Comparing communities in South Africa, the overweight prevalence among young white (23%) and Indian populations (25%) were higher than that among young Africans (17%). In industrialized, economically developed countries, children in the lowest socioeconomic status groups and children in specific racial or ethnic groups may be at the greatest risk for overweight/obesity (Wang & Lobstein, 2006).

The enormous direct and indirect costs of adult obesity in the United States have been well-documented (Wang & Lobstein, 2006; Finkelstein, Fiebelkorn & Wang, 2003). Adult obesity often begins during childhood and adolescence. The epidemic of childhood obesity, if not reversed, warns of increasing medical and financial obesity-related costs (Finkelstein, Fiebelkorn & Wang, 2003). The next generation of adults will have to confront these problems at an even earlier age (Wang & Lobstein, 2006), especially members of our most vulnerable populations. Obesity-related co-morbidities include dyslipidemia, obstructive sleep apnea, disordered sleep, joint pain, hypertension, insulin resistance, diabetes, erosive tooth wear, and depression (Barlow and the Expert Committee, 2007) and children living in ethnic minority or low-socioeconomic communities are at greatest risk. These conditions have the potential to adversely affect the quality of life for obese children.

Previous research has presented various conclusions regarding the prevalence of overweight/obesity among individuals living in ethnic minority and low socioeconomic communities. These conclusions have included such findings as: (1) obesity is viewed more positively by individuals living in ethnic minority and low socioeconomic communities than by individuals in more affluent communities; (2) overweight/obesity resulted in less adverse psychosocial influence; and (3) overweight/obesity was perceived to cause less undesirable health impact. These conclusions may be problematic as they may reflect culture values that may be difficult to change and could represent insurmountable obstacles to the development of effective interventions. They may also serve as defense mechanisms for warding off adverse psychosocial complications (Bennett & Wolin, 2006).

Over the past decade public awareness of the adverse effects of obesity has increased and most individuals have become more knowledgeable of the benefits of healthier lifestyles. This increased awareness and knowledge should result in positive lifestyle changes, especially among at-risk populations. Therefore, the questions we must now ask are: (1) "Will more recent studies provide any new insight on the disparate prevalence of childhood obesity?' and (2) Will the former conclusions about the at-risk communities require any modifications?"

The specific aim of this chapter is to review some of the recent scientific evidence on the prevalence and impact of childhood obesity among communities of diverse ethnicity and low-socioeconomics and to review the changes associated with crucial factors that may affect the quality of life of overweight/obese children. By reviewing the prevailing data, we hope to answer the above questions. The chapter will look at (1) the prevailing obesity prevalence disparity; (2) the frequency of the misperception of weight status among adults in communities of diverse ethnicity/low-socioeconomics and its impact on their children; (3) the effect of the mother's perceptions of their children's weight ; (4) the role of behavioral and social factors such as family involvement, frequency of family dinners, television watching, physical inactivity and healthful eating; (5) the built environment concept, especially the role of parental perception of neighborhood safety and their willingness to allow their children to participate in outside physical activity; (6) the significance of "food deserts" and "food insecurity"; (7) the relationship between economics and attitudes toward health; (8) the critical medical and psychosocial consequences of childhood obesity that influence the quality of life for obese children; and (9) the self-image of obese children, especially data from recent studies among obese African American children.

The chapter is based on a PubMed literature search conducted by focusing on the major topic of "childhood obesity". Several different subtitles were incorporated including: "obesity disparity", "misperception of weight among adults", "mothers' weight perception of children", "behavioral and social factors", family involvement", "built community", "food deserts", "economics and health", school environment", "faith organizations", and "psychosocial consequences". The search was limited to English-language and foreign-languages articles with English abstracts published between 2006-2011. In addition, a number of studies identified in the course of reading were included.

2. Quality of life

The quality of life (QOL) model consists of subjective evaluations of positive and negative aspects of life (http://www.cdc.gov/hrqol/concept.htm; http://en.wikipedia.org/wiki/Quality_of_life). Quality of life refers to the personal satisfaction or dissatisfaction with the cultural or intellectual conditions of our living conditions and is distinct from the basic tangible belongings we need for comfort (http://www.cdc.gov/hrqol/concept.htm; http://en.wikipedia.org/wiki/Quality_of_life). Key domains of the overall quality of life include health, job, housing, school and neighborhood. In addition, culture, values, and spirituality are vital aspects of overall quality of life (http://www.cdc.gov/hrqol/concept.htm; http://en.wikipedia.org/wiki/Quality_of_life).

Health-related quality of life (HRQOL) provides a measure of the burden of preventable disease, injuries, and disabilities (http://www.cdc.gov/hrqol/concept.htm; http://en.wikipedia.org/wiki/Quality_of_life). The concept of health-related quality of life and its determinants cover the features of overall quality of life that affect physical and or mental health (http://www.cdc.gov/hrqol/concept.htm; http://en.wikipedia.org/wiki/Quality_of_life) and can offer a better understanding of the relationships between health-related quality of life and risk factors. On the individual level, determinants of health-related quality of life include physical and mental health perceptions and other correlates such as health risks and conditions, functional status, social support and, socioeconomic status. Health surveillance frequently includes health-related quality of life questions about perceived physical and mental health and function. These questions are important components of health surveillance and are commonly regarded as compelling markers of service needs and intervention outcomes (http://www.cdc.gov/hrqol/concept.htm; http://en.wikipedia.org/wiki/Quality_of_life).

Intuitively, there should be general consensus that obesity affects the quality of life for adults and children. One health-related quality of life measurement tool is the Impact of Weight on Quality of Life-Kids. It is a 27-item questionnaire assessing weight-specific health-related quality of life. It provides scores on physical comfort, body esteem, social life, family relations, and a total score. Higher scores indicate better health-related quality of life. A study to examine the health-related quality of life in adolescents with extreme obesity, i.e., body mass index greater than 40 kilogram per meter-squared, concluded that generic and weight-specific measurement tools, as assessed by the Pediatric Quality of Life Inventory and Impact of Weight on Quality of Life-Kids, respectively, indicated global health-related quality of life impairment and that the impairment differed significantly by race (Modi et al., 2008). Physical, emotional and social scores on the Pediatric Quality of Life Inventory and the physical comfort and body esteem scores of the Impact of Weight on Quality of Life-Kids were significantly higher for black compared to white adolescents with extreme obesity. The authors acknowledged that although racial differences in adolescent body image/esteem had been previously reported it was unknown why black adolescent with extreme obesity reported less impact of weight on their physical functioning. Interestingly, health-related quality of life did not differ for extremely obese adolescents based on type of treatment sought as extremely obese adolescents seeking bariatric surgery reported similar health-related quality of life compared to adolescents requesting behavioral treatment. The data suggested that health-related quality of life was not homogenous in adolescents with extreme obesity (Modi et al., 2008).

The association between obesity and obesity-related co-morbidities is well document (Barlow, 2007; Daniels, 2006) and we are witnessing the impact of these co-morbidities on health-related quality of life throughout the world. The overall prevalence of overweight and obesity in urban children in New Delhi increased from 16% in 2002 to 24% in 2006-2007 with 29% of children in private schools and 11.3% of children in government funded schools

(Bhardwaj et al., 2008) affected. India has the highest number of patients with type 2 diabetes mellitus globally and the rapid rise of obesity in children is the prime reason for increasing insulin resistance, the metabolic syndrome, dyslipidemia, polycystic ovarian syndrome and elevated C-reactive protein. (Bhardwaj et al., 2008). As compared to other ethnic groups, children with ancestral origin in South Asia manifest adiposity, insulin resistance and metabolic perturbations earlier in life; and the metabolic syndrome and obesity track into adulthood (Bhardwaj et al., 2008).

The Treatment Options for Type 2 Diabetes in Adolescents and Youth cohort represents the largest and best-characterized national sample of American youth with recent-onset type 2 diabetes (Copeland et al., 2011). Analysis of the cohort at baseline revealed that 64.9% were female; mean age was 14.0 years; mean diabetes duration was 7.8 months; mean body mass index Z-score was 2.15; 89.4% had a family history of diabetes; 41.1% were Hispanic; 31.5% were non-Hispanic black; 38.8% were living with both biological parents; 41.5% had a household annual income of less than $25,000; 26.3% had a highest education level of parent/guardian less than a high school degree; 26.3% had a blood pressure at the 90th percentile or great; 13.6% had a blood pressure at the 95th percentile or greater; 13.0% had microabluminuria; 79.8% had a low high-density lipoprotein level; and 10.2% had high triglycerides. Alarmingly, the clinical and biochemical abnormalities and comorbidities were prevalent within 2 years of diagnosis (Copeland et al., 2011).

Adenotonsillectomy is the first-line treatment for sleep-disordered breathing (Amin et al., 2008). Three clinical markers have been found to be independent risk factors for recurrence of sleep-disordered breathing after adenotonsillectomy: the velocity of increased body mass index, obesity, and being African American (Amin et al., 2008). In the children with recurrence of disordered-sleep, systolic blood pressure at 1 year post surgery was higher than baseline and higher than in children who did not experience recurrence (Amin et al., 2008). Another study of health-related quality of life for children with sleep-disordered breathing who underwent adenotonsillectomy demonstrated similar findings in that it documented these children were more likely to be obese than children seen in a general pediatric clinic and that African American children who were obese were more likely to have sleep-disordered breathing (Rudnick et al., 2007).

Among first and second generation United States immigrant children and adolescents from Central and South American and the Caribbean basin the prevalence of the metabolic syndrome was 29% overall (Messiah et al., 2009). Boys were significantly more likely than girls to have abnormal systolic blood pressure and Hispanics were significantly more likely than blacks to have abnormal triglycerides and HDL cholesterol (Messiah et al., 2009). Additionally, obese 13-19 year-old children have increased odds of erosive tooth wear compared to similar aged healthy weight children (McGuire et al., 2009).

Weight-related teasing is an increasing problem, especially for children overweight or obese and negative outcomes have been associated with weight-based teasing (McCormack & Laska, 2011). Specifically, body satisfaction was lower among children being teased by family or peers than those who were not teased. Stigmatization of overweight children is extremely prevalent and stereotypes about low intelligence may contribute to weight stigma (Latner et al., 2007). In 2007 a study was completed to determine the weight-based stigmatization of Mexican overweight and non-overweight children by their mothers and peers (Bacardi-Gascon et al., 2007). Four hundred and thirty-two fifth and sixth graders and 342 mothers participated. Children were given a questionnaire displaying six drawings; participants' responses were numbered in order of preference from 1 to 6 (most to least well liked). Participants were divided into categories based on socioeconomic status, ethnicity, and current body mass index. The majority of the children chose the child in a wheelchair as the preferred friend. Boys and girls, Indian and non-Indian, with and without risk of overweight chose the obese peer as the least-preferred friend. Non-overweight girls and their mothers liked the obese child less than non-overweight boys and their mothers. Based on their data, the authors concluded that the negative attitude of mothers toward the obese child was projected to their children and influenced their children's decisions (Bacardi-Gascon et al., 2007).

Chinese children's perceptions of self-competence and their coping strategies varied based on gender and weight (Chen et al., 2007). Higher body mass index was related to lower athletic competency in boys and lower social competence in girls. Better behavioral conduct competence contributed to better global self-worth in boys while in girls, better behavioral conduct competence and physical appearance competence contributed to better global self-worth (Chen et al., 2007). Eating and drinking were reported as one of the most frequently used coping strategies by children, but the children felt that this strategy was not effective (Chen et al., 2007).

Ecological models of health suggest that lower individual and environmental socioeconomic status may be related to health attitudes and behaviors that contribute to obesity (McAlexander et al., 2009). After examining the role of social relationships and negative emotional traits in the development of central adiposity and arterial stiffness in healthy adolescents, it appears that psychosocial variables may be important in the development of central adiposity and arterial stiffness in adolescence and that adolescents with less supportive relationships and higher anger had increased waist-to-hip ratios, i.e., increased risk of central adiposity, overtime (Medie & Matthews, 2009).

The question has been asked as to whether overweight and obesity may eventually be associated with premature death. Proportional hazards analysis and data from the National Health Interview Survey Linked Mortality Files were used to estimate life expectancies for each body mass index strata and quantified years-of-life-lost by comparing differences between age, race, smoking status and gender and the normal body mass index reference group (Finkelstein et al., 2010). The evidence suggested that overweight and mild obesity were not associated with a reduction in life expectancy. However, higher body mass index categories were associated with lower expected survival. In aggregate, excess body mass index is responsible for approximately 95 million years-of-life lost. White females accounted for more than two-thirds of the aggregate years-of-life-lost. The authors concluded that unless something is done to reduce the rising prevalence of those with body mass indexes greater than 35, or to diminish the impact of obesity or its correlates on years-of-life-lost, expected life expectancy for United States adults may decrease in the future (Finkelstein et al., 2010). This prediction is even more concerning when we recall that adult obesity begins in childhood/adolescence. Clearly, we must evaluate the impact on quality of life in the process of identifying effective weight management programs (Fullerton et al., 2007).

2.1 Socioeconomic status or position

Socioeconomic position has been shown to be related to obesity and weight gain (Baltrus et al., 2007). Specifically, (1) long-term weight gain in adulthood was associated with childhood socioeconomic position and education in women and education and income in men; (2) low childhood socioeconomic position was associated with increased weight among women 17-30 years old; (3) and low educational status was associated with increased weight gain among women 13-30 years and men 17-30 years (Baltrus et al., 2007). Socioeconomic status/race variable explains approximately 24% of geographic variability in childhood obesity and childhood obesity is significantly associated with lower household income, lower home ownership, less educated women, single parent household, and non-white residents (Grow et al., 2010). Daily priorities are affected by the reality of household finances. Local community leaders in the south-side of Chicago felt awareness was higher for acute health conditions than for obesity, and though parents were concerned about their children's health parents were stressed by competing priorities and constrained by lack of knowledge, parenting skills, time, and financial resources (Burnet & Plaut, 2008).

Distinct socioeconomic status dimensions can differentially predict obesity across race/ethnicity (Scharoun-Lee M, Adair L et al., 2009). After studying the effect of social advantage, schooling, employment and economic hardship, the authors concluded that the association of social advantage and economic hardship factors with obesity differed by race/ethnicity in females (Scharoun-Lee M, Adair L et al., 2009). High social advantage was inversely associated with obesity in white and Hispanic females (9-20% lower) while high scores on economic hardship were positively associated with obesity in white and Asian females. In contrast, no significant racial/ethnic differences were observed in males. The schooling factor was significantly positive for females of all racial/ethnic groups (Scharoun-Lee M, Adair L et al., 2009).

The racial/ethnic disparities in obesity escalate from childhood to adulthood in the United States and may be attributed to the differences in socioeconomic status (Scharoun-Lee M, Kaufman J et al., 2009). Males with a disadvantaged background who experienced an early transition into the labor force, marriage and residential independence have the highest risk for developing obesity while females exposed to persistent adversity were at highest risk. Socioeconomic status has a stronger relationship with the persistence of obesity than its incidence and ethnic minorities have the highest obesity risk across socioeconomic status groups (Scharoun-Lee M, Kaufman J et al., 2009).

Race/ethnicity, socioeconomic status, and behavior factors were independently related to childhood and adolescent obesity (Singh et al., 2008). Among children in the United States, aged 10-17 years, who participated in the 2003 National Survey of Children's Health, ethnic minority status, non-metropolitan residence, lower socioeconomic status, lower social capital, higher television viewing and higher physical inactivity were all independently associated with higher obesity prevalence (Singh et al., 2008). Compared to affluent white children, the odds of obesity were 2.7, 1.9 and 3.2 times higher for poor Hispanics, whites and black children, respectively (Singh et al., 2008).

While the social disparities in body mass index trajectories may vary across adulthood by gender, race/ethnicity and lifetime socio-economic position the body mass index scores are consistently higher for women, racial/ethnic minority groups and those from a lower socioeconomic position (Clarke et al., 2009). However, body mass index scores for socially advantaged groups in recent years are actually higher than those for their socially disadvantaged counterparts who were born 10 years earlier. Social status and socio-economic resources are important for maintaining optimal weight (Clarke et al., 2009). Although those in advantaged social positions have experienced an increase in body mass index recently (Clarke et al., 2009) overall, poor children with a sedentary lifestyle have a 3.7 times higher odds of obesity than their active, affluent counter parts (Singh et al., 2008).

2.1.1 Prevailing obesity prevalence disparity

Pediatric obesity has reached critical levels and a worrisome trend has been identified worldwide (Lieb et al., 2009). There is a greater prevalence of obesity in ethnic and racial minorities than in non-Hispanic whites (Clarke et al., 2009; Lieb et al., 2009; Scharoun-Lee M, Kaufman J et al., 2009). The reason for this disparity is multifactorial, with culture, environment, and genetics playing a role (Calzada, Anderson-Worts, 2009). Of note, the higher availability of obesigenic diets and poor dietary behavior world-wide have created an increasingly urban Asian childhood obesity epidemic, which coupled with persistent undernutrition, present a complex double burden of malnutrition (Guldan, 2010). Some dietary patterns associated with overweight include snacking, eating out, fast food, sweetened beverages and excessive meat; unhealthy macronutrient energy proportions and a preference for refined grains (Guldan, 2010). Among White and South Asian children age 5-7 years, born between 1991 and 1999, and included in the East Berkshire Child Health System, overweight and obesity among South Asian boys were significantly higher than that among South Asian girls and the boys may be at greater risk of morbidity and mortality (Balakrishnan et al., 2008).

A cross-sectional study to examine factors associated with health behaviors, including physical activity and dietary intake of Chinese women who had immigrated to the United States and their children revealed that approximately 37% of the children were overweight with body mass index greater the 85th percentile (Chen, 2009). A high household income was related to low maternal body mass index, higher maternal fat intake, and high maternal intake of sweets while a high level of maternal acculturation was related to low body mass index in children (Chen, 2009). In contrast, among 3 to 5 years old Canadian Inuit children across the Canadian High Arctic the overall prevalence of overweight was 50.8% with significantly more boys (57.1%) than girls (45.2%) in the overweight category (Galloway et al., 2010). Yet, an examination of biological, socio-economic and dietary factors, including birth weight, breastfeeding, day care attendance, traditional and market food consumption and sweetened beverage intake revealed no significant associations that could explain the development of obesity in this population (Galloway et al., 2010).

In a study of Norwegian adolescents, aged 15-16 years, the prevalence of overweight was 11.8% and obesity was 2.4%, higher in boys (Groholt et al., 2008). Further analysis revealed that the northernmost counties were 70% to 90% more likely to be overweight and obese compared with adolescents in Oslo, the capital and southernmost county. Other factors that were significantly associated with overweight and obesity included lower educational plans, poor family economy and physical inactivity. Eating breakfast was positively associated with not being overweight or obese (Groholt et al., 2008). A nationwide representative survey of New Zealand schoolchildren demonstrated a 2.7% incidence of extreme obesity compared to 4% in the United States but ethnic differences in prevalence with 0.8% in New Zealand European, 5.1% in Maori, and 10.9% in Pacific Island groups (Goulding et al., 2007). Data from the Reports on School Health Survey, Ministry of Education, Culture, Sports, Science and Technology, revealed no evidence of any major rise in prevalence of obesity as expressed by mean body mass index for Japanese children 5-17 years old between 1948-2003 (Hermanussen et al., 2007). The authors concluded that Japanese children and adolescents may be more resistant against environmental factors that have caused obesity in affluent western societies (Hermanussen et al., 2007). However, a previous study using data from the cross-sectional annual National Nutrition Survey, Japan, from 1976 to 2000 of children between the ages of 6 and 14 revealed an increasing trend in obesity prevalence in Japanese school children (Matsushita et al., 2004). The prevalence of obese boys and girls increased from 6.1% and 7.1%, respectively, between 1976 and 1980, to 11.1% and 10.2% in 1996 to 2000. The increasing trend was most evident among 9- to 11-year old children of both sexes living in small towns, whereas no changes were observed in girls in metropolitan areas (Matsushita et al., 2004).

In the United States, one of the states with the highest prevalence rates of obesity is Mississippi. The prevalence and trends of obesity among Mississippi public school students, 2005-2009 were published in 2010 (Molaison et al., 2010). The data revealed that in 2009 the prevalence of obesity for all students in K-12 was 23.9% as compared to 23.5%in 2007, and 25.5% in 2005. However, the disparity between races appeared to be increasing over time with the prevalence remaining level for non-white students while decreasing each year for white students (Molaison et al., 2010).

2.2 Misperception of weight status among adults

Misperception of weight has been defined as viewing self as being about the right weight when actually overweight or obese (Bennett & Wolin, 2006). Adults frequently misperceive their weight and the level of misperception appears to vary based on ethnicity/race and gender (Bennett & Wolin, 2006). According to Bennett & Wolin misperception was present among 43% of overweight white men and 9% among obese white men versus 21% among overweight white women and 3% among obese white women compared to 66% for overweight black men and 26% for obese black men versus 41% for overweight black women and 11% for obese black women compared to 64% for overweight Hispanic men and 17% for obese Hispanic males versus 29% for overweight Hispanic women and 7% for obese Hispanic women (Bennett & Wolin, 2006). The high level of misperception among blacks may be a function of several factors: (1) weight satisfaction versus a lack of awareness about the extent of their overweight; (2) lack of awareness about clinical thresholds for overweight and obesity; or (3) a reliance on social comparisons to make judgment about their weight status (Bennett & Wolin, 2006).

Despite greater self-reported prevalence of certain risk factors for poor health, African Americans may have a more optimistic view of their overall health and weight status and lack of an awareness of their actual risk (Burroughs et al., 2008). Surprisingly, 72% of African Americans reported "good to excellent" health compared to 62% of Hispanics even though 56% of African Americans compared to 34% of Hispanics who self-described as "slightly" overweight met criteria for obesity based on body mass index (Burroughs et al., 2008). Additionally, 33% of the African Americans reported high blood pressure, 20% arthritis, 18% high cholesterol, and 15% diabetes compared to 17% of Hispanics who reported high cholesterol, 15% high blood pressure, and 12% sleep difficulty. Misperception of their weight may cause parents to misperceive the children's weight and delay corrective intervention.

2.3 Effect of the mother's perceptions of their children's weight

Parents frequently define overweight in functional terms while children will define it based on physical appearance (Burnet & Blaut, 2008). In a study examining maternal perception of their overweight children among participants in an urban Special Supplemental Nutritional Program for Women, Infants and Children serving primarily Hispanic families, (Hackie &

Bowles, 2007), 61% of mothers did not recognize their children, ages 2-5 years, as overweight. Perception of the child's overweight was independent of age and educational level of the mother. Fifty percent of mothers had taken no steps to control what their child ate. The authors concluded that Hispanic mothers of overweight children may not perceive their children as being overweight and interventions will need to be based on the mother's belief system and cultural background (Hackie & Bowles, 2007).

In a similar study, of 192 African-American and Hispanic 4-5 year old children, most mothers perceived their children to be thinner than actual size (Killion et al., 2006). Approximately 66% of mothers of overweight and obese children were satisfied with their children's existing body size or wanted them to be heavier while 50% of the mothers of obese children wanted their children to be thinner (Killion et al., 2006).

The agreement between adolescent and caregiver on body size satisfaction varies by body mass index category (Mitola et al., 2007). Among normal weight adolescents, 61% of adolescent-caregivers agreed that current body size was ideal. Among adolescents at risk for overweight, 38% of adolescent-caregivers agreed that current body size was ideal, and 38% were discordant with adolescents wanting to be thinner and caregivers satisfied with current body size. Among overweight adolescents, adolescent-caregiver agreement was 67%; 52% agreed the adolescent should be thinner and 15% agreed current body size was ideal. Body size satisfaction is related to body mass index category for adolescents and caregivers, but adolescents have a lower threshold for satisfaction therefore, encouraging caregivers to discuss their adolescents' views on body size satisfaction may allow caregivers to support their adolescents in addressing weight-related issues (Mitola et al., 2007).

2.3.1 Body image discrepancy

Body image discrepancy reflects the difference between ideal and current body images (Banitt et al., 2008). In a cross-sectional study to investigate the relationship between body image discrepancy and weight status among adolescents, participants were asked to select body imagines from a 13-figure rating scale. There was an increase in body image discrepancy with the increasing prevalence of obesity (Banitt et al., 2008). Overall, half of the females and one third of males wanted a thinner body (Banitt et al., 2008). Body image discrepancy was positively related to body mass index percentile. A one-unit increase in body image discrepancy was observed with a 4.84 unit increase in body mass index percentile among females and a 3.88-unit increase in males. Both male and female adolescents reported body image discrepancy at a body mass index percentile that corresponded to normal weight. While black and white differences existed in body image discrepancy, black female adolescents were similar to their white counterparts and reported body image discrepancy at a weight range that was within the normal range (Banitt et al., 2008). The authors stressed the need for interventions that will help adolescents develop a healthy and realistic body image and healthy ways to manage their weight (Banitt et al., 2008).

Whether satisfaction with overweight and obesity contribute to greater weight gain in African American women than men remains debatable; yet little data is available for younger adult African Americans on their perceived and ideal body image (Gilliard et al., 2007). In a survey of 509 self-identified African American freshmen in 2003 and 669 in 2006 at a historically black university, the data did not suggest that greater weight gain in women than men is driven by a desire to be heavier. The high proportion of overweight women with a normal perceived body image may contribute to the greater weight gain. Of concern, nearly half of men with normal body mass index wanted to be heavier, while approximately 5/8 of overweight men were satisfied with being overweight or wanted to be heavier (Gilliard et al., 2007).

2.4 Role of behavioral and social factors

Ethnicity is associated with differences in food-related beliefs, preferences, and behaviors; and cultural influences may contribute to the higher than average risk of obesity among children and youth in United States ethnic minority populations (Kumanyika, 2008). Evidence indicates that ethnic differences along several pathways may increase the risk of obesity. Development of useful interventions in the future requires a better understanding of which causes of obesity might be more prevalent or intensified in low-income and diverse communities; understanding of how the social, cultural and economic environments might magnify these factors; and determining which changes in those environments would help the most to reduce obesity (Kumanyika & Greer, 2006). Parents' weight is among the strongest correlate for child weight (Elder & Arredondo, 2010).

The social and structural environment in which Hispanic children are reared may play an essential role in uncovering their risk for obesity and related behaviors (Elder & Arredondo, 2010). Overweight children were less active compared to normal weight children; parents of overweight children provided less instrumental support to engage in activity and set fewer limits on their child's activities; parents of overweight children were less likely to control, but more likely to set limits on their child's diet compared to normal weight children; parents who rated their health more positively and were less acculturated were more likely to have overweight children (Elder & Arredondo, 2010). Foreign-born Hispanic men and women have a substantially lower likelihood of being overweight or obese than Hispanics born in the United States; and the likelihood of obesity/overweight increases the longer foreign-born individuals remained in the United States (Akresh, 2008).

Racial discrimination may be an important factor related to weight gain among ethnic minorities (Gee et al., 2008). Findings from an analysis of data from the 2002 to 2003 National Latino and Asian American Study revealed that: (1) racial discrimination was associated with increased body mass index and obesity; (2) the association between racial discrimination and body mass index strengthened the longer the time spent in the United States (Gee et al., 2008).

Cultural attitudes and belief are not the only potential sources of ethnic variation in childhood obesity prevalence and should not be studied in isolation (Kumanyika, 2008). Demographic, socio-structural and environmental variables must also be considered. Attitudes about and environmental contexts for physical activity are relevant. Individual behavior and lifestyle are responsive to the ecological contexts in which they are practiced (Kumanyika, 2008).

A secondary analysis of cross-sectional data from the 2004-2005 School Physical Activity and Nutrition study examined the prevalence rates of five types of beverage consumption (fruit-flavored drinks, regular sodas, diet sodas, milk, and 100% fruit juice) by sociodemographic factors among fourth, eighth, and eleventh grade public school students in Texas (Evans et al., 2010). The data revealed that the most commonly consumed beverage by all students was milk. More than 50% of students also had consumed regular soda and fruit-flavored drink during the previous day. Milk and fruit juice intake decreased with increasing grade level. By the eleventh grade, the prevalence of any beverage consumption, including milk and juice was significantly greater among boys. Ethnic differences in sugar-sweetened beverage consumption were most prevalent in eighth and eleventh grades, with the highest estimated prevalence of sugar-sweetened beverages (fruit-flavored drink and regular soda) consumption among African Americans (Evans et al., 2010).

Evidence linking restaurant food with overweight and the role of different types of restaurants among Latinos demonstrated that both child and parent body mass index scores were lowest in families selecting Mexican restaurants (Duerksen et al., 2007). The authors suggested that eating at fast-food chains and other Anglo-oriented restaurants may contribute to higher obesity rates linked to acculturation among Mexican Americans (Duerksen et al., 2007).

2.4.1 Family involvement

Home and family variables such as parenting styles, female-headed households, parental education, teen parenting, obese adults and economic insecurity may contribute to childhood obesity (Kumanyika & Grier, 2006). Parenting interventions have produced changes in factors associated with childhood obesity (Ayala et al., 2010). In 2008, researchers examined the intervention effect on (1) parenting strategies, including limit setting, monitoring, discipline, control, and reinforcement related to children's diet and physical activity; (2) parental support for physical activity; (3) parent-mediated family behaviors such as family meals eaten together and television viewing during family dinners; and (4) perceived barriers and other parent cognitions related to children's eating and activity. After 2 years, significant improvements were observed in three of five parenting strategies, parental support, and two of four parent-medicated family behaviors among parents receiving monthly visits by the promotora and monthly mailed newsletters as compared with those in the interventions targeting the school and community environments via physical and social changes such as training school personnel to promote healthy eating or modifying child menus in local restaurants) and control conditions (Ayala et al., 2010).

To determine the self-efficacy and dietary fat reduction behaviors in obese African-American and white mothers recruited from the Special Supplemental Nutrition Program for Women, Infants and Children in Wisconsin, Chang et al., 2008 designed a study to examine the influence of weight management and education on five types of fat reduction behaviors mediated through three task-specific domains of self-efficacy (negative mood, positive mood, and food availability) among young, low-income obese African-American and white mothers. The study also investigated the interaction of race with the relationships between weight management, education, self-efficacy, and fat reduction behaviors. For both racial groups, weight management status predicted low-fat food substitution and meat modifications behaviors; education predicted meat modification behavior. Three task-specific domains of self-efficacy predicted different types of fat reduction behaviors and differed by race. Weight management influenced behaviors of low-fat food substitution, meat modification and fried-food avoidance, mediated partially through self-efficacies of negative mood (African Americans), positive mood (African Americans, whites), and food availability (African Americans). Race affected the relationships between weight management, education, three task-specific domains of self-efficacy, and five types of fat reduction behaviors. Self-efficacies operated differentially for African Americans and whites (Chang et al., 2008).

The efficacy of an interactive, child-centered and family-based program in promoting healthy weigh and health behaviors in Chinese American children has been demonstrated (Chen et al., 2010) and significantly decreased body mass index, diastolic blood pressure and fat intake while increasing vegetable and fruit intake, actual physical activity and knowledge about physical activity. The authors concluded that interactive child-centered and family-based behavioral programs were feasible and effective and could be modified for other minority ethnic groups who are at high risk for overweight and obesity and have limited access to programs that promote healthy lifestyles (Chen et al., 2010).

Ellis et al., 2010 conducted a pilot randomized clinical trial to determine whether participation in an intensive, home- and community-based 6-months intervention could increase family support for healthy eating and exercise in obese African-American adolescents. Results demonstrated that participation was associated with significantly greater improvements in family encouragement for healthy eating and family participation exercise and greatly decreased discouraging behavior from family members. Increased family participation in exercise was significantly related to lower youth body mass index, percent overweight, and body fat composition (Ellis et al., 2010).

2.4.2 Frequency of family dinners

The recommendation for reducing childhood obesity from the expert committee (Barlow et al., 2007) included limiting eating out at restaurants, particularly fast food restaurants and other kinds of restaurants that serve large portions of energy-dense foods. They also included encouraging family meals in which parents and children eat together. Studies have indicated that family meals may be a protective factor against childhood obesity (Rollins et al., 2010). As limited evidence is available for children with different racial, socioeconomic and individual characteristics, Rollins' team (Rollins et al., 2010) examined data from the 2003 National Survey of Children's Health (n=16,770). This study revealed that: (1) non-Hispanic white children who consumed family meals every day were less likely to be obese than those eating meals zero to a few days per week; (2) a moderate effect for sex was observed in non-Hispanic black children, as meal frequency was marginally protective in boys but not in girls; and (3) a higher frequency of meals was a marginal risk factor for obesity in Hispanic boys from low-education households but not in girls from similar households (Rollins et al., 2010).

A similar study determined that for whites, higher frequency of family dinners was associated with (1) reduced odds of being overweight in 1997; (2) reduced odds of becoming overweight, and (3) increased odds of ceasing to be overweight in 2000 (Sen, 2006). No such associations were found for blacks and Hispanics. The author suggested that the reasons for racial and ethnic differences in the relationship between frequency of family dinners and overweight may include differences in the types and portions of food consumed at family meals.

2.4.3 Television watching

The imbalance between energy intake and energy expenditure forms the foundation for childhood obesity (Cillero & Jago, 2010). There is escalating public health concern regarding the effects of sedentary lifestyles on children and adolescents (Marshall, Gorely & Biddle, 2006). Many studies have proposed that the increased sedentary lifestyle among children and adolescents is associated with obesity (Crespo et al., 2001). Television viewing, playing digital games and using computers constitute critical sedentary activities (Rey-Lopez et al., 2008). It has been argued that not all forms of sedentary behavior contribute equally in the development of obesity. The effect of sedentary lifestyle on the risk for obesity may depend on genotype. For example, a higher risk of obesity was found among girls carrying the 27Glu allele of the ADRB2 gene, even when they spent less than 12.5 hour per week viewing television (Ochoa et al., 2006); and blunting of meal-related changes in active ghrelin and PYY in obese Hispanic youth (Mittelman et al., 2010).

Stamatakis and colleagues (Stamatakis, Hamer & Dunstan., 2011) demonstrated that recreational sitting, as reflected by television/screen time, is related to mortality and CVD risk in adults regardless of physical activity participation. Acknowledging that the precise pathways linking sitting and cardio-metabolic disease are unclear, they proposed that metabolic mechanisms e.g., disturbed lipid metabolism, might partly explain the links. A dramatic reduction of lipoprotein lipase activity by 80% to 90% during sitting compared with standing or ambulating has been reported (Stamatakis, Hamer & Dunstan, 2011).

Lipoprotein lipase is a key enzyme for the catabolism of triglyceride-rich lipoproteins in the endothelium. A reduction in its activity might raise the possibility of other metabolic actions being impaired. It has been suggested that metabolic and inflammatory pathways may partially explain the association between sitting and CVD risk (Stamatakis, Hamer & Dunstan, 2011). C-reactive protein was 3-fold higher in participants spending more than 4 hours per day in screen time. Similarly, 5 days of bed rest, which represents an extreme form of sedentary behavior, had profound effects on various metabolic risk (including insulin resistance and vascular dysfunction) but not on inflammation. Thus, low-grade inflammation might only result from chronic exposure to sedentary lifestyle (Stamatakis, Hamer & Dunstan, 2011).

To develop effective strategies to prevent and treat obesity, we must delineate and understand the relationships among childhood obesity and health behaviors such as dietary intake and sedentary lifestyles. Sedentary lifestyle has been described as "the absence of health-enhancing physical activity" (Marshall, Gorely & Biddle, 2006). Increasing the percentage of activity for children and adolescents is important for at least two reasons: (a) reallocating small amounts of sedentary time to more active behavior significantly improves energy balance and fitness and (b) epidemiologic data suggest that some sedentary behaviors track better than physical activity from childhood to adolescence (Marshall, Gorely & Biddle, 2006).

In 1985 the first assertion that television viewing may lead to obesity in some children and adolescents was published (Dietz & Gortmaker, 1985). The authors reported that the prevalence of obesity in adolescents increased 2% for each additional hour of television watched (Yen et al., 2010). They suggested that this relationship may be mediated by a direct displacement of physical activity, as well as, an increase in caloric consumption induced by food advertisements and snacking time (Dietz & Gortmaker, 1985).

The displacement hypothesis suggests that sedentary lifestyle decreases physical activity as a result of the increasing availability of high-tech devices in an industrialized lifestyle (Yen et al., 2010). Some studies on the association between sedentary behaviors and adolescent obesity have demonstrated only a weak association or no association at all. Many of these studies are not comparative and the results are not conclusive (Rey-Lopez et al., 2008). The absence of consensus has been suggested to be due to the lack of controls for confounding variables such as socioeconomic status and age (Yen et al., 2010).

During the late 1950s, sedentary behavior included an array of activities such as listening to the radio/vinyl records, reading books/comics, and television viewing (Stamatakis, Hamer & Dunstan, 2011). Contemporary activities include television viewing, Internet, compact disc/MP3 players and cellular phones. Screen time, especially television viewing, seems to be the primary indicator of "non-occupational sitting" among adults (Stamatakis, Hamer & Dunstan, 2011) and aside from sleeping, television viewing comprises most of the "domestic setting" time (Stamatakis, Hamer & Dunstan, 2011).

Previous studies have demonstrated that adolescents and young adults from racial and ethnic minority groups watch more television and are less physically active (Richmond et al., 2010; Kimbro et al., 2011). However, several studies of children and young adults have demonstrated that television viewing and weight were not statistically related in black girls (Richmond et al., 2010; Lowry et al., 2001). Limitations of previous studies include: small sample size, localized to a few cities, and study design inconsistency that prevented study comparison (Richmond et al., 2010).

"Problematic sedentary behavior" has been defined as viewing television more than 2 hours per day, using the internet more than 20 hours per week; and using the cellular phone more than 1 hour per day (Yen et al., 2010; American Academy of Pediatrics, 2001). Interestingly, not all sedentary behavior has the same potential to increase the risk of obesity. According to Yen (Yen et al., 2010) adolescents who had high television viewing had higher BMI after controlling for the effects of socio-demographic characteristics and exercise level. While the associations between BMI and television viewing and exercise level became insignificant, the interaction between television viewing and exercise level was significantly associated with BMI. Among adolescents who had a *high exercise level*, no significant difference in BMI was found between those with high and low television viewing (Yen et al., 2010). Among adolescents who had a *low exercise level*, those who had high television viewing had higher BMI than those who had low television viewing. Adolescents who had *high Internet* use had higher BMI after controlling for the effects of sex, age, residential background, parental education level and exercise level. Interactions between Internet use and sex, age, parental education and exercise level were not significantly associated with BMI (Yen et al., 2010). Among Internet use, visiting erotic websites, viewing online films and reading online news were significantly associated with increased BMI. The amount of *cellular phone* use was not significantly associated with BMI after controlling for the effects of sex, age, residential background, parental education level and exercise level. Adolescents who used cellular phones to play electronic games had increased BMI. However, sending text messages, taking pictures, accessing the Internet and transmitting music/images were not associated with BMI (Yen et al., 2010).

Marshall and colleagues (Marshall, Gorely & Biddle, 2006) completed a systemic review to (a) estimate the prevalence and dose of television viewing, video game playing and computer; (b) assess age-related trends in television viewing; and (c) secular trends in television viewing among children 18 years old and younger. Their results suggested that over the past five decades children have not had a significant increase in the number of hours they watch television (Marshall, Gorely & Biddle, 2006). In 1948 US children and teenagers viewed television approximately 3.1 hour per day for 6 to 12 year olds and 2.6 hours per day for 13 to 19 year olds. In 1949, the average viewing time was 3.4 hours per day. In 1950s the average time was 2.6 hours per day. The television viewing times increased between 6-11 years, decreased between 11 to 15 years and peaked between 9-12 years (Marshall, Gorely & Biddle, 2006).

Today, children and adolescents watch 1.8 to 2.8 hours of television per day; 66% are "low users" (less than 2 hours per day); 28% watch more than 4 hours per day; boys and girls with access to video games spend approximately 60 minutes and 23 minutes per day, respectively playing video games (Marshall, Gorely & Biddle, 2006). Computers are used an additional 30 minutes per day and, on average, television viewing decreases during adolescence. However, high television users at a young age tend to remain high users when older (Marshall, Gorely & Biddle, 2006).

A meta-analysis found that a statistically significant relationship exists between obesity and television viewing among children and youth; but, the relation was too small to be of substantial clinical relevance (Gorely, Marshall, & Biddle, 2004). Television viewing is often associated with lower levels of physical activity among girls (Gorely, Marshall & Biddle, 2004) and it appears to have an independent relationship with weight status even after controlling for levels of physical activity (Richmond et al., 2010; Eisenmann et al., 2008).

After controlling for confounding variables Yen and colleagues (Yen et al., 2010) found adolescents with high television viewing or high Internet use had increased BMI. The relationship between BMI and television viewing and Internet use were statistically significant. Yet, they cautioned that similar to other studies, television viewing and Internet use only accounted for a very small variance in BMI. They also raised a provocative question as to whether the Internet and cellular phones may provide overweight adolescents who have low self-esteem alternatives through which they can reduce social interaction and feel more comfortable (Yen et al., 2010).

There is evidence that adolescents and young adults from racial and ethnic minority groups watch more television and are less physically active than their white peers (Crespo et al., 2001; Richmond 2010).

Yet, some studies have found that television viewing and weight are not statistically related in preadolescent to young adult black females (Richmond et al., 2010). Richmond and colleagues suggested that the lack of a relationship between television viewing and BMI among black girls may be one reason why some studies using racially heterogeneous populations have had not demonstrated a positive association (Richmond et al., 2010). In the study by Richmond et al (Richmond 2010), black females reported watching television 15 hours per week compared to 11 hours per week for both Hispanic and white females; BMI increased with greater time spent watching television; those who watched 8 to 14 hours per week had BMIs that were on average 0.8kg/meter-squared higher and those who watched greater than 14 hours per week had BMIs that were on average 1.2 kg/meter-squared higher than those who watched 7 hours of less per week. Having at least one obese parent was associated with a 3.7 kg/meter-squared increase in BMI relative to those without an obese parent. Overall all, black, Mexican-American, and Puerto Rican females were all significantly heavier than their white peers (Richmond et al., 2010). When data was stratified by race/ethnicity, they found similar results among white females between television viewing and BMI as in the overall population. Among both black and Hispanic females, they found no association between television viewing and BMI. They proposed that these differences may represent the fact that: (1) the majority of blacks are beyond some threshold effect for television exposure (Richmond et al., 2010); (2) blacks interact with television media differently than whites (Richmond et al., 2010); (3) blacks are less susceptible to the effects of television advertising than whites [16]; (4) the television is more likely to be on throughout the day in black homes so reported television viewing hours may not have their full attention and thus have less of an impact (Richmond et al., 2010; Henderson, 2007); and (5) television is such a small factor in the lives of black Americans relative to other obesity-prone aspects of their environment (Richmond et al., 2010).

2.4.4 Healthful eating

The childhood obesity expert committee (Barlow et al., 2007) recommended that families adopt and maintain healthy habits that may help prevent excessive weight gain. These recommendations included eating diets with the recommended quantities of fruits and vegetables, rich in calcium, high in fiber and with a balanced source of energy from fat, carbohydrates and protein as well as limiting portion size, limiting consumption of sugar-sweetened beverages and eating breakfast daily.

Breakfast consumption has been a frequent focus of studies exploring dietary intake among adolescents and overall health (Merten et al., 2009). Analysis of the relationship between breakfast and obesity over time and in relation to weight outcome in young adulthood (Merten et al., 2009) revealed that adolescent regular breakfast consumption significantly predicted young adult regular breakfast consumption and an important factor associated with adolescents eating breakfast was having at least one parent home in the morning. Regular consumption during both adolescence and young adulthood prevented obesity in both periods. Living in disadvantaged communities decreased the odds adolescents would eat breakfast during adolescence and increased their chances for chronic obesity (Merten et al., 2009).

The role of sugar-sweetened beverages in obesity remains a source of research. In a representative sample of 365 low-income African-American preschool 3-5-year-old children investigators sought to determine the association between sugar-sweetened beverage consumption (soda, fruit drinks, and both combined) and overweight and obesity (Lim et al., 2009). After two years, the prevalence of overweight increased from 13% to 19% and the prevalence of obesity increased from 10% to 20%. The authors concluded that high consumption of sugar-sweetened beverages was significantly associated with an increased risk of obesity (Lim et al., 2009).

The Memphis Girls health Enrichment Multi-site Studies tested the effectiveness of a 2-year family-based intervention to reduce excessive increase in body mass index by promoting healthy eating habits and increasing physical activity in 303 healthy African-American girls, ages 8-10 years old along with one parent/caregiver. It was a randomized, controlled trail conducted at community centers. The main outcome measure was the difference in body mass index between the control and intervention groups. At the end of the 2-year trial the body mass index increased in all girls and no significant treatment effect was noted. However, positive effects were observed with a reduction of daily consumption of sweetened beverages and an increased consumption of water and vegetables. Nonetheless, the authors concluded that this particular intervention alone was insufficient for obesity prevention (Klesges et al., 2008; Klesges et al., 2010).

2.5 Built environment concept

The built environment consists of the neighborhoods, roads, buildings, food sources, and recreational facilities in which people live, work, are educated, eat, and play (Sallis & Glanz, 2006). The debate is ongoing as to whether recent changes in the built environment have promoted sedentary lifestyles and encouraged less healthful diets (Sallis & Glanz, 2006). The physical design and quality of neighborhoods may determine where and how often children and adolescents participate in physical activity and parents may restrict their children's outdoor activities if neighborhood safety is a concern (Kumanyika & Grier, 2006). Additionally, family work schedules, discretionary time, money, and car ownership may adversely affect the ability of parents and caregivers in low-income communities to transport children to sports and other activities (Kumanyika & Grier, 2006).

While these arguments may be logical, research on the link between neighborhood socioeconomic status and obesity in child and adolescents is mixed, with some studies showing strong correlations among neighborhood, obesity, and physical activity and others showing little to no effect (Kimbro et al., 2011). Contrary to expectations, one study demonstrated some interesting findings among 5-year old children living in public housing (Kimbro et al., 2011). The authors showed that the poorest and wealthiest children had the lowest BMIs, while children in the middle of the socioeconomic distribution had the highest body mass indices; that the hours of outdoor play and television watching were both associated with body mass index, as was the ratio of outdoor play to television watching; that children living in public housing and those living in the neighborhoods with higher levels of physical disorder were playing outdoors more often than other children; and that children of mothers who perceived a high level of collective efficacy in their neighborhoods were playing outside for longer periods of time daily, watching television less and visiting the park or playground more often each week (Kimbro et al., 2011). Neighborhood safety may be modified by the mother's perceived neighborhood cohesiveness and social support as neighborhood cohesiveness had little to do with the actual physical state of the neighborhood environment (Kimbro et al., 2011).

Scientific evidence as to whether the built environment can directly affect childhood obesity and whether improvements to the built environment can encourage more physical activity and more healthful diets is limited (Sallis & Glanz, 2006; Kumanyika & Grier, 2006). Researchers have found many links between the built environment and children's physical activity but have not provided conclusive evidence that aspects of the built environment promote obesity. Obviously, barriers such as an absence of sidewalks, living long distances from schools, and the need to cross busy streets can discourage walking and biking to school. However, while removing these barriers may increase rates of "active commuting", there is no scientific evidence that more "active commuting" reduces the rates of obesity (Sallis & Glanz, 2006). Although research into the link between the built environment and childhood obesity is relative new, it is reasonable to assume that individuals who live in safe neighborhoods that enhance walking, and offer local markets with healthful food are likely to be more active and to eat more healthful foods (Sallis & Glanz, 2006).

2.6 Significance of food deserts and food insecurity

Food deserts describe areas that do not have easy access (within walking distance in cities or a reasonable driving distance in rural areas) to healthy foods, usually in the form of a supermarket. In urban areas, food desert also implies that the area is low income and residents may not own or have easy access to a vehicle, therefore, access to healthy foods must be within reasonable walking distance. Food security refers to the availability of food and one's access to it. A household is considered food-secure when its occupants do not live in hunger or fear of starvation (http://en.wikipedia.org/wiki/Food_security). More than

23% of American households with children did not have enough money to buy food in 2010 (http://www.upi.com/Health_News/2011/08/11).

For parents poor food quality and discrimination affect parent's food choices and their perceptions of food availability in their neighborhood (Sealy, 2010). Within communities with lower than average availability of healthful foods, higher than average availability of fast food restaurants, and increased exposure to ethnically-targeted food marketing may result in dependency on high calorie foods and beverages which are valued both socially and culturally. (Kumanyika, 2008).

Food-related parenting attitudes may influence children's dietary intake and weight. In food-insecure families, attitudes toward making healthful foods available were inversely associated with children's daily energy intake and body mass index among fifth grade Mexican-American students (Matheson et al., 2006). In food-secure families, attitudes about making healthful foods available were positively associated with children's fruit intake and percentage of energy from fats. Additionally, parental modeling of healthful food behavior was inversely associated with the energy density of foods (Matheson et al., 2006).

2.7 Relationship between economics and attitudes toward health

An analysis of data from the National Survey of Children's Health collected from 2003 to 2004 revealed that poverty impacts body mass index in at least two specific ways: unsafe neighborhoods and the cost and availability of healthy foods in low income communities (Lutfiyya et al., 9220). Overweight children were more likely to be African American and Hispanic than white; be males; live in households with incomes below 150% of Federal poverty level; watch television three hours or more daily; and not have received preventive care in the past 12 months. Overweight children were less likely to get minimum levels of moderate physical activity or have participated on a sports team (Groholt et al., 2008).

Utilizing data from the National Ambulatory Medical Care Survey and the National Hospital Ambulatory Medical Care Survey from 2001 to 2004, the frequency of clinician-reported delivery of obesity-prevention counseling at well-child visits was assessed (Branner et al., 2008). The results revealed that of 55,695,554 (weighted) visits, 24.4% included obesity prevention counseling; 15.4% of Hispanic patients received obesity prevention counseling compared to 28.8% of non-Hispanics. Frequencies of counseling were similar between whites and blacks, 25% and 27.1% respectively. Disparity was noted between frequency of counseling and insurance as 26.9% of patients with private insurance received more counseling compared to 19.1% of Medicaid patients and 15.1% of self-pay patients (Branner et al., 2008).

3. Conclusion

Obesity should be addressed through a comprehensive approach across multiple settings and sectors that can change individual nutrition and physical activity behavior and the environments and policies that affect these behaviors. New and continued national, state, and community-level surveillance of obesity, its behavioral risk factors, and the environment and polices that affect these behaviors is critical (MMWR 2010; 59(30):951-955).

Based on this review of several recent studies, some of the previously published findings on childhood obesity in communities of diverse ethnicity and low-socioeconomics must be refuted, supported or recommended as areas for further reach. Specifically, this review did not identify any theories that can be unequivocally refuted for all low-income and ethnically diverse communities. The review supports the findings of the prevailing overweight/obesity prevalence disparity and has identified several areas where further research is warranted. The areas for future research include:

1. Is there a "critical body mass index" at which the number of hours of watching television is no longer effective in preventing obesity?
2. Are the adverse psychosocial effects of overweight/obesity in low-income and ethnically diverse communities age-independent?
3. Would correction of the child-parent/caretaker body image dissatisfaction discrepancy be an effective means of reducing overweight/obesity?
4. Does the frequency of family meals prevent overweight among blacks and Hispanics?
5. Are child-centered, family based interventions effective in all low-income and ethnically diverse settings?
6. As neighborhood safety is an important but not the only factor that will determine parental willingness to allow their children to participate in outdoor physical activity what other factors should be explored and enhanced?

It was not the aim of this review to be an exhaustive review of the literature. We hoped to provide an up-to-date summary of some of the more recent studies and to stimulate discussion among researchers focused on the quality of life impact of childhood obesity for members of low-socioeconomic and diverse communities based on more recent data. The review confirms the need for ongoing research in several areas relative to childhood obesity and hopefully will be a useful resource for future researchers and funders. The primary limitation of this review includes the fact that the review was limited and utilized only one major data source, PubMed. Additionally, there may have been selection bias on the part of the author. As we continue to search for effective interventions to reduce the prevalence of overweight and obesity among children living in low-income and diverse communities, it will be critical to have evidence-based data generated from comparative studies using multiple data sources.

4. Acknowledgement

Special thanks to Misa Mi, PhD, former medical librarian, at The University of Toledo Medical Center, for her assistance with the literature review.

5. References

Akresh, I. (2008). Overweight and obesity among foreign-born and U.S.-born Hispanics. *Biodemography & Social Biology*. Vol. 54, No2, (Fall, 2008), pp.183-199, ISSN 1948-5565.

American Academy of Pediatrics. (2001). Children, adolescents, and television. *Pediatrics*. Vol.107, No.2, (Feb, 2001), pp.423-426, ISSN 0031-4005.

Amin, R., Anthony L., Virend, S., Fenchel, M., McConnell, K., Jefferies, J., Willging, P., Kalra, M. & Daniels, S. (2008). Growth velocity predicts recurrence of sleep-disordered breathing 1 year after adenotonsillectomy. *American Journal of Respiratory & Critical Care Medicine*. Vol.177, No.6 (Jan., 2008), pp. 654-659, ISSN 1073-440X.

Ayala, G., Elder, J., Arredondo, E., Ayala, G., Slymen, D. Campbell, N. & Slymen, D. (2010). Longitudinal intervention effects on parenting of the Aventuras para Ninos study. *American Journal of Preventive Medicine*. Vol.38, No.2, (Feb., 2010), pp.154-162, ISSN 0749-3797.

Bacardi-Gascon, M., Leon-Reyes, M. & Jimenez-Cruz, A. (2007). Stigmatization of overweight Mexican children. *Child Psychiatry Human & Development*. Vol.38, No.2, (Aug., 2007), pp.99-105, ISSN 0009-398X.

Balkrishnan, R., Webster, P. & Sinclair, D. (2008). Trends in overweight and obesity among 5-7-year-old white and South Asian children born between 1991 and 1999. *Journal of Public Health (Oxford)*. Vol.30., No.2, pp.139-144, ISSN 1741-3842.

Baltrus, P., Everson-Rose, S., Lynch, J., Raghunathan, T. & Kaplan, G. (2007). Socioeconomic position in childhood and adulthood and weight gain over 34 years: the Alameda County Study. *Annals of Epidemiology*. Vol.17, No.8, (Aug., 2007), pp.608-614, ISSN 1047-2797.

Barlow, S. and the Expert Committee (2007). Expert Committee recommendations regarding the prevention, assessment, andtreatment of child and adolescent overweight and obesity: summary report. *Pediatrics*. Vol.120. Supplement 4, (Dec., 2007), ppS164-S192, ISSN0031-4005.

Banitt, A., Kaur, H., Pulvers, K., Nollen, N., Ireland, M. & Fitzgibbon, M. (2008). BMI percentiles and body image discrepancy in black and white adolescents. *Obesity (Silver Spring)*. Vol.16, No.5, (May, 2008), pp.987-991, ISSN 1930-7381.

Bennett, G. & Wolin, K. (2006). Statisfied or unaware: racial differences in perceived weight status. *International Journal of Behavioral Nutrition & Physical Activity*. Vol.3, No. 1, pp.40, ISSN 1479-5868.

Bhardwaj, S., Misra, A., Khurana, L., Gulati, S., Shah, P. & Vikram, N. (2008). Childhood obesity in Asian Indians: a burgeoning cause of insulin resistance, diabetes and sub-clinical inflammation. *Asia Pacific Journal of Clinical Nutrition*. Vol.17 Suppl1, pp.172-175, ISSN 0964-7058.

Branner, C., Koyama, T. & Jensen, G. (2008). Racial and ethnic differences in pediatric obesity-prevention counseling: national prevalence of clinician practices. *Obesity (Silver Spring)*. Vol.16, No.3, (Mar, 2008), pp.690-694, ISSN 1930-7381.

Burroughs, V., Nonas, C., Sweeney, C., Rohay, J., Harkins, A., Kyle, T. & Burton, S. (2008). Self-reported comorbidities among self-described overweight African-American and Hispanic adults in the United States: results of a national survey. *Obesity (Silver Spring)*. Vol.16, No.6, (Jun., 2008), pp.1400-1406, ISSN 1930-7381.

Burnet, D., Plaut, A., Ossowski, K., Ahmad, A., Quinn, M., Radovick, S. Gorawara-Bhat, R. & Chin, M. (2008). Community and family perspectives on addressing overweight in urban, African-American youth. *Journal of General Internal Medicine*. Vol.23, No.2, (Feb., 2008), pp. 175-179, ISSN 0884-8734.

Calzada, P. & Anderson-Worts, P. (2009). The obesity epidemic: are minority individuals equally affected? *Primary Care*. Vol.36, No.2, (Jun., 2009), pp.307-317, ISSN 0095-4543.

Centers for Disease Control & Prevention. (2010). Vital signs: state-specific obesity prevalence among adults—United States, 2009. *Morbidity Mortality Weekly Report*. Vol.59, No.30, (Aug, 2010), pp.951-955.

Centers for Disease Control & Prevention. (2011). Grand Rounds: Childhood obesity in the United States. *Morbidity Mortality Weekly Report* . Vol.60, No.2, pp.42-46.

Chang, M., Brown, R., Baumann, L., & Nitzk, S. (2008). Self-efficacy and dietary fat reduction behaviors in obese African-American and white mothers. *Obesity (Silver Spring)*. Vol.16, No.5, (May, 2008), pp.992-1001, ISSN 1930-7381.

Chen, J. (2009). Household income, maternal acculturation, maternal education level and health behaviors of Chinese-American children and mothers. *Journal Immigrant & Minority Health*. Vol.11, No.3, (Jun, 2009), pp.198-204, ISSN 1557-1912.

Chen, J., Weiss, S., Heyman, M. & Lustig, R. (2010). Efficacy of a child-centered and family-based program in promoting healthy weight and healthy behaviors in Chinese American children: a randomized controlled study. *Journal of Public Health (Oxford)*. Vol.32, No.2, (Jun., 2010), pp.219-229, ISSN 1741-3842.

Clarke, P., O'Malley P., Johnston, L. & Schulenberg, J. (2009). Social disparities in BMI trajectories across adulthood by gender, race/ethnicity and lifetime socio-economic position: 1986-2008. *International Journal of Epidemiology*. Vol.38, No.2, pp.499-509, ISSN 0300-5771.

Copeland, K., Zeitler, P., Geffner, M., Guandalini, c., Higgins, J., Hirst, K., Kaufman, F., Linder, B., Marcovina, s. McGuigan, P., Pyle, L., Tamborlane, W. & Willi, S. (2011). Characteristics of adolescents and youth with recent-onset type 2 diabetes: the TODAY cohort at baseline. *Journal of Clinical Endocrinology Metabolism*. Vol.96, No.1, (Jan., 2011), pp.159-167, ISSN 0021-972X.

Crespo, C., Smit, E., Troiano, R., Bartlett, S., Macera, C. & Andersen, R. (2001). Television watching, energy intake and obesity in US children. *Archives of Pediatrics & Adolescent Medicine*. Vol.155, No.3, (Mar., 2001), pp.360-365, ISSN 1072-4710.

Daniels, S. (2006). The consequences of childhood overweight and obesity. *Future of Children*. Vol.16, No.1 (Spring, 2006), pp47-67, ISSN 1054-8289..

Dietz, W. & Gortmaker, S. (1985). Do we fatten our children at the television set? Obesity and television viewing in children and adolescents. *Pediatrics*. Vol.75, No. 5, (May, 1985), pp.807-812, ISSN 0031-4005.

Duerksen, S., Elder, J., Arredondo, E., Ayala, G., Slymen, d. Campbell, N. & Baquero, B. (2007). Family restaurant choices are associated with child and adult overweight status in Mexican-American families. *Journal of the American Dietetic Association*. Vol.107, No.5, (May, 2007), pp.849-853, ISSN 0002-8233.

Eisenmann, J., Bartee, R., Smith, D., Welk, G. & Fu, Q. (2008). Combined influence of physical activity and television viewing on the risk of overweight in US youth. *International Journal of Obesity*. Vol.32, No.4, (Apr., 2008), pp.613-618, ISSN 0307-0565.

Elder, J., Arredondo, E., Campbell, N., Baquero, B., Duerksen, S., Ayala, G., Crespo, N. slymen, D. & McKenzie, T. (2010).

Individual, family, and community environmental correlates of obesity in Latino elementary school children. *Journal of School Health*. Vol.80, No.1, (Jan., 2010), pp.20-30, ISSN 0022-4391.

Ellis, D., Janisse, H., Naar-King, S., Kolmodin, K., Jen, K., Cunningham, P. & Marshall, S. (2010). The effects of multisystemic therapy on family support for weight loss among obese African-American adolescents: findings from a randomized controlled trial. *Journal of Developmental & Behavioral Pediatrics*. Vol. 31, No.6, (Jul/Aug., 2010), pp.461-468, ISSN 0196-206X.

Evans, A., Springer A., Evans, M., Ranjit, N. & Hoelschner, D. (2010). A descriptive study of beverage consumption among an ethnically diverse sample of public school students in Texas. *Journal of the American College of Nutrition*. Vol.29, No.4, (Aug., 2010), pp.387-396, ISSN 0731-5724.

Finkelstein, E., Brown, D., Wrage, L., Allaire, B. & Hoerger, T. (2010). Individual and aggregate years-of-life-lost associated with overweight and obesity. *Obesity (Silver Spring)*. Vol.18, No.2, (Feb., 2010), pp.333-339, ISSN 1930-7381.

Finkelstein E, Fiebelkorn, I. & Wang, G. National medical spending attributable to overweight and obesity: how much, and who's paying. Accessed 07/19/2011. Available from <http://content.healthaffairs.org/content/suppl/2003/12/05/hlthaff.w3.219.v1.DC1.>

Food security. Accessed Aug 10, 2011. Available from <http://en.wikipedia.org/wiki/Food_security>.

Fullerton, G., Tyler, C., Johnston, C., Vincent, J., Harris, G. & Foreyt, J. (2007). Quality of life in Mexican-American children following a weight management program. *Obesity (Silver Spring)*. Vol.15, No.11, (Nov., 2007), pp.2553-2556, ISSN 1930-7381.

Galloway, T., Young, T. & Egeland, G. (2010). Emerging obesity among preschool-aged Canadian Inuit children: results from the Nunavut Inuit Child Health Survey. *International Journal of Circumpolar Health*. Vol.69., No.2, pp.151-157, ISSN 1239-9736.

Gee, G., Ro, A., Gavin, A. & Takeuchi, D. (2008). Disentangling the effects of racial and weight discrimination on body mass index and obesity among Asian Americans. *American Journal of Public Health*. Vol.98, No.3, (Mar 2008), pp.493-500, ISSN 0090-0036.

Gilliard, T., Lackland, D., Mountford, W. & Egan, B. (2007). Concordance between self-reported heights and weights and current and ideal body images in young adult African American men and women. *Ethnicity & Disease*. Vol.17, No.4, pp.617-623, ISSN 1049-510X.

Gorely, T., Marshall, S. & Biddle, S. (2004). Couch kids: Correlates of television viewing among youth. *International Journal of Behavioral Medicine*. Vol.11, No.3, (Sep., 2004), pp.152-163, ISSN 1070-5503.

Goulding, A., Grant, A., Taylor, R., Williams, S., Parnell, W., Wilson, N. & Mann, J. (2007). Ethnic differences in extreme obesity. *Journal of Pediatrics*. Vol.151, No.5, (Nov., 2007), pp.542-544, ISSN 0022-3476.

Greves-Grow, H., Cook, A., Arterburn, D., Saelens, B., Drewnowski, A. & Lazano, P. (2010). Child obesity associated with social disadvantage of children's neighborhoods. *Social Science & Medicine*. Vol.71, No.3, (Aug., 2010), pp.584-591, ISSN 0277-9536.

Groholt, E., Stigum H. & Nordhagen, R. (2008). Overweight and obesity among adolescents in Norway: cultural and socio-economic differences. *Journal of Public Health (Oxford)*. Vol.30, No.3, pp.258-265, ISSN 1741-3842.

Grund, A., Krause, H., Siewers, M., Rieckert, H., Muller, M. (2001). Is TV viewing an index of physical activity and fitness in overweight and normal weight children? *Public Health Nutrition*. Vol.4, No.6, (Dec., 2001), pp.1245-1251, ISSN 1368-9800.

Guldan, G. (2010). Asian children's obesogenic diets-time to change this part of the energy balance equation? *Research in Sports Medicine*. Vol.18., No.1, (Jan-Mar., 2010), pp.5-15, ISSN 1543-8627.

Hackie, M. & Bowles, C. (2007). Maternal perception of their overweight children. *Public Health Nursing*. Vol.24, No.6, (Nov., 2007), pp.538-546, ISSN 0737-1209.

Hancox, R. & Poulton, R. (2006). Watching television is associated with childhood obesity: but is it clinically important? *International Journal of Obesity*. Vol.30, No.1, (Jan., 2006), pp.171-175, ISSN 0307-0565.

Hanson, M. & Chen, E. (2007). Socioeconomic status, race and body mass index: The mediating role of physical activity and sedentary behaviors during adolescence. *Journal of Pediatric Psychology*. Vol.32, No.3, (Apr., 2007), pp.250-259, ISSN 0146-8693.

Health-Related Quality Of Life Concepts. Accessed 06/24/2011. Available from < http://www.cdc.gov/hrqol/concept.htm>.

Henderson, V. (2007). Longitudinal associations between television viewing and body mass index among white and black girls. *Journal of Adolescent Health*. Vol.41, No.6, (Dec., 2007), pp.544-550, ISSN 1054-139X.

Hermanussen, M., Molinari, L., Satake, T. (2007). BMI in Japanese children since 1948: no evidence of a major rise in the prevalence of obesity in Japan. *Anthropologischer Anzeiger*. Vol.65, No.3, (Sep., 2007), pp.275-283.

Hoyos-Cillero, I., & Jago, R. (2010). Systematic review of correlates of screen-viewing among young children. *Preventive Medicine*. Vol.51, No.1, (Jul., 2010), pp.3-10, ISSN 0091-7435.

Klesges, R., Obarzanek, E., Klesges, L., Stockton, M., Beech, B., Murray, D., Lanctot, J. & Sherrill-Mittleman, D. (2008). The Memphis Girls health Enrichment Multi-site Studies (GEMS): phase 2: design and baseline. *Contemporary Clinical Trials*. Vol.29, No.1, (Jan., 2008), pp42-55, ISSN 1551-7144.

Klesges, R., Obarzanek, E., Kumanyika, S., Murray, D., Klesges, L., Relyea, G., Stockton, M., Lanctot, J., Beech, B., McClanahan, B., Sherrill-Mittleman, D. & Slawson, D.. (2010). The Memphis Girls health Enrichment Multi-site

Studies (GEMS): an evaluation of the efficacy of a 2-year obesity prevention program in African American girls. *Archives of Pediatric & Adolescent Medicine*. Vol.164, No.11, (Nov., 2010), pp1007-1014, ISSN 1072-4710.

Killion, L., Hughes, S, Wendt, J., Pease, D. & Nickas, T. (2006). Minority mothers' perceptions of children's body size. *International Journal of Pediatric Obesity*.Vol.1., No.12, (Apr., 2006),pp96-102, ISSN 1747-7166.

Kimbro, R., Brooks-Gunn, J. & McLanahan, S. (2011). Young children in urban areas: Links among neighborhood characteristics, weight status, outdoor play, and television watching. *Social Science & Medicine*. Vol.72, No.5, (Mar., 2011), pp.668-676, ISSN 0277-9536.

Kumanyika, S. (2008). Environmental influences on childhood obesity: ethnic and cultural influences in context. *Physiology & Behavior*. Vol.94, No.1, (Apr., 2008), pp.61-70, ISSN 0031-9384.

Kumanyika, S. & Grier, S. (2006). Targeting interventions for ethnic minority and low-income populations. *Future of Children*. Vol.16, No.1, (Spring 2006), pp.187-207, ISSN 1054-8289.

Latner, J., Simmonds M., Rosewell, J. & Stunkard, A. (2007). Assessment of obesity stigmatization in children and adolescents: modernizing a standard measure. *Obesity (Silvery Spring)*. Vol.15, No.12, (Dec., 2007), pp.3078-3085, ISSN 1930-7381.

Latner, J. & Stunkard, A. (2003). Getting worse: The stigmatization of obese children. *Obesity Research. Vol.*11, No.3, (Mar., 2003), pp.452-456.

Lieb, D., Snow, R. & DeBoer, M. (2009). Socioeconomic factors in the development of childhood obesity and diabetes. *Clinics in Sports Medicine*. Vol.28, No.3, (Jul., 2009), pp.349-378, ISSN 0278-5919.

Lim, S., Zoellner, J., Lee, J., Burt, B., Sandretto, A., Sohn, W., Ismail, A. & Lepkowski, J. (2009). Obesity and sugar-sweetened beverages in African-American preschool children: a longitudinal study. Obesity (Sliver Spring). Vol 17.,No.6 (Jun 2009),pp1262, ISSN 1262-1268.

Lowry, R., Wechsler, H., Galuska, D., Fulton, J. & Kann L. (2002). Television viewing and its associations with overweight, sedentary lifestyle, and insufficient consumption of fruits and vegetables among US high school students: differences by race, ethnicity, and gender. *Journal of School Health*. Vol.72, No.10, (Dec., 2002), pp.*413-421, ISSN 0022-4391.*

Lutfiyya, M., Garcia R., Dankwa, C., Young, T. & Lipsky, M. (2008). Overweight and obese prevalence rates in African American and Hispanic children: an analysis of data from the 2003-2004 National survey of Children's Health. *Journal of the American Board Family Medicine*. Nol.21, No.3, (May-Jun., 2008) pp.191-199, ISSN 1557-2625.

Marshall, S., Biddle, S., Gorely, T., Cameron, N. & Murdey, I. (2004). Relationships between media use, body fatness and physical activity in children and youth: A meta-analysis. *International Journal of Obesity & Related Metabolic Disorders*. Vol.28, No.10, (Oct., 2004), pp.1238-1246, ISSN 0307-0565.

Marshall, S., Gorely, T. & Biddle S. (2006). A descriptive epidemiology of screen-based media use in youth; A review and critique. *Journal of Adolescence*. Vol.29, No.3, (Jun., 2006), pp.333-349, ISSN 0140-1971.

Matheson, D., Robinson, T., Varady, A. & Killen, J. (2006). Do Mexican-American mothers' food-related parenting practices influence their children's weight and dietary intake. *Journal of American Dietetic Association*. Vol.106, No.11, (No., 2006), pp.1861-1865, ISSN 0002-8223.

Matsushita, Y., Yoshiike, N., Kaneda, F., Yoshita, K. & Takimoto, H. (2004). Trends in childhood obesity in Japan over the last 25 years from the National Nutrition Survey. *Obesity Research*. Vol.12, No.12, (Feb 2004).

McAlexander, K., Banda J., McAlexander, J. & Lee, R. (2009). Physical activity resource attributes and obesity in low-income African Americans. *Journal of Urban Health*. Vol.86, No.5, (Sep., 2009), pp.696-707, ISSN 1468-2869.

McCormack, L., Laska, M., Gray, C., Veblen-Mortenson, S., Barr-Aderson, D. & Story, M. (2011). Weight-related teasing in a racially diverse sample of sixth-grade children. J*ournal of American Dietetic Association*. Vol.111, No.3, (Mar., 2011), pp.431-436, ISSN 0002-8223.

McGuire, J., Szabo, A., Jackson, S., Bradley, G. & Okunseri, C. (2009). Erosive tooth wear among children in the United States: relationship to race/ethnicity and obesity. *International Journal of Paediatric Dentistry*. Vol.19, No.2, (Mar. 2009), pp.91-98, ISSN 0960-7439.

Merten, M., Williams, A. & Shriver, L. (2009). Breakfast consumption in adolescence and young adulthood: parental presence, community context, and obesity. *Journal of the American Dietetic Association*. Vol.109, No.8, (Aug., 2009), pp.1384-1391, ISSN 0002-8223.

Messiah, S., Carrillo-Iregui, A., Garibay-Nieto, N., Lopez-Mitnik, G., Cossio, S. & Arheart, K. (2009). Prevalence of metabolic syndrome in US-born Latin and Caribbean youth. *Journal of Immigrant & Minority Health*. Vol.11, No.5, (Oct., 2009), pp.366-371, ISSN 1557-1912.

Midie, A., & Matthews, K. (2009). Social relationships and negative emotional traits are associated with central adiposity and arterial stiffness in healthy adolescents. *Health Psychology*. Vol.28, No.3, (May, 2009), pp.347-353, ISSN 0278-6133.

Mitola, A., Papas, M., Le, K., Fusillo, L. & Black, M. (2007). Agreement with satisfaction in adolescent body size between female caregivers and teens from a low-income African-American community. *Journal of Pediatric Psychology*. Vol.32, No.1, (Jan., 2007), pp.42-51, ISSN 0146-8693.

Mittelman, S., Klier, K., Braun, S., Azen, C., Geffner, M., Buchanan, T. (2010). Obese adolescents show impaired meal responses of the appetite-regulating hormones ghrelin and PYY. *Obesity*. Vol.18, No.5, (May, 2010), pp.918-925, ISSN 1930-7381.

Modi, A., Loux, T., Bell, S., Harmon, C., Inge, T. & Zeller, M. (2008). Weight-specific health-related quality of life in adolescents with extreme obesity. *Obesity (Sliver Springs)* Vol.16, No.10 (Oct., 2008), pp. 2266-2271, ISSN 1930-7381.

Molaison, E., Kolbo, J., Zhang, L., Harbaugh, B., Armstrong, M., Rushing, K., Blom, L. & Green, A. (2010). Prevalence and trends in obesity among Mississippi public school students, 2005-2009. *Journal Mississippi State Medical* Association. Vol.51, No.3, (Mar., 2010), pp.67-72, ISSN 0026-6396.

More than 23 percent went hungry in the U.S. in 2010. Available from <http://www.upi.com/Health_News/2011/08/11/More-than-23-percent-went-hungry-in-the-US-in-2010/UPI-64421313119188/. Accessed Aug 12, 2011.

Munter, P., He, J., Cutler, J., Wildman, R. & Whelton, P. (2004). Trends in blood pressure among children and adolescents. *Journal of the American Medical Association*. Vol.291, No.17, (May, 2004), pp.2107-2113, ISSN 0098-7484.

Ochoa, M., Moreno-Aliaga, M., Martinez-Gonzalez, M., Martinez J. & Marti, A. GENOI Members. (2006). TV watching modifies obesity risk linked to the 27GLU polymorphism of the ADRB2 gene in girls. *International Journal of Pediatric Obesity*. Vol.1, No.2, (Apr., 2006), pp.83-88, ISSN 1747-7166.

Proctor, M., Moore, L., Gao, D, Cupples, L., Bradlee, M., Hood, M. & Ellison R. (2003). Television viewing and change in body fat from preschool to early adolescence: The Framingham Children's study. *International Journal of Obesity and Related Metabolic Disorders*. Vol.27, No.7, (Jul., 2003), pp.827-833, ISSN 0307-0565.

Quality of Life. Accessed 06/24/2011. Available from <http://en.wikipedia.org/wiki/Quality_of_life>.

Rey-Lopez, J., Vicente-Rodriguez, G., Biosca, M. & Moreno, L. (2008). Sedentary behavior and obesity development in children and adolescents. *Nutrition, Metabolism and Cardiovascular Diseases*. Vol.18, No. 3, (Mar., 2003), pp.242-251, ISSN 0939-4753.

Richmond, T., Walls, C., Gooding, H. & Field, A. (2010). Television viewing is not predictive of BMI in Black and Hispanic young adult females. *Obesity (Silver Spring)*. Vol. 18, No.5, (May, 2010), pp.1015-1020, ISSN 1930-7381.

Rollins, B., Belue, R. & Francis, L. (2010). The beneficial effect of family meals on obesity differs by race, sex, and household education: the national survey of children's health, 2003-2004. *Journal of the American Dietetic Association*. Vol.110, No.9, (Sep., 2010), pp.1335-1339, ISSN 0002-8223.

Rudnick, E., Walsh, J., Hampton, M. & Mitchell, R. (2007). Prevalence and ethnicity of sleep-disordered breathing and obesity in children. *Otolaryngology Head Neck Surgery*. Vol.137, No.6 (Dec., 2007), pp. 878-882, ISSN 0194-5998.

Sallis, J. & Glanz, K. (2006). The role of built environments in physical activity, eating and obesity in childhood. *Future of Children*. Vol.16., No.1, (Spring, 2006), pp.89-108, ISSN1054-8289.

Scharoun-Lee, M., Adair, L., Kaufman, J. & Gordon-Larsen, P. (2009). Obesity, race/ethnicity and the multiple dimensions of socioeconomic status during the transition to adulthood: a factor analysis approach. *Social Science & Medicine*. Vol.68, No.4, (Feb 2009), pp.708-716, ISSN 0277-9536.

Scharoun-Lee, M., Kaufman, J., Popkin, B. & Gordon-Larsen, P. (2009). Obesity, race/ethnicity and life course socioeconomic status across the transition from adolescence to adulthood. *Journal of Epidemiology & Community Health*. Vol.63, No.2, (Feb, 2009), pp.133-139.

Sealy, Y. (2010). Parents' perceptions of food availability: implications for childhood obesity. *Social Work Health Care*. Vol.49, No.6, pp.565-580, ISSN 0098-1389.

Sen, B. (2006), Frequency of family dinner and adolescent body weight status: evidence from the national longitudinal survey of youth, 1997. *Obesity (Silver Spring)*. Vol.14, No.12, (Dec., 2006), pp.2266-2276, ISSN 1930-7381.

Singh, G., Kogan, M., Van Dyck, P. & Siahpush, M. (2008). Racial/ethnic, socioeconomic, and behavioral determinants of childhood and adolescent obesity in the United States: Analyzing independent and joint associations. *Annals of Epidemiology*. Vol.18, No.9, (Sep., 2008), pp.682-695, ISSN 1047-2797.

Stamatakis, E., Hamer, M. & Dunstan, D. (2011). Screen-based entertainment time, all-cause mortality, and cardiovascular events: Population-based study with ongoing mortality and hospital events follow-up. *Journal of the American College of Cardiology*. Vol.57, No.3, pp.292-299, ISSN 0735-1097.

Steinberger, J. & Daniels, S. (2003). Obesity, insulin resistance, diabetes and cardiovascular risk in children: an American Heart Association Scientific Statement from the Atherosclerosis, Hypertension, and Obesity in the Young Committee (Council on Cardiovascular Disease in the Young) and the Diabetes Committee (Council on Nutrition, Physical Activity, and Metabolism). *Circulation*. Vol.107, No.10, (Mar., 2003), pp.1448-1453, ISSN 0009-7322.

Viner, R., Cole, T. (2005). Television viewing in early childhood predicts adult body mass index. *Journal of Pediatrics*. Vol. 147, No.4, (Oct., 2005), pp.429-435, ISSN 0022-3476.

Wang , Y. & Lobstein, T. (2006). Worldwide trends in childhood overweight and obesity. *International Journal of Pediatric Obesity, Vol.*1,No 1.,(Jan., 2006), pp.11-25, ISSN 1747-7166.

Yen, C., Hsiao, R., Ko, C., Yen, J., Huang, C., Liu, S. & Wang, S. (2010). The relationships between body mass index and television viewing, Internet use and cellular phone use: The moderating effects of socio-demographic characteristic and exercise. *International Journal of Eating Disorders*. Vol.43, No.6, (Sep., 2010), pp.565-571, ISSN 0276-3478.

10

Childhood Obesity: The Need for Practice Based Solutions – A South African Perspective

A.E. Pienaar and G.L. Strydom
North-West University, Potchefstroom
Republic of South Africa

1. Introduction

Obesity is a complex problem with no simple solutions. In the quest to find possible solutions for this growing problem among children, literature has already indicated a gap between evidence-based research and practice-based intervention (Robert Wood Johnson Foundation, 2008). This chapter will provide a focus on childhood obesity in South Africa, and will discuss the extent of this problem within the complex context of the South African demographics. It often happens that when researchers have published the results of intervention studies or clinical trials, they may walk away totally satisfied with positive and promising results. The challenge however, remains to translate these research results for practitioners to be used as "tools" in addressing the existing problem. This chapter, therefore, intends to deal with practice-based solutions and recommendations suggesting some strategies in this part of the world.

In order to understand the problem of childhood obesity better in the context of this country (South Africa) it is important to shortly review the socio-economic conditions that currently prevail in this part of the continent as demographic background information.

2. Demographic background

Human growth and development do not take place in a biological vacuum, but in an environmental context where several factors, including genetic potential can affect the development of the child (Cameron, 2005). It is also proved that many so called "developing countries" around the world, of which South Africa is one, at present, are undergoing epidemiological transition (Goedecke et al., 2006). This process is associated with some typical health risks, not only for the adult population, but also for children (Cameron, 2005). Although South Africa is a country with high potential, and many efforts are made to improve the health and well-being of the people living here, many challenges exist to the health and optimal development of children growing up in this country. This country with 50 million people is described as a developing and middle-income country with high socio-economic disparities (46.3% low socio-economic, 53.7% in middle to high socio-economic) (Zere & McIntyre, 2003), where more than 14 million people were beneficiaries of income support in 2010 and 24.8% were living below the food poverty line in 2008 (Millenium Development Goals, Country Report, 2010). Statistics show that 40% (18.3 million) of the South African population are 18 years and younger. African children accounted for 84% of the total child population, while white (5%) coloured (9%) and Indian (2%) children comprise the rest (South African Child Gauge, 2008/2009). In 2007, two thirds of these children lived in income poverty and about 40% in a household where no adult is employed.

Another health burden is HIV, the epidemic that affects health, livelihoods, economic growth, demographic futures, as well as impacting on the lives of individuals, families and workplaces (Millenium Development Goals, Country Report, 2010). HIV and AIDS have had a significant negative impact on life expectancy in South Africa, and have left many families and children economically vulnerable and often socially stigmatized and continue to leave South Africa with a legacy of young adult deaths. AIDS orphans are socially and economically vulnerable children (South African Child Gauge, 2008/2009). The adult incidence of HIV and AIDS for sub-Saharan Africa was 5.2% compared to a global total incidence of 0.8% in 2008. The proportion of HIV positive babies in 2009-2010 was 9.4% and statistics further show that the HIV prevalence among pregnant women aged 15- 24 years is 22.8%, with an overall national transmission rate of 11% of HIV to babies born to HIV-infected mothers. HIV is also associated with other life threatening conditions, with tuberculoses being the most common opportunistic infection, with rates exceeding 70% (Millenium Development Goals, 2010). All of the above contribute to South Africa having a high <5 years child mortality rate that is reported to be still much higher than the set target for South Africa by 2015. It is, therefore, not strange that the main priorities of this country are to alleviate poverty and improve primary health care among children in an effort to decrease early childhood mortality.

3. Obesity – A health burden

Recent statistics obtained by the National Health and Nutrition Examination Survey in the USA indicate 21.5% overweight and 10.4% obesity among 2-5 year olds (Ogden et al., 2010a), while increasing tendencies are also reported in this age group in Europe and Australia (Baur, 2001; Maffeis et al., 2006; Apfelbacher, 2008; Cretikos et al., 2008). Even bigger increases are reported in developing countries such as Thailand (WHO, 2010) and Chili (Kain et al., 2002). Although this disease is not life threatening during the childhood years, and mainly the result of lifestyle related habits, it is prevalent among affluent and less affluent families and has lifelong consequences with an increasing burden on the healthcare system of a country as the child grows older. This growing epidemic of childhood obesity can, therefore, not be ignored in the health care focus of any country. The Medical Research Council of South Africa (Steyn, 2007) reported that health services spend 8 billion rand per annum involving direct and indirect costs resulting from lifestyle related diseases such as heart disease and stroke (Steyn, 2007). Pienaar (2009) argues that disease prevention is as important as the treatment thereof and should receive high priority in the country. This researcher recommends that strategies should be put in place to prevent diseases from a very young age as research indicates that exposure to health risks due to physical inactivity, which is one of the main causes of childhood obesity, already start in childhood, although the consequences or clinical symptoms may only occur in mid- to later life when the individual reaches the clinical horizon (Rowland, 1990). Kruger et al. (2005) also highlight that obesity needs to be viewed as a disease in its own right and one that warrants intervention even when co-morbidities are not present.

Furthermore recent data in the USA, where the national obesity rates have tripled among children and adolescents over the last 30 years, suggest that obesity is now responsible for more disability and activity limitations than smoking. As a direct result of this obesity epidemic, doctors are noticing a significant rise in chronic illnesses among children. Obese children are also more than twice as likely to develop type 2 diabetes than children of normal weight (CDPH, 2010). In California, cost attributable to physical inactivity, obesity and overweight in 2006 was estimated at $41.2 billion. This suggests, however, that a 5% improvement in each risk factor could result in annual savings of nearly $2.4 billion (CDPH, 2010). This burden is also indicated in many other countries around the world, viz: Australia and UK. In South Africa it is estimated that 30% of ischaemic heart disease, 27% of colon cancer, 22% of ischaemic stroke and 20% of type 2 diabetes were attributable to physical inactivity (Joubert et al., 2007). Thus, considering the major burden/health concern of obesity in child and adulthood as well as the complex co-morbidities originated from obesity, it is imperative that more focus should be directed on the developing child to reinforce healthy lifestyles in order to reduce the burden of non-communicable diseases of adulthood.

Kruger et al. (2005) indicated that obesity prevention initiatives should be focused on children to ensure the adoption of a healthy lifestyle from an early age. The challenge to deal with this epidemic should, therefore, rather be to prevent it, highlighting childhood as a critical developmental phase. It is agreed that besides genetic predisposition, lifestyle habits are determined in the first years of a child's life. During this critical phase of human development some developmental "windows of opportunity" occur (Gabbard 1998). When optimal stimulation is not received during these critical periods, the opportunity passes, leaving the individual in many cases with some developmental restrictions. Intervention later in life can improve the situation but the individual may never reach his/her optimal potential in the specific area. The words of the previous Surgeon General of the USA, Dr. Everette Koop, sum up this situation viz. (1996): *"Everything we have ever done in health education, as good as it might be, always has one fault: It's too late."*, again emphasizing that the period of childhood is a critical phase on which to focus.

4. Prevalence of childhood obesity in South Africa

A worldwide increase in childhood obesity is reported, including in South Africa. Kruger et al. (2005) reported in this regard that earlier South African studies (1996-1998) showed a prevalence of about 10% of overweight and obesity among children in this country. More recent statistics indicate higher incidences that are similar to that of developing countries a decade ago (Steyn et al., 2005; Armstrong et al., 2006). Differences are also reported between urban and rural environments, indicating that urbanisation plays a role in the prevalence of obesity, while ethnic and gender differences are also evident from reported statistics.

The results of a nationally representative study ("National Food Health Consumption Survey" (Labadarios, 1999) of 1-9 year old children indicated that 6.7% of them were overweight and 3.7% were obese. When international BMI standards as proposed by Cole et al. (2000) were applied to these results, 17.1% of the children were classified as overweight and obese (Steyn et al., 2005). Another comprehensive study among 6 and 13 year old children and also based on the same cut-off values indicates a prevalence of 14% and 3.2% of overweight and obesity among boys, while 17.9% and 4.9% of girls were overweight and obese respectively (Armstrong et al., 2006). Statistics in a regional representative sample of

7-year old children in one of the nine provinces of South Africa, the North West Province, indicates an overweight and obesity prevalence of 11.64 % (overweight =7.84%; obesity =3.80%) (Kemp et al., 2011), with significant differences between gender and children growing up in different socio-economic environments. The prevalence of obesity is reported to vary between rural and non-rural communities (Monyeki et al., 1999) with higher percentages reported in the non-rural areas. Monyeki et al. (1999) reported the prevalence of overweight in 3 to 10 year old children in disadvantaged communities in the Limpopo Province as low (0% - 2.5% and 0% - 4.3% among boys and girls respectively) while Steyn et al. (2005) reported the highest prevalence of overweight (20.1%) in urban areas and the lowest in farming communities.

Studies on overweight and obesity among boys and girls show a gradual increase as girls get older, with significant differences between genders. Statistics on 10-12 year old girls living in the North West Province of SA, indicating 16.52% to be overweight and 4.93% to be obese (Pienaar et al., 2007). The "International Obesity Task Force" reported that 25% of all SA girls in the 13-19 year age group are overweight, compared to 7% of boys (Somers et al., 2006). Somers et al. (2006) further indicated that overweight among 10-16 year old girls (21.1%) was significantly higher than among boys (8.4%), with no significant differences with regard to obesity. A possible explanation is that girls are more prone to overweight and obesity, especially before the onset of the growth spurt at about 10-years of age and after menarche has commenced (Armstrong et al., 2006).

Differences are also reported between ethnic groups and those living in different socio-economic conditions (McVeigh et al., 2004 & Armstrong et al., 2006). These researchers reported that White boys and girls showed the highest BMI values, although after the age of 11 years, black girls presented with the highest BMI values. The incidence of overweight and obesity among Black girls increased from 12% at the age of 6-years to 22% at the age of 13-years, while a decreasing trend from 25% to 15% was found among White girls. The "South African Youth Risk Behaviour" study reported the incidence of overweight and obesity among Black, White and Indian girls in the 13-19 year old group as 30%, 34% en 41% respectively (Steyn, 2005). Pienaar et al. (2007) found ethnical differences in a representative sample of 10-12 year old girls living in the North West Province of South Africa, where White girls showed the highest percentage of overweight (21.28%), followed by Indian (17.39%), Black (15.81%) and Coloured girls (9.10%). Indian girls showed the highest prevalence of obesity (8.7%) followed by White (8.51%) and Black girls (4.35%), with no obesity found among coloured girls in this age group. Somers et al. (2006) investigated the prevalence of overweight and obesity among 10-16 year old children in rural environments in the Western Cape Province of South Africa, and found that 15.7% of the children were overweight and 6.2% obese. The prevalence of overweight was also much higher among Black children (21.8%) than Coloured children (13.7%), with similar trend regarding obesity in the two ethnic groups (5.8% versus 6%). Black girls showed the highest percentage (30.8%) of overweight especially in the 16-year old children.

5. Causes of childhood obesity in South Africa

The problem of childhood obesity is very complex in this country due to some historical, socio-economic and other circumstances. Kruger et al. (2005) suggested that various socio-economic and cultural factors may contribute to the obesity epidemic in South Africa. It is, therefore, not limited to a specific ethnic, age or socio-economic group, indicating that cultural, environment and genetic factors should also be taken into consideration when causes of childhood obesity are analysed. Further some of the major factors that may be relevant in this regard will be outlined briefly.

5.1 Poverty

Obesity in the general population is much more likely to result from excess calories consumption and sedentary lifestyle than from any other factors (Kimm, 2004). Most commonly, obesity (overnutrition) leads to an accelerated growth rate and tall stature during childhood with early achievement of normal adult height. Poverty and unemployment on the other hand, generally result in poor levels of nutrition, increased levels of food insecurity and incidences of malnutrition (Millenium Development Goals, 2010). A reasonable proxy for income poverty and hunger is child under-nutrition. It is reported that 2.7 million children live in households that reported child hunger (South African Child Gauge, 2008/2009). The underweight-for-age incidence rate (a weight less than 60% of estimated 'normal' weight-for-age) is generally higher than the severe malnutrition incidence rates of a country. Severe malnutrition is reported to average over the period 2001 to 2010 to be between 4.4% and 13.3% for the <5 year old in the different provinces of South Africa (District Health Information System in the Department of Health). These poor levels of nutrition contribute to growth deficiencies such as stunting (retarded growth) and wasting (low weight-for- age). In this regard the Barker hypotheses implicates the fetal in-utero environment as a significant determinant of risk for major chronic diseases such as cardiovascular disease, hypertension, type 2 diabetes and obesity, later in life (Kimm, 2004). In a study done on a Fillipino group of children, low birth weight was associated with higher blood pressure and heavier bodyweight during adolescence (Kimm, 2004). Small stature associated with obesity during child and adulthood can, however, result from a diverse set of conditions (Kimm, 2004). These include being born small for gestational age, postnatal malnutrition, hormone abnormalities such as deficiencies of growth hormone or thyroid hormone, late effects after childhood, cancer, certain medications, and genetic syndromes. Common features of growth disorders in the context of obesity include limited growth hormone or thyroid hormone or their action, or limited sensitivity to insulin. Abnormalities of leptin and newly identified appetite-regulating peptides may also lead to poor growth and overweight. Popkin et al. (1996) were the first to highlight that the prevalence of childhood obesity was greater in children who were stunted in communities undergoing nutritional transition. In this regard Naude et al. (2008) reported higher BMI, fat percentages and intra-abdominal fat storage among stunted children compared to non-stunted children in South Africa. From the previous discussion it is obvious that children born under these difficult conditions suffer a high risk of stunting during infancy, and that growth retardation during early childhood is associated with significant dysfunctional improvement during adulthood (Cameron, 2005) including obesity (Popkin et al., 1996). This phenomenon was also supported by a study of Ravelli et al. (1976) on the importance of adequate nutrition during the prenatal period in children born under famine conditions. The most famous of these was the "Dutch Hunger Winter" beginning in October 1944 when food suppliers to the Dutch cities were reduced due to German occupation of the Western Netherlands (Cameron, 2005). During this time the average per capita daily ratio of approximately 1800 kcal/day dropped to 600kcal/day. In the follow-up

study of Ravelli et al. (1976) it was indicated that in men (Dutch military conscripts) exposed to famine in the first two trimesters of pregnancy, the prevalence of obesity was dramatically increased compared to those exposed to famine in the third trimester or post-natally. A possible mechanism underpinning this phenomenon is not yet well established but may be linked to the so-called "intra-uterine programming" (Cameron, 2005). Following birth this programming caused them to respond adversely to changes in lifestyle that may result in obesity in later life (Cameron, 2005).
Other indicators of overweight and obesity are mothers that smoke and the absence of breastfeeding (Burke, 2006). To minimize mother-to-baby transmission of the HIV virus, breastfeeding practices are not recommended among HIV positive mothers. A link was also confirmed between low educational level and a higher BMI in a group of economically active South Africans representing four different ethnic groups in the country (Senekal et al., 2003).

5.2 Urbanisation and diet

Kruger et al. (2005) reported that the obesity epidemic in South Africa reflects globalization which is the primary driving mechanism towards nutritional transition. These researchers indicated that more freedom of movement of especially the black population and an increase in exposure to the global market economy led to a shift from traditional foods, low in fat and rich in fibre, towards meat and diary products containing high levels of saturated fats and more highly refined foods. Globalization may, therefore, increase the risk amongst the urban population by creating an evironment which is conducive to the consumption of food rich in fat and sugar (Bourne et al., 2002; MacIntyre et al., 2002). Urbanisation is also linked to a higher income which contributes to a higher fat intake and an increase in sedentary behaviour (Kain et al., 2004; Van der Merwe, 2004). It is further indicated that in townships and among street vendors, cheap fatty meat and snacks and few fruit and vegatables are sold (Kruger et al., 2005).

5.3 Cultural differences

The diverse culture of the 4 major ethnic groups in South Africa (Asian, black, coloured and whites/Caucasian) contributes to deepen the complexity of the problem. Kruger et al. (2005) indicate that culture shapes eating habits. In some cultures social gatherings encourage overeating and certain foods (luxurious foods rich in fat and energy) are associated with social status and become more acceptable among urban South Africans. In some of the groups, overweight (and obesity) reflects the "good" life viz, wealth, good standing, attractiveness and absence of HIV/AIDS, which is associated with respect, dignity and affluence, therefore, a bigger body size is more acceptable (Senekal et al., 2001; Puoane & Hughes, 2005). In this scenario a paradigm shift is necessary to convince individuals about the health consequences of obesity and overweight.

5.4 Sedentary behaviour and physical inactivity

Sedentary behaviour is identified as one of the most important contributing factors of childhood obesity (Steyn, 2005). Dodd (2007) reported that the increased prevalence among children can mainly be attributed to a decrease in energy expenditure and increased sedentary behaviour. Although South Africa has high percentages of children living in poor socio-economic circumstances, 53.7% are brought up in middle to high socio-economic conditions (Zere & McIntyre, 2003). Children growing up in such households are more likely to participate in passive pastimes such as TV watching and computer games. Television viewing of more than 3 hours per day and the absence of Physical Education in SA schools are reported to contribute to more sedentary behaviour and obesity among school going children (Medical Research Council, 2002). In addition, Van der Merwe (2004) indicated that 40% of all advertisement during TV programmes for children, is about food products with a high fat and or suger content, which encourage a higher energy intake. Trends have also changed where in most households, both parents are working and children have to stay at daycare centres or in after-school programmes, which restrict them to participate in after school activity programmes (Pienaar, 2009). High crime rates, unsafe environments and stranger fear is a reality in South Africa with a profound effect on children moving freely and unrestricted around and playing outside (Bourne et al., 2002; Sabin et al., 2004). This contributes to parents being afraid of using public transport which decreases walking and bicycling activities among children.

In South Africa 17% of primary school children and 29% of secondary school children have to travel more than 30 minutes to reach the school nearest to them. Many children in low socio-economic situations have to walk to school by necessity, and benefit from this activty, but this is associated with hardship and when such children have an option later in their life, they will choose easier options to commute, contributing to a more sedentary lifestyle (Lennox et al., 2007). Very high percentages of TV watching (especially watching soap operas) is also reported among adolescents living in poor socio-economic circumstances, especially girls. This behaviour provides an easy escape from their daily reality, but contributes to sedentary lifestyles (Lennox et al., 2007). This trend is similar in America which indicates the highest percentages of obesity among children living in poor socio-economic conditions (Ogden et al., 2010b).

5.5 Familial obesity

Studies indicate that parental overweight and obesity are the biggest risk factor for overweight and obesity among children (Van der Merwe, 2004). The "American Academy of Child and Adolescent Psychiatry" indicates that when both parents are obese, the risk for the child to be also obese is 80%, and 50% when one parent is obese (AACAP, 2010). This relationship is also reported to be higher with the mother (Padez et al., 2005). The cultural perception of overweight and obesity as acceptable, make this factor an important contributing factor to overweight in this country.

6. Evidence-based practice to intervention-based practice

This part will focus on a summary of research findings regarding the success of different intervention strategies and the knowledge that practitioners can gain from these results in order to treat childhood obesity more effectively. Successful strategies, barriers and challenges will be further identified in the treatment process of childhood obesity.

Before commencing with this discussion it is, however, important to provide a conceptualization of the health paradigms. In order to understand the roles of various health disciplines in illness, health and well-being, and to understand how the treatment of childhood obesity and the manifestations of this condition fits into the illness/well-being continuum and health paradigm, it is important to discuss the illness/well-being continuum briefly and its position in the various health paradigms viz. the pathogenic and fortogenic paradigm. This will provide the reader with a better understanding of where practitioners that treat childhood obesity are positioned in this health paradigm and of the specialized training and skills that such practitioners need to treat this condition effectively.

6.1 The health paradigms – A conceptualisation

The World Health Organisation (WHO) already postulated a definition of health in 1947 indicating that "Health is a condition of optimal physical, psychological and social well-being and not merely the absence of disease". From this definition it is clear that illness and well-being focus on two different entities in the individual's health and well-being. This is clearly illustrated in the illness/well-being continuum as illustrated by Robbins et al. (1991)(Fig 1.).

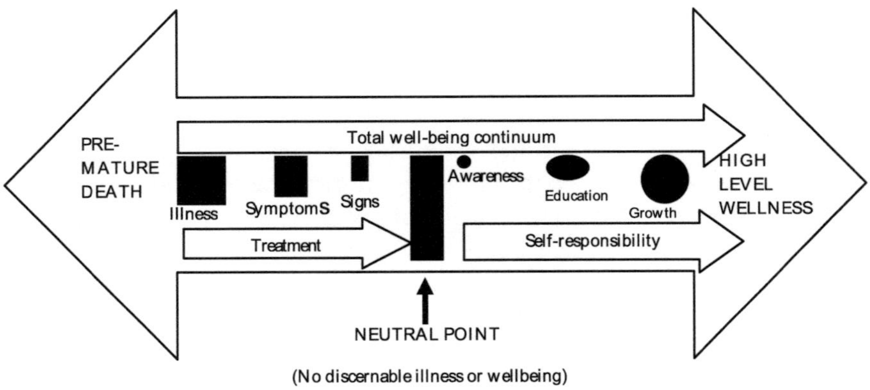

Fig. 1. The illness/well being continuum (Robbins et al., 1991)

In the past the responsibility for the individual's health was solely the responsibility of the doctor. When any signs, symptoms and illness occurred the patient went to the doctor for medical attention in order treat the signs/symptoms and to restore life to the neutral point where no signs of the illness is noticeable. However, in this scenario no effort is being made from the patient's side to improve his own health and well-being by embracing a healthy lifestyle such as healthy eating habits and regular exercise.

To combat the problem of obesity among children, the primary focus should be on the right hand side of the continuum (Fig. 1). This comprises of providing the child with the necessary developmentally appropriate motor skills and creating an understanding of healthy behaviour and convert the knowledge and behaviour into effective strategies for health enhancement (Crawford, 2008), hereby educating the child and allowing him/her to grow to eventually accept self-responsibility for his/her own well-being. It is in this respect that Dr Koop, former Surgeon General of the USA, suggested that this health and well-being "message" should reach the very young child in order to develop healthy lifestyle habits. It is, therefore, clear that the main focus of a profession dealing with childhood obesity should fall on the right hand side of the continuum, which is focused on health promotion and, therefore, primarily can be described in the fortogenic paradigm which seeks "strong" (healthy) points to be enhanced ('Forte' means 'strong'). To understand the role of pediatric exercise science in the various health paradigms, the following conceptualisation (Fig. 2) may be useful.

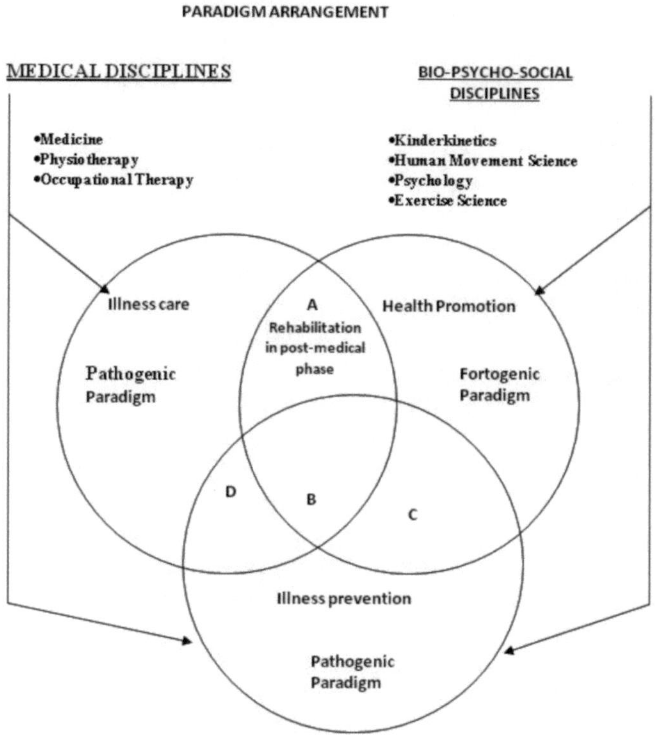

Fig. 2. The role of kinderkinetics in the various health paradigms (Adapted from Strydom et al., 2009)

In Fig. 2, the three constructs regarding health, viz, *illness care, illness prevention* and *health promotion* are arranged into the two paradigms namely the pathogenic and fortogenic paradigm. In the concept *"illness care"* it is suggested that a pathology is already present and the main focus is to cure the problem. In the case of *illness prevention* no pathology existed, only the threat of a pathology is present (immunisation against a certain illness such as polio is a typical example). In both constructs, because pathology forms the main focus of the treatment, the traditional health care professionals such as doctors, nurses and physiotherapists may be mainly responsible for treatment. In the *health promotion* construct no pathology or threat is present, and the aim is purely to improve health and well-being. This construct falls exclusively within the fortogenic paradigm where the aim is primarily to improve health and well-being by taking self-responsibility. As stated earlier the primary focus of Kinderkinetics falls in this paradigm. However, it is important to understand that the application of this discipline is also relevant in the pathogenic paradigm where the actions may be more of therapeutic value indicated by areas that overlap (Fig 2).

Area A (Fig 2) would, therefore, suggest the rehabilitation or improvement of a pre-diagnosed condition. A child suffering from type 1 diabetes mellitus (which is associated with obesity) is a typical example in this scenario. While the pathology is medically treated and managed by the traditional health care professionals, the young child is motivated to participate in scientifically designed exercise programmes, tailored for his/her developmental needs, taking into account the barriers imposed on the child by the specific pathological condition. By participating in physical activity the pathology (type 1 diabetes) will not be totally cured but the benefits of exercise for this condition are already well described. It may also motivates the child to lead a physically active life into adulthood, preventing various health threats associated with a sedentary lifestyle (hypokinetic diseases) and strive to improve quality of life. It may also be during this phase when the young child is introduced to physical activity that the perception that the illness which is present (diabetes) need not be an ordeal but that the child may lead a 'normal' and productive life and that it is his/her responsibility to follow the necessary precautions to manage the disability. In many cases the perception of the child being a "disabled" as a result of the illness is a major obstacle for the parents to overcome, as they tend to be overprotective of such a child. Participating in a specialized environment and in programmes conducted by specialised trained health professionals, the parents may have peace of mind that the person who is working with the child is adequately trained.

Area B (Fig. 2) suggests a situation where the child may suffer from a pre-diagnosed condition that may be positively affected by physical activity so that it may lead to a possible improvement of the condition. An example here is the obese child. An increase in physical activity may improve the condition and also lead to improvement of the child's well-being. In Area C no pathology is currently present but the threat existed, which may lead to health consequences if the problem is ignored. An example in this case is the clumsy child. If such children are not exposed to activity provided by a trained professional who can assess their developmental barriers and can treat them effectively by equipping them with appropriate motor skills, a love for activity and an understanding of the importance of an active lifestyle, the clumsy child may continue to withdraw himself from movement and physical activity, eventually suffering from various hypokinetic diseases later in life.

6.2 Evidence-based intervention – Successes, challenges and principles

6.2.1 Successes

In this section the outcomes of different obesity intervention studies on children with regard to the nature, the extent, the successes and the challenges will be discussed briefly, after which important principles that can guide the intervention process will be highlighted. Campbell et al. (2001) reported a research environment that is still void of current statistical power to set clear guidelines for the prevention of obesity across a variety of risk groups. Obesity prevention is, however, recommended as the best strategy in the combatting of obesity among children (Bosch et al., 2004; Boon & Clydesdale, 2005), although in reality this strategy is not always possible. The literature describes obesity treatment in prevention or curative settings, and as treatment based on singular (physical activity, diet or behaviour modification) or multi-component aspects (combinations of the aforementioned three components). Furthermore, studies report the results of childhood obesity treatment in clinical, family or school based settings.

A systematic review of 7 studies (4 shorter and 3 over a longer period) by Campbell et al. (2001) and 28 studies by Connelly et al. (2007) (11 successfull, 17 unsuccessful) indicated mixed success rates. However, it was concluded by Connoly et al. (2007) that the factor that contributed most to the effectivenes of the treatment was compulsory physical activity with a moderate to high intensity. An overview by Jerum and Melnyk (2001) of randomised controlled studies that focused on the prevention of childhood obesity indicated that health workers such as doctors and nurses should play a more prominent role in the prevention of obesity and that multi-component treatments are more successful than single component treatment. The importance of parent involvement is also highligted over the whole spectrum of obesity intervention (Jerum & Melnyk, 2001; Golan et al., 2006).

It seems that multi-disciplinary interventions that include physical activity, diet and behaviour modification, contributed to better results in comparison to studies that only focused on singular aspects. School-based programmes are found to be effective in combatting obesity by increasing the physical activity levels of the children and improving healthy eating habits. It can, therefore, be concluded that physical activity plays an important role in the prevention and treatment of overweight and obesity and the the type of treatment as well as the intensity and duration of the activity are very important.
The treatment of established obesity is, however, more complex and needs more intensive treatment. Clinical intervention based on a multi-disciplinary approach seems to be succesful (Eliakim et al., 2002; Nemene et al., 2005; Sacher et al., 2005; Korsten-Reck et al., 2005; Dreimane, et al., 2007; Eneli et al., 2008; Knöpfli et al., 2008; Weigel et al., 2008). It is also reported that interventions are more successful when the child is motivated to lose weight (Boon & Clydesdale, 2005), and that interventions on obese children with concerned parents are more successful than for instance school-based multi-disciplinary interventions where children sometimes are not even aware of the fact that they have a weight problem. Studies indicated that at least 12 weeks and a frequency of 3-5 times per week are required to provoke positive effects. Most studies use weight loss as a precursor of the success of the treatment. However, it is reported that obesity intervention has more advantages than only a positive change in body composition. An overall decrease of the metabolic syndrome was for instance reported among 10 to 17-year old children with a mean body fat percentage of 37.5%, after an intensive 2-week in-patient intervention in which no changes were found in the body fat percentage (Chen et al., 2006). A literature review by Eneli et al. (2008) showed similar results with only a small change in BMI, although improvements were seen in the lipid profile, blood pressure and insulin resistance.

6.2.2 Challenges

Obesity treatment requires considerable lifestyle related modifications which has to be sustainable in order to be successful. The sustainability of the effects of childhood obesity treatment is however reported as poor. The maintenance of the effects after the treatment phase is therefor a major challenge to overcome (Crawford, 2008). It often happens that when a controlled treatment ends, which is usually in the form of research, children are expected to follow a home programme by themselves. A main challenge for obese children is then to stay committed to make time to participate in the prescribed regular daily physical activity of moderate to high intensity level for at least 30 minutes, on their own, and sometimes in an unsympathetic environment. In addition, their expectations and setting of realistic goals are usually unrealistic, and because of this they can easily become frustrated. A possible reason for this might be that children younger than 12 years are still in the pre-operational and concrete mental-operations stages of cognitive development as described by Piaget (Sherrill, 2004). This implies less mature stages of thinking and reasoning without abstract thought. With regard to health behaviour, Crawford (2008) states that children in these stages of cognitive development will experience barriers to plan for the future because they cannot form mental images of the positive and negative consequences of certain health behaviours. These reasoning skills are in turn, needed to assume a more internal locus of control regarding their own personal health management choices. Children thus require different techniques to get them to take responsibility for their health. In addition they also tend to be more extrinsically motivated in general and it is not clear when they shift to a more internal motivation with regard to health goals (Crawford, 2008). As obese children are often negative towards participation in physical activities, this is a major challenge to overcome because of the importance of physical activity in their treatment. The content of the physical activity program should therefore be scientifically grounded but delivered in such a manner that the child will associate movement with enjoyment in order for this part of their treatment to provide enough external motivation to them to persist with it. Without a positive attitude towards participation in physical activity, it will be hard to motivate obese children to increase their activity levels and to stay active.

Furthermore, obese children with co-morbidities are at risk for contra-indications and should not participate in unsupervised physical activity programmes with high intensities which is required for weight loss. In addition, the development of age appropriate motor skills, strength, fitness and proper body posture are important goals in the treatment of obese children in order to equip them with the necessary motor repertoire based on their developmental level and abilities to be able to participate in sports programmes and recreational activities with their peers. They should therefore be assessed and a programme should be described to them based upon this assessment which is tailored to their specific needs. It is therefore imperative that the health care professional should have a thorough scientific background and understanding of the obese child regarding the physical, emotional, cognitive and physiological barriers these children have to deal with and which they have to overcome in order for an intervention to be sustainable and to contribute to permanent lifestyle changes. In this regard high levels of social support (network of family, friends, health professionals and community resources by providing appropriate information and encouragement) and self efficacy are indicated to be important predictors in adherence (Crawford, 2008).

6.2.3 Principles of prevention programmes

Kruger et al. (2005) provide important recommendations and discussed various principles for the treatment of obesity in South Africa. However, the applicability of some of the recommendations will be more challenging and will need some adaptations to be effective when applied to children. They reported that at the first WHO Expert Consultation on Obesity, the development and implementation of effective obesity prevention strategies were identified as an immediate action priority. To guide this process, these researchers indicated that South African researchers and health workers should take note of the proposed principles upon which obesity prevention should be based. These principles will be used as a guide in the discussion of the way forward.

1. Interventions should focus on education and address environmental and social factors to promote and support behaviour change.
2. Increased physical activity.
3. Sustainability of programmes is crucial to ensure positive change in diet, activity and obesity levels over time.
4. Political support, inter-sectoral collaboration and community participation are essential for success.
5. Local actions within the context of national initiatives allow programmes to meet needs, expectations and opportunities.
6. All parts of the population must be reached.
7. Programmes must be adequately resourced.

8. Integration of new programmes within existing initiatives.
9. Programme planning should be evidence-based.
10. Programmes should be properly monitored, evaluated and documented to ensure dissemination and transfer of experience.

Kruger et al. (2005) also report that the US Institutes of Medicine suggested three levels of prevention to ensure the correct focus for obesity prevention which include:

1. *Universal prevention* interventions, focused on everyone in an eligible population irrespective of their current level of risk. This may be family-based, school-based, work site-based or community-wide. Secondly, *selective prevention* interventions, focusing on the prevention of obesity in selected high-risk groups, based on known biological, psychological or social/ cultural risk factors, which will focus on the development of lifetime behavioural patterns that will prevent obesity, and thirdly, *targeted prevention* that focuses on individuals who are overweight and aims to prevent weight gain, as well as the development of co-morbidities.

Different modes of delivery of prevention programmes are also reported by Kruger et al. (2005). These include:

1. *Do-it-yourself in self-initiated or group settings.* This self-help programmes are seen as low-intensity, cheaper intervention methods, associated with better longer term compliance but poorer weight loss outcomes than higher-intensity methods.
2. *Non-clinical programmes* provided to individuals/groups by trained professionals, not necessarily registered healthcare professionals. Information on diet, exercise and behaviour modification is provided at regular meetings. These programmes are popular and often commercially franchised.
3. *Clinical programmes* provided by registered healthcare professionals with specialized training in weight management. These could involve a consultation with a dietician, medical doctor or a multi-disciplinary team.

Kruger et al. (2005) finally stressed that all obesity treatment programmes should aim to empower individuals/groups to take responsibility for making permanent lifestyle changes towards healthy dietary intake and physical activity through behaviour modification, and recommend the inclusion of the following essential components in such programmes.

Component	Description/guidelines
Reasonable weight goals Healthful eating component	Individualised, realistic, maintainable, contribute to general well-being. Based on the 2004 South African food-based dietary guidelines. Limiting energy, fat and alcohol intakes.
Physical activity component	Accumulate 45–60 min of moderate-to-vigorous activity on most days - accumulating 10 min here and there is acceptable. Increased physical activity of daily living, fitness and recreational activity, strength and flexibility exercises.
Behavioural and psychological component	Long-term lifestyle (dietary and physical activity) changes; self-concept, body image, stress management, communication and environment management, cognitive behavioural skills necessary to bring about change. To ensure success the 'stage of change' of the individual/ target group needs to be considered.

For effective implementation of the above treatment principles among children, specific recommendations should, however, be *added* with regard to the *weight goals and eating habits* and *physical activity components* because children have developmental limitations on different levels. With regard to weight goals and healthy eating patterns, it should be remembered that children's bodies are in a growing phase and that weight loss will not necessarily be the most suitable goal, depending on the extent of the obesity problem. Although individual differences and circumstances should always be taken into consideration, it is suggested that the eating habits and patterns of young children should rather be managed by lifestyle changes which incorporate changing of eating habits rather than they being expected to follow a strict diet. Steyn (2007) reports in this regard the National guidelines of the Department of Health which states that the weight of children aged between 2 and 7 years who have no complications should be maintained, because there will be weight loss as a result of an increase in length. If there are however, complications such as high blood pressure, insulin resistance or orthopaedic problems, weight loss will be necessary. In children over 7 years, weight loss should be started when the BMI of the child' lies above the 95th percentile, or otherwise the international age specific cut-off values for obesity of Cole et al. (2000) can be used as a quick screening method. The AED (2011) also recommends that interventions should aim for the maintenance of individually appropriate weights, that is, that children will continue to grow at their natural rate and follow their own growth curve, underscoring that a healthy weight is not a fixed number but varies for each individual. The South African version of the stoplight (robot) diet is suggested for use among children towards healthier dietary intake (Steyn, 2007). Foods are categorised in this diet in categories of use, in limited, moderate or restricted amounts, and parents and children are asked to keep record of all that is eaten, which makes them aware of the quantity and quality of foods being consumed. The guidelines of the ACSM (2000) for the structuring of obesity programmes are also valuable with regard to the weight and eating management of obese children. This includes a recomendation of maintaining a minimal intake of about 1200 calories per day, and engaging in a daily exercise program that expends 300 or more calories per day. For weight-loss goals, exercise of long duration /moderate intensity is generally considered best (ACSM, 2000). The AED (2011) highlights that weight is not a behaviour and therefore not an appropriate target for behaviour modification in school and community based intervetions. They recommend that interventions should be weight-neutral, thus not have specific goals for weight change but aim to increase healthy living at any size. Children across the weight spectrum benefit from limiting time spent watching television and eating a healthy diet.Children therefore need education to understand what realistic goals are with regard to weight management and that they will have to make a commitment to adhere to their goals, also with regard to participating in physical activity.

Regarding the guidelines for physical activity component of treatment programmes, the developmental needs of obese children regarding their motor skills development or the lack of it because of their overweight problem, should receive attention. This is a unique requirement of childhood treatment programmes in comparison to adult programmes. The activities included in a programme, therefore, need to focus on increased levels of participation in conjunction with opportunities to enhance basic motor skills that are needed for sport participation or recreational activities. Weight bearing activities which can improve bone health should also be included in the activity programme. Guidelines as suggested by Short et al. (1999) for aerobic functioning among 6-17 year old children can be use as a guideline in determining the intensity level of the physical activity programme of obese children or with regard to daily physical activity that is expected from them, depending on their age (Table 1). Parizkova (2005) report in this regard that exercise must be vigorous enough to impose an adequate training load on the cardiorespiratory system, and stress that this part of a programme should be adequately monitored.

Lastly with regard to the behavioural and psychological component of treatment programs, the immature cognitive understanding and reasoning skills of children as described earlier, might influence children's commitment to changes in their personal health management. The Academy for Eating disorders (2011) recommend that the ideal intervention should be based on an integrated approach that addresses risk factors for the spectrum of weight-related problems, including screening for unhealthy weight control behaviours; and promotes protective behaviours, such as decreasing dieting, increasing balanced nutrition, encouraging mindful eating, increasing activity, promoting positive body image and decreasing weight-related teasing and harassment. Behavioural changes that are expected from them should, therefore, be carefully managed. The AED (2011) also recommend that interventions should also be created and led by qualified health care providers who acknowledge the importance of a health focus over a weight focus when targeting lifestyle and weight concerns in youth. In this regard, the modes of delivery of prevention programmes as suggested by Kruger et al. (2005), will also be challenging for children because they are mostly based on self-help programmes and the implementation of knowledge gained from regular meetings. Delivery of programmes in this way will be challenging for children to comply with or to understand. Sustainable programmes, especially with regard to physical activity, managed by a trained health care professional who understands the limitations of children and who can adress it appropriately within a supportive family environment (Steyn 2007), might be the only workable solutions to adress these developmental deficiencies of children.

Group	Frequency	Intensity	Duration
Adolescents (13-17)	3-5 days per week	55-90% HR max (115-180 beats/min) 12-16 RPE 10-15METs	20-60min per day (accumulated: >10 min per bout)
Older children (10-12)	4-7 days per week	55-70% HR max (115-145 beats/min) 12-13 RPE 5-7METs	30-60+min per day (accumulate, intermittent)
Younger children (6-9)	4-7 days per week	De-emphasized; participants is encouraged	30-60min+min per day (accumulate, intermittent)
Adjustments for youngsters with diabetes	No change unless disability can be exacerbated by regular activity	Reduced as a function of fitness level; adjust THRZ for individuals using arms-only activity and for individuals with SCI quadriplegia	Accumulate more intermittent activity or reduce total time if necessary

*These values represent moderate physical activity; ideally, this level will be exceeded to vigorous levels at times.

Table 1. Guidelines for developing aerobic functioning

Reprinted, by permission, from F.X. Short, J. McCubbin, and G. Frey, 1999, Cardiorespiratory endurance and body composition. In *The Brockport physical fitness training guide,* edited by J.P. Winnick and F.X. Short (Champaign, IL: Human Kinetics).

7. Practice-based solutions – The way forward

As described, childhood obesity is a challenging problem to combat especially in a country like South Africa where the health care system is challenged with numerous complexities. From the above discussion it is clear that it is important to intervene at a young age in order to establish a healthy lifestyle among children. However, children cannot be treated as mini-adults, because of their developmental needs and limitations on various levels that have to be taken into consideration when addressing this problem. Intervention of childhood obesity (prevention and treatment), therefore, calls for comprehensive and innovative strategies. A few practice-based solutions that are implemented successfully in this country will be discussed in the following section.

7.1 Paediatric exercise science – The development of a new health care profession in South Africa

In combating the obesity epidemic among children, an increase in physical activity plays an important role, both in primary and secondary intervention. A real challenge is to provide evidence-based physical activity intervention to children during early childhood (3-12 years). For the very young child, a physical activity intervention should be age and developmentally appropriate. Therefore, the professional who administers the intervention during this stage should be thoroughly trained in childhood development and paediatric exercise science. The literature has already indicated a gap between evidence-based research and practice-based intervention (Robert Wood Johnson Foundation, 2008). It is often seen that when researchers have published the results of their intervention studies or clinical trials, they walk away totally satisfied with positive and promising results. The challenge, however, remains for somebody to translate these research results for practitioners to be used as "tools" in addressing the existing problem.

The treatment offered should be based on an individual assessment of each child and then tailored to the requirements of the developmental stage and the severity of the problem. This should *i.a* include the following: obtaining a medical and family history, a physical activity profile and information about the eating habits of the child to determine possible reasons for his overweight problem. Situational influences relevant to the health behaviour such as cultural influences should also be taken into consideration. Secondly, his body composition (weight, height, hip and waist-circumferences, skinfolds and BMI), current motor and physical abilities (strength, strength endurance, cardiovascular endurance and flexibility) and basic motor skills needed for sport participation as well as his body posture should be assessed to determine individual goals for treatment. Thirdly, the baseline principles of intervention strategy with regard to frequency, duration, mode of delivery and type of activities should be followed (Parizkova, 2005). Older children may be requested to select preferred sporting activities that can be included as a part of their treatment regime in order to make it more enjoyable for them making them feel part of the decision making process of their treatment. Such a programme should be offered in a controlled and child-friendly environment with considerable support from the health care professional who conducts the programme. The basic and underlying philosophy of treatment in this regard is to expose the young child to physical activity adapted to his/her individual needs while creating a child-friendly atmosphere. In this environment professionally trained individuals have to support and motivate the child to participate and enjoy the prescribed activities within a scientifically based programme. If any health risks associated with obesity such as hypertension or other cardiovascular risks are identified during the initial screening process, such a child should be referred to a medical practitioner who has to clear the child clinically for participation in an exercise programme.

This approach calls for a comprehensive strategy managed by an appropriately qualified professional. In South Africa a new field of study has developed over the past 2 decades, seeking to bridge the gap between research and implementation. From this field of study a "new health profession" has emerged, called "Kinderkinetics" - derived from the terms "kinder" as in "children" and "kinesis" as in "movement". The focus of this profession primarily falls on the field of pediatric exercise science - using exercise/activity as a therapeuticum, profilaticum and health promotion modality.

Students in this profession are trained at 4 South African Universities/tertiary institutions following a 4 year degree integrated with laboratory and practical experience in various centres, which requires hands-on experience in order to obtain professional registration. At present, qualified professionals are registered by a professional body, the South African Professional Institute for Kinderkinetics (SAPIK) to practice as Kinderkineticists. The scope of this discipline falls primarily within the health promotion paradigm (fortogenic), providing scientifically-based exercise programmes to stimulate the young child according to his/her psycho-physical developmental stage in order to obtain optimal development. However, the scope also includes children with pre-diagnosed clinical problems such as obesity, diabetes mellitus, HIV, Down Syndrome and other ailments where children may have special needs and/or barriers regarding their physical activity and motor development, hence overlapping in the pathogenic paradigm.

This fairly new discipline (Kinderkinetics) has already gained substantial recognition as a potential health discipline and more than 150 practitioners are already working in this field, ranging from self-employment in private practices to employment in school and pre-school environment. In practice many referrals are received from other health professionals, such as paediatricians, general practitioners, occupational therapists, teachers and parents. The SAPIK is currently in the process of applying for official recognition of this profession from a Statutory Health Professions Council in South Africa in order to ethically legalise referrals from other health practitioners mentioned, as ethical rules of those health professionals prohibit mutual referral and cooperation between registered versus unregistered practitioners. These negotiations with the Statutory Health Professions Council are already in an advance stage and will hopefully be successful.

7.1.1 Applied research

The profession of Kinderkinetics is guided by applied research where the growth and motor development and physical activity of children, as well as interventions to improve shortcomings that are identified in this regard, have already been extensively researched within the field of pediatric exercise science. In this regard obesity among children of different age groups and from different perspectives for a better understanding of the

problem have been published. This *i.a* include the prevalence of childhood obesity in different age groups (Du Toit & Pienaar, 2003), relationship of childhood obesity with the motor (Du Toit & Pienaar, 2003); fitness, (Truter et al., 2010); psychological (Pienaar & Eggar, 2007; Kemp & Pienaar, 2010), physiological (Kemp & Pienaar, 2010) and academic abilities (Du Toit et al., 2011), as well as relationships of obesity with diagnosed motor delays such as Developmental Coordination Disorder among children (Pienaar et al., 2007). The most recent study that will be published shortly indicates significant relationships between hypertension, overweight and obesity among a representative group of 7-year old children in this country (Kemp et al. 2011, in press).
After accumulating all this evidence, the next action taken was the planning of research in which an obesity intervention programme could be developed and assessed. A programme based on the principles of physical activity participation, behaviour modification and dietary guidelines was then compiled and the outcomes evaluated. The energy expenditure of the group was monitored by Actical software in order to determine the effectiveness of the intensity of the physical activity part of the programme, but also to analyse the activity patterns of the children during the week and weekend and to determine possible changes in their activity patterns resulting from the programme. This intervention on 9-12 year old children was conducted over a period of 13 weeks at a frequency of three times per week with a home program and parent meetings regarding school lunch boxes and physical activity guidelines. The physical activity intervention was delivered on two days of the week, while behaviour modification regarding their eating patterns, self perception and physical activity habits was the focus of the third day of the week. Dietary modification by means of empowering the children with knowledge of different foods, healthy eating patterns, improvement of self-perception and goal setting strategies to improve physical activity were addressed through play and activity themes on this day. A home program was provided to them that they had to follow for the two additional days of the week. Significant improvement was found in the children's body composition (body fat percentage) while, waist- and upper arm-circumferences decreased significantly. A non-significant decrease of 2.9 kg was also found in body weight. The self-perception of the group improved significantly as assessed by the Harter Scale (Kemp & Pienaar, 2010). The compliance to the programme decreased when the supervised part ended, again highlighting the need for professional supervision and sustained motivation of children in obesity treatment regimens. This protocol is now implemented as an obese intervention by Kinderkineticists, with specific adjustments with regard to age appropriateness of the level, selection and inclusion of motor activities and the intensity level of physical activities. The treatment programme can also be used effectively for inactive children by only modifying the intensity of the programme, as it incorporates all the necessary fitness components such as strength and strength endurance, cardiovascular endurance, flexibility and the development of basic motor skills needed for sport participation.

7.1.2 Implementation

The need for the expertise, provided by this discipline in this country with its extreme diversity, not only in population and ethnic groupings, but also in socio-economic status, is substantial. Challenges to bring this service to the deep-rural and remote areas of the country still ask for innovative thinking. A first step in childhood obesity treatment will have to be national initiatives acknowledging the severity of the problem, policy support and community engagement on the level of implementation. The training of mid-level professionals, who can assist the Kinderkineticist in the screening and recruiting process and in the sustainability of programmes by supervising and monitoring it is essential. The training of such workers is envisaged as a sub-register that will be part of the professional registration of Kinderkinetics in the future. The training of multi-skilled professionals who can work multi-disciplinary with the Kinderkineticists such as nurses in health care clinics or in the school system or of Life Orientation teachers who can do screening for abnormalities, is also a possibility to ensure early identification and referral of obese children, as well as of other children at-risk for developmental problems.

7.2 Obesity prevention

The important message of obesity prevention by embracing a healthy lifestyle should be echoed through the school system, as most children can be reached through the school curriculum. The AED (2011) recommends that interventions should not be marketed as "obesity prevention", but rather interventions should be referred to as "health promotion," as the ultimate goal is the health and well-being of all children, and health encompasses many factors besides weight. Physical education (PE) was, however, phased out of South African schools to make more time available for the "so-called" academic subjects, and with that, teachers with the necessary training to make children aware of the importance of a healthy lifestyle and to provide them with the necessary skills and physical activity, also declined. Since 2010 PE was reinstated in the school curriculum where this message can be portrayed, and screening for overweight can be done with the necessary education or referral for help. Interventions should focus on making children's environments healthier rather than focusing solely on personal responsibility, which include serving healthy meals, providing opportunities for fun physical activities, implementing a no-teasing policy, and providing students and school staff with educational sessions about body image, media literacy, and weight bias (AED, 2011). However, this is going to be a long process as teachers for this profession have to be trained from scratch and schools have to be equipped with the necessary resources to teach this subject effectively.

7.3 Improved sustainability of obesity intervention

Kruger et al. (2005) report that lifestyle modification as an isolated tool for weight management has a high drop-out rate with less than 5% of patients remaining successful after 5 years. If lifestyle modification is this challenging to adults, young children will need much more encouragement, support and supervision to change their lifestyle because of their poorer cognitive understanding of the consequences of the problem of overweight and hence the lack of self-responsibility and commitment to do something about it. It can, therefore, hardly be expected from overweight and obese children to comply with a treatment programme which includes lifestyle modifications including physical activity, dietary and behaviour modification on different levels, on their own. Health promotion awareness campaigns that urge children to be more active because of the health consequences of physical inactivity will hence not be enough to motivate them to become more active and stay active. Practitioners need to design programmes and apply it in such a way that it is attractive to these children and thereby motivate them to participate as part of their understanding and commitment to a lifestyle change. Obese children are normally not keen to be active for various reasons such as physical discomfort, previous negative experiences, anxiety and a low self-esteem (Parizkova, 2005). Obesity treatment also requires many changes on different levels which make it difficult for children to stay motivated while engaging in such programmes, especially the part that requires high levels of physical exertion. All these changes that are required from them, can thus be overwhelming and will require several emotional coping responses from the child to deal with it. Boon and Clydesdale (2005) recommend in this regard that changes should be introduced one at a time because the ability of children to concentrate on one change will then be easier as fewer rules have to be remembered. Continuous support of children by means of re-assessment and the setting of realistic goals is therefore imperative. The younger the child the bigger the challenge will be for results because of their developmental limitations and the higher the need for a ongoing and supervised treatment programme will be. Interventions should also focus on making children's environments healthier rather than focusing solely on personal responsibility (AED, 2011). It is also recommended that obese children should participate in small groups as this is conducive to the need for group activities with peers of a similar size and shape, and provide support and opportunity for social interaction. In so doing such children do not feel isolated or different from their peers as they are matched with children with similar abilities and problems which make it easier to participate in activities that are strenuous.

Research experience (Kemp & Pienaar, 2010; Truter et al., 2010) indicate that although many children were identified as obese and invited to participate in an obesity intervention, free of charge, parents were still hesitant to provide permission for their children to benefit from this opportunity. It is understandable that parents want to protect their children from unnecessary labels that could affect their emotional development or self-confidence negatively. Main obstacles are, therefore, the acknowledging of the problem of childhood obesity by parents as well as the urgency to address it, and further to support the child once overweight or obesity is established as a health concern that needs to be addressed. Family involvement on various levels is considered to be critical in the treatment of childhood overweight. Practitioners must remember that when parents provide informed consent for their child to participate in a treatment programme, it should not necessarily be considered as active involvement on the part of the parent. Parental involvement is considered to be critical to influence the home environment (dietary modification) and to monitor and motivate children to comply with programmes and to support them to change their lifestyle behaviour and physical activity modification. It is reported in this regard that if the family is not ready to support the programme, success will be unlikely (Kain et al., 2004; Crawford, 2008).

The accessibility of facilities where treatment programmes are offered is important for the sustainability of programs. In the USA it is already indicated that clinical options at hospitals are not effective in the challenge of childhood obesity among children living in poor socio-economic environments (California Department of Public Health, 2010). They claimed that the service should rather be delivered in the environment of the child living in lower socio-economic circumstances. Nearby community centres, churches or school yards are recommended as possible venues with mid-level workers who can assist in non-clinical programmes. Health care facilities in remote areas can also be used for basic screening and to provide education and referral help for the parents.

Specific knowledge of the target populations and the best way to engage them in change is essential, therefore, specific issues, and social and cultural values (cultural view of 'ideal body image') need to be taken into consideration. The question of what will increase the probability of the group to be motivated to participate or comply with changes is essential to be answered in this regard.

Awareness campaigns that stress the urgency of dealing with this problem by taking action and the responsibility of the parent in this decision are, therefore, much needed priorities. Kruger et al. (2005) indicated that stakeholders from government (Departments of Education, Health and Safety and Security) need to understand the factors contributing to decreased physical activity among children and the effects of inactivity on health and should initiate programmes to increase physical activity among South Africans, while stakeholders from the health professions, non-government organisations and communities should also become involved in these efforts.

7.4 Community engagement

The majority of children in South Africa live in environments that are not conducive to their health and well-being and it is, therefore, a challenge to reach these children who are in many areas considered at-risk and in need of developmental help. Statistics show that nearly 40% of children live a long distance from their nearest primary health care clinic (South African Child Gauge, 2008/2009). Strategies to improve community engagement for the purpose of primary prevention should, therefore, be implemented. Expanding high quality preventative services in both clinical and community settings are, therefore, important for successful prevention. In this scenario it is anticipated that a qualified practitioner can make a significant contribution as he/she is specifically trained. Mid-level workers that can assist this healthcare professional in providing more basic services for the obese child, and multi-skilled workers such as nurses who can be trained to do basic screening and risk field analysis and to refer the child for help in remote areas is recommended. In this regard it is indicated that in all interventions aimed at preventing and managing overweight and obesity, systematic assessment and evaluation should form a routine procedure. The incorporation of BMI and waist-circumference as part of a risk factor analysis to be used at primary healthcare level may be the first step in the recognition of chronic, non-communicable diseases by the Department of Health (Kruger et al., 2005). Traditional and community leaders should be involved in providing strategies and support. The AED recommend in this regard that representatives of the community should be included in the planning process to ensure that interventions are sensitive to diverse norms, cultural traditions, and practices. Furthermore, clinical training grants should be provided by the government for in-service training and non-governmental initiatives should be seek to obtain resources, to ensure successful service delivery at community level. These also include commitments from the government to making neighborhoods safer, providing access to nutritious foods, constructing sidewalks and bicycle lanes, building safe outside play areas, and encouraging parents to serve regular family meals, create a non-distracting eating environment, and provide more active alternatives to TV viewing (AED, 2011).

8. Conclusion

Pienaar (2009) stated that the 20st century will challenge movement specialists worldwide, to not only provide services and support to children who are diagnosed with serious activity/movement deficiencies and who meet the legal requirements to be classified as disabled, but also to address other individual needs of children that require professional help. Therefore, children who are not identified by government for special assistance, but who have individual needs that require specialized assistance, should also be able to acquire the specialised knowledge of trained health care professionals such as Kinderkineticists in SA. These will include children with poor fitness levels, overweight and obese, insufficient motor development, poor motor skills or individuals with poor functional posture, injuries or specific medical conditions.

Childhood obesity will never be easy to address, but passionate and specialised professionals who understand the level of problems of children who battle with overweight and who can support them on a scientific and professional level in their quest to overcome the problem, may make a considerable contribution to improve the health burden. The need of children in South Africa for this important impetus in their overall development as a human being inspires professionals to keep on convincing government and other officials to take national action, and hopefully to get the necessary policies and resources in place, to ensure the implementation of a scientifically-based service to a very vulnerable population.

9. References

Academy for Eating Disorders (AED). (2011). Guidelines for Childhood Obesity Prevention Programs, 27/08/2011, Available from: <http://www.aedweb.org/AM/Template.cfm?Section=Advocacy&Template=/CM/ContentDisplay.cfm&ContentID=1659>

American Academy of Child and Adolescent Psychiatry (AACAP). (2010). *Obesity In Children And Teens, 06/02/2010, Available from http://www.AACAP.Org*

American College of Sports Medicine (ACSM). (2000).ACSM's guidelines for exercise testing and prescription *(6th ed), Lippincott, Williams, & Wilkins, Philadelphia*

Apfelbacher, C.J., Cairns, J., Bruckner, T., Möhrenschlager, M., Behrendt, H., Ring, J. & Krämer, U. (2008). Prevalence of Overweight and Obesity in East and West German Children in the Decade After Reunification: Population-Based Series of Cross-Sectional Studies. *Journal of Epidemiology and Community Health,* Vol.62, No.2, (Feb 2008), pp.125-130

Armstrong, M.E.G., Lambert, M.I., Sharwood, K.A. & Lambert, E.V. (2006). Obesity and Overweight in South African Primary School Children - The Health of the Nation Study. *The Official Journal of The Society for Endocrinology, Metabolism and Diabetes of South Africa,* Vol.11, No.2, (Nov 2006), pp.52-63

Baur, L.A. (2001). Obesity: Definitely a Growing Concern. *Medical Journal of Australia,* Vol.174, (Jun 2001), pp.553-554

Boon, C.S. & Clydesdale, F.M. (2005). A Review Of Childhood and Adolescent Obesity Interventions. *Critical Reviews in Food Science and Nutrition,*Vol.45, No.7-8, (2005), pp.511-525

Bosch, J., Stradmeijer, M. & Seidell, J. (2004). Psychosocial Characteristics of Obese Children/Youngsters and their Families: Implications for Preventive and Curative Interventions. *Patient Education and Counseling,* Vol.55, No.3, (Dec 2004), pp.353-362

Bourne, L.T., Lambert, E.V. & Steyn, K. (2002). Where does the Black Population of South Africa stand on the Nutrition Transition? *Public Health Nutrition,* Vol.5, No.1a, (Feb 2002), pp.157-162

Burke, V. (2006). Obesity in Childhood and Cardiovascular Risk. *Clinical and Experimental Pharmacology and Physiology,* Vol.33, No.9, (Aug 2006), pp.831-837

Cameron, N. (2005). Childhood Obesity in Developing Countries. *Journal of Human Ecology.* Vol.13, pp.53-59

Campbell, K., Waters, E., O'meara, S. & Summerbell, C. (2001). Interventions for Preventing Obesity in Childhood. A Systematic Review. *Obesity Reviews,*Vol.2,No.3, (Aug 2001), pp.149-157

California Department of Public Health (CDPH) (2010). California Obesity Prevention Plan: a Vision for Tomorrow, Strategic Actions for Today. California Obesity prevention program, Sacramento, CA. Available at www.cdph.ca.gov/obesityprevention

Chen, A.K., Roberts, C.K. & Barnard, R.J. (2006). Effect of a short-term diet and exercise intervention on metabolic syndrome in overweight children, *Journal of metabolism,* Vol. 55, pp. 871-878

Cole, T.J., Belizzi, M.C., Flegal, K.M. & Dietz, W.H. (2000). Establishing a standard definition for Child Overweight and Obesity Worldwide: International Survey. *British Medical Journal,* Vol.320, No.7244, (May 2000), pp.1240-1243

Connelly, J.B., Duaso, M.J. & Butler, G. (2007). A Systematic Review of Controlled Trials of Interventions to Prevent Childhood Obesity and Overweight: A Realistic Synthesis of the evidence. *Journal of The Royal Institute of Public Health,* Vol.121, No.7, (Jul 2007), pp.510-517

Crawford, M.A. (2008). Marathoners: A childhood obesity prevention program. College of Nursing, *M.Sc dissertation, The University of Arizona, USA*

Cretikos, M.A., Valenti, L., Britt, H.C. & Baur, L.A. (2008). General Practice Management of Overweight and Obesity in Children and Adolescents in Australia. *Medical Care,* Vol.46, No.11, (Nov 2008), pp.1163-1169

Dodd, C.J. (2007). Energy Regulation in Young People. *Journal of Sport Science and Medicine,* Vol.6, (Sept 2007), pp.327-336

Dreimane, D., Safani, D., Mackenzie, M., Halvorson, M., Braun, S., Conrad, B. & Kaufman, F. (2007). Feasibility of a Hospital-Based, Family-Centered Intervention to Reduce Weight Gain in Overweight Children and Adolescents. *Diabetes Research and Clinical Practice,* Vol.75, No.2, (Feb 2007), pp.159-168

Du Toit, D. & Pienaar, A.E. (2003). Overweight and Obesity and Motor Competence of 4-5 Year Old Preschool Children. *South African journal for Research in Sport, Physical Education and Recreation,* Vol.23, No.2, pp.51-62

Du Toit, D & Pienaar, A.E., Truter, L. (2011). Relationship Between Physical Fitness and Academic Performance in South African Children. *South African Journal for Research in Sport, Physical Education and Recreation,* Vol.33, No.3, pp.

Koop, C.E. (1996). Exclusive: Worksite Health Interviews C. Everett Koop. *AWHP'S Worksite Health Spring 1996,* Vol.3, No.8, pp.10-13

Eliakim, A., Kaven, G., Berger, I., Friedland, O., Wolach, B. & Nemet, D. (2002). The Effect of a Combined Intervention on Body Mass Index and Fitness in Obese Children and Adolescents - A Clinical Experience. *European Journal of Pediatrics,* Vol.161, No.8, (Aug 2002), pp.449-452

Eneli, I.U., Cunningham, A. & Woolford, S.J. (2008). The Pediatric Multidisciplinary Obesity Program: An Update. *Progress in Pediatric Cardiology,* Vol.25, No.2, (Sept 2008), pp.129-136

Gabbard, C. (1998). Windows of opportunity for early brain development. *Journal of Physical Education, Recreation and Dance,* Vol.69, No.4, (Oct 1998), pp.52-54

Goedecke, J.H.; Jennings, C.L.; Lambert, E.V. (2006). Obesity In South Africa. In *Chronic Diseases Of Lifestyle In South Africa:1995–2005;* Steyn, K., Fourie, J., Temple, N.Z., Eds.; Medical Research Council: Cape Town, South Africa, 2006; (May 2006), pp. 65–79

Golan, M., Kaufman, V. & Shadar, D.R. (2006). Childhood Obesity Treatment: Targeting Parents Exclusively Vs. Parents And Children. *British Journal of Nutrition,* Vol.95, No.5, (May 2006), pp.1008-1015

Jerum, A. & Melnyk, B.M. (2001). Effectiveness of Interventions to Prevent Obesity and Obesity-Related Complications in Children and Adolescents. *Pediatric Nursing,* Vol.27, No.6, (Nov-Dec 2001), pp.606-610

Joubert, J, Norman, R, Bradshaw, D, Goedecke, J.H., Steyn, N.P., Puoane, T. & the South African Comparative Risk Assessment Collaborating Group. (2007). Estimating the Burden of Disease Attributable to Excess Body Weight in South Africa in 2000. *South African Medical Journal,* Vol.97, No.8, (August 2007), pp.683-690

Kain, J., Uauy, R., Vio, F. & Albala, C. (2002). Trends in Overweight and Obesity Prevalence in Chilean Children. *European Journal of Clinical Nutrition,* Vol.56, No.3, (Mar 2002), pp.200-204

Kain, J., Uauy, R., Albala, A., Vio, F., Cerda, R. & Leyton, B. (2004). School-Based Obesity Prevention in Chilean Primary School Children: Methodology and Evaluation of a Controlled Study. *International Journal of Obesity,* Vol.28, No.4, (Apr 2004), pp.483-493

Kemp, C. & Pienaar, A.E. (2010). The Effect of a Physical Activity, Diet and Behaviour Modification Intervention on the Self-Perception of 9 to 12 Year Old Overweight and Obese Children. *African Journal for Physical, Health, Education, Recreation and Dance,* Vol.16, No.1, (Mar 2010), pp.98-112

Kemp, C. & Pienaar, AE. (2011). Physical Activity Levels and Energy Expenditure of 9 to 12 Year Old Overweight and Obese Children. *SA Health/SA Gesondheid,* Vol.16, No.1, (Mar 2011), pp.1-6 557

Kemp C., Pienaar, A.E. & Schutte, A. (2011). The Prevalence of Hypertension and the Relationship with Body Composition in grade 1 learners in the North West province of South Africa. *South African Journal of Sports Medicine*, Vol.23, No.4, page nr not yet available

Kimm, S.Y.S. (2004). Fetal Origins of Adult Disease: The Barker Hypothesis Revisited-2004. *Endocrinology and Diabetes*. Vol.11, No.4, (Aug 2004), pp.192-196

Korsten-Reck, U., Kromeyer-Hauschild, K., Wolfarth, B., Dickhuth, H.H. & Berg, A. (2005). Freiburg Intervention Trial for Obese Children (Fitoc): Results of a Clinical Observation Study. *International Journal of Obesity*, Vol.29, No.4, (Apr 2005), pp.356-361

Kruger, H.S., Puoane, T., Senekal, M. & Van Der Merwe, M.T. (2005). Obesity in South Africa: Challenges for Government and Health Professionals. *Public Health Nutrition*, Vol.8, No.5, (Aug 2005), pp.491-500

Knöpfli, B.H., Radtke, T., Lehmann, M., Schätzle, B., Eisenblätter, J., Gachnang, A., Wiederkehr, P., Hammer, J & Wildhaber, J.B. (2008). Effects of a Multidisciplinary Inpatient Intervention on Body Composition, Aerobic Fitness, and Quality of Life in Severely Obese Girls and Boys. *Journal of Adolescent Health*, Vol.42, No.2, (Feb 2008), pp.119-127

Labadarios D. (1999). The National Food Consumption Survey (NfCS): Children Aged 1-9 Years, South Africa, 1999. Pretoria: National Department Of Health; 2000, Vol.8, No.5, (Aug 1999), pp.533-543

Lennox, A., Pienaar, A.E., Coetzee. M. (2007). Barriers, motivators, sport participation and perceptions of physical activity among adolescents living in semi urban surroundings. *African Journal for Physical, Health, Education, Recreation and Dance*, Vol.13, No.1, (Sept 2007), pp.289-303

MaCintyre, U.E., Kruger, H.S., Venter, C.S. & Vorster, H.H. (2002). Dietary Intakes of an African Population in Different Stages of Transition in the North-West Province, South Africa: The Thusa-Study. *Nutrition Research*, Vol.22, No.3, (Mar 2002), pp.239-256

Maffeis, C., Consolaro, A., Cavarzere, P., Chini, L., Banzato, C., Grezzani, A., Silvagni, D., Salzano, G., De Luca, F. & Tato, L. (2006). Prevalence of Overweight and Obesity in 2- to 6-Year-Old Italian Children. *Obesity*, Vol.14, No.5, (May 2006), pp.765-769

Mcveigh, J.A., Norris, S.A., Cameron, N. & Pettifor, J.M. (2004). Associations Between Physical Activity and Bone Mass in Black and White South African Children at Age 9 Yrs. *Journal of Applied Physiology*, Vol.97, No.3, (May 2004), pp.1006-1012

Medical Research Council. (2002). Umthente Uhlaha Usamila: The 1st South African National Youth Risk Behaviour Survey, 11/05/2010, Available from: <http://www.Mrc.Ac.Za/Healtpromotion/Reports.Htm>

Millenium Development Goals. (2010) Country Report, 22/08/2011, Available from: www.Statssa.Gov.Za/News_Archive/Docs/Mdgr_2010.Pdf

Monyeki, K.D., Lenthe, F.J. & Steyn, N.P. (1999). Obesity: Does it Occur in African Children in a Rural Community in South Africa? *International Journal of Epidemiology*, Vol.28, No.2, (1999), pp.287-292

Naudé, D. Kruger, H.S. & Pienaar, A.E. (2009). Differences in body composition, body proportions and timing of puberty between stunted and non-stunted adolescents. *African Journal for Physical, Health, Education, Recreation and Dance,* Vol.15, No.4, (Dec 2009), pp.678-689

Nemene, D., Barkan, S., Epstein, Y., Friedland, O., Kowen, G. & Eliakim, A. (2005). Short- and Long-Term Beneficial Effects of a Combined Dietary-Behavioral-Physical Acivity Intervention for the treatment of Childhood Obesity. *Pediatrics,* Vol.115, No.4, (Apr 2005), pp.443-449

Ogden, C.L., Carroll, M.D., Curtin, L.R., Lamb, M.M. & Flegal, K.M. (2010a). Prevalence of High Body Mass Index in US Children and Adolescents, 2007-2008. *Journal of The American Medical Association,* Vol.303, No.3, (Jan 2010), pp.242-249

Ogden, C.L., Lamb, M.M., Carroll, M.D. & Flegal, K. (2010b). Obesity and socioeconomic status in children: United States 1988-1994 and 2005-2008, NCHS data brief no. 51, MD: National Center for Health Statistics, Hyattsville

Padez, C., Mourao, I., Moreira, P. & Rosado, V. (2005). Prevalence and Risk Factors for Overweight and Obesity in Portugese Children. *Acta Paediatrica,* Vol.94, No.11, (Nov 2005), pp.1550-1557

Parizkova, J. (2005). *Practical Programs for Weight Management during the Growing Years. In:* Childhood obesity: prevention and treatment, Parizkova, J. & Hills, A.P., pp.271-345, *CRC Press*

Pienaar, A.E., Bell, G.J. & Dreyer, L.I. (2007). The Incidence of Obesity And Developmental Coordination Disorder (DCD) Among 10-12 Year-Old Girls Of Different Race Groups In The North-West Province: Thusa Bana Study. *African Journal of Physical, Health Education, Recreation And Dance,* Supplement Edition, (Sept 2007), pp.221-237

Pienaar A.E & Eggar, N. (2007). Perception of Physical Competence, Physical Appearance And Weight Control: Is There A Relationship With DCD? *African Journal For Physical, Health, Education, Recreation And Dance,* Vol.13,No.3, (Sept 2007), pp.306-318

Pienaar, AE. 2009. Kinderkinetics: an investment in the total well-being of children. *South African Journal for Research in Sport, Physical Education and Recreation,* Vol.1, No.1, (2009), pp.49-67

Puoane, T & Hughes, G. (2005). "Impact Of The Hiv/Aids Pandemic On Non-Communicable Disease Prevention."*South African Medical Journal,* Vol.95, No.4, (2005), pp.228-230

Popkin, B. M.; Richards, M. K. & Monteiro, C.A., (1996). Stunting is associated with Overweight in Children of Four Nations that are Undergoing the Nutrition Transition. *Journal of Nutrition,* Vol.126, No.12, (Dec 1996), pp.3009-3016

Ravelli, G. P.; Stein, Z. & Susser, M., (1976). Obesity in Young Men after Famine Exposure in Utero and Early Infancy. *New England Medical Journal,* Vol.259, No. ,(1976), pp.349-353

Robbins, G; Powers, D & Burgess, S. (1991). *A Wellness Way of Life WMC,* Brown Publisher, Dubuque

Robert Wood Johnson Foundation. (2008). F as in Fat. How obesity policies failing in America. Preventing epidemics. Protecting people, Robert Wood Johnson Foundation. Issue report, (Aug 2008)

Rowland, T.W., (1990). *Exercise and Children's Health,* Human Kinetics Books, Champaign, Illinois

Sabin, M.A., Crowne, E.C. & Shield, J.P.H. (2004). The Prognosis in Childhood Obesity. *Current Paediatrics,* Vol.14, No.2, (Apr 2004), pp.110-114

Sacher, P.M., Chadwick, P., Wells, J.C.K., Cole, T.J. & Lawson, M.S. (2005). Assessing the Acceptability and Feasibility of The Mend Programme in a Small Group of Obese 7-11-Year-Old Children. *Journal of Human Nutrition And Dietetics,* Vol.18, No.1, (Feb 2005), pp.3-5

Senekal, M., Steyn, P.N., Mashego T.B., & Helena, J.N. (2001). Evaluation of Body Shape, Stice, E., Hayward, C., Cameron, R.P., Killen, J.D., & Taylor, C.B. (2000). *Journal of Abnormal Psychology,* Vol.109, (2001), pp.438-444

Senekal, M., Steyn, N.P., Nel, J.H. (2003). Factors Associated with Overweight/Obesity in Economically Active South African Populations. *Ethnicity & Disease,* Vol.13, (2003) pp.109-116.

Sherrill, C. (2004). *Adapted physical activity, recreation and sport. Cross disciplinary and lifespan.* (6th ed.), McGraw Hill, New York

Short, F.X., J. McCubbin, J. & Frey, G. (1999), Cardiorespiratory endurance and body composition. In *The Brockport physical fitness training guide,* Human Kinetics, Champaign

Somers, A., Hassan, M.S., Rusford, E. & Erasmus, R.T. (2006). Overweight and Obesity in Learners Residing in the Belhar, Delft and Mfuleni Communities of Cape Town, Western Cape, South Africa. Medical Technology South Africa, Vol.20, *No.1, (Jun 2006), pp.11-20*

South African Child Gauge, (2008/2009). Edited by Pendlebury, S., Lake, L., & Smith, C., Children's institute, University of Cape Town

Steyn, N.P. (2005). Managing Childhood Obesity: A Comprehensive Approach. Continuing *Medical Education, Vol.23, No.11, (Nov-Dec 2005), pp.540-544*

Steyn, N.P., Labadarios, M.B., Mauder, E., Nel, J. & Lombard, C. (2005). Secondary Anthropometric Data Analysis of The National Food Consumption Survey in South Africa: The Double Burden. *Nutrition,*Vol. 21, No.1, (Jan 2005), pp.4-13

Steyn, C., (2007). *All South Africans at risk of dying young, says new report,* 15/10/2008, Available from: <www.heartfoundation.co.za/doc/releases/SAREPORT>

Strydom, G.L., Wilders, C.J., Moss, S.J. & Bruwer, E. (2009). A conceptual framework of Biokinetic procedures and referral system: An integrated protocol for the various health paradigms. *African Journal for Physical, Health Education, Recreation and Dance.* Vol.15, No.4 (Dec 2009), pp.641-649

Truter, L., Pienaar, A.E. & Du Toit D. (2010). Relationship between overweight, obesity and physical fitness of 10 to 12-year old South African children. *South African Family Practice,* Vol .52, No.3, pp. 227-233

Van Der Merwe, M.T. (2004). Childhood Obesity. *South African Family Practice,* Vol.46, No.6, (2004), pp.16-19

Weigel, C., Kokocinski, K, Lederer, P., Dotsch, J., Rascher, W. & Knerr, I. (2008). Childhood Obesity: Concept, Feasibility, and Interim Results Of A Local Group-Based, Long-Term Treatment Program. *Journal of Nutrition Education and Behaviour,* Vol.40, (2004), pp.369-373

World Health Organisation (WHO). *(2010). Obesity. 08/09/2010,* Available from: *<Http://Www.Who.Int >*

Zere, E & Mcintyre, D. (2003). Inequities in Under-Five Child Malnutrition in South Africa. *International Journal For Equity In Health.* Vol.2, No.7, (Sept 2003), pp.1-10

11

"Jugando a Ganar Salud" ("Playing to Gain Health"): A Summer-Vacation Physical Activity and Correct Eating Workshop for School-Aged Children – A Pilot Study

Karime Haua-Navarro[1], Luz Irene Moreno-Landa[1], Marcela Pérez-Rodríguez[2], Guillermo Meléndez[2] and Ana Bertha Pérez-Lizaur[1]

[1]*Health Department, Universidad Iberoamericana (UIA), Mexico City,*
[2]*FUNSALUD, Mexico City,*
Mexico

1. Introduction

According to the most recent data on nutritional evaluation in Mexican population, one of every four children between 5 and 11 years of age (26%) presents overweight or obesity, dramatically surpassing the estimate calculated for 2010 for childhood obesity at the worldwide level of 6.7% (Olaiz-Fernández G, 2006). This problem acquires great relevance not only because of the prevalence of obesity, but also due to the consequences associated with this condition, such as high risk of adult-age obesity and chronic diseases such as diabetes mellitus, high blood pressure, dyslipidemias, obstructive apnea sleep disorder syndrome, and non-alcoholic steatosis (Pimenta AM, 2010; Elizondo-Montemayor L, 2010). Conclusive evidence has been established that physical activity is a promoter of healthy lifestyle promoter and a preventer of excessive weight gain (Summerbell CD, 2005) and other diseases. In particular, habitual physical activity at early ages increases the probability of exerting an impact on the mortality and longevity of persons, as well as improving some cardiovascular risk indicators (Hills AP, 2007; Balas-Nakaxh M, 2010). Generality in existing consensuses for the prevention and treatment of childhood obesity cites the promotion of physical activity as an imperative strategy. The different guidelines that exist on physical activity in children recommend 60 min of physical activity daily of at least moderate intensity, including vigorous aerobic activity at least 3 days a week (Jasen I, 2010; O'Donovan G, 2010). Unfortunately, in Mexico, the reality concerning the time devoted to physical activity in children lies very far from these recommendations. An observational study conducted in Mexico quantified the physical activity engaged in within the school environment, identifying that children have few opportunities to participate in moderate- and vigorous-intensity physical activity, scarcely achieving one half of the time recommended by international guidelines for this age group (Jennings-Aburto N ,2009). A large proportion of the reports on studies examining the promotion of physical activity in this age group are hardly encouraging in terms of the results obtained regarding body weight modification, eating habits, and a sedentary lifestyle at the long term (Jennings-Aburto N, 2009). The lack of available physical and environmental spaces that promote physical activity within the inter- as well as the extra-academic environment could also contribute to the problem. In addition, the amount of physical activity carried out by children in the school environment is diminishing over time; a study conducted with Mexican children reported that moderate-to-vigorous physical activity decreased 40% from kindergarten to second grade of primary school (Jáuregui A, 2011).

The increase of overweight and obesity has been associated with multiple factors such as the genetic factor, the social factor, and those of behavior and ecology (Jennings-Aburto N, 2009). Only some of these factors can be modified at a certain percentage; the development of overweight and obesity are the consequence of changes in dietary patterns: the increase of the availability of food; the consumption of foods with greater energetic density, and less consumption of fruits and vegetables. In Mexico, in the last 14 years, the purchase of vegetables and fruits has diminished by 29.3%. The consumption of vegetables and fruits in Mexican children stands at one portion (100 g) (Ramírez-Silva I, 2009); this is considered insufficient for maintaining a healthy diet and for preventing chronic degenerative diseases. The purchase of high-energetic-.density industrialized foods has increased by 6.3% and the purchase of sweetened beverages has increased by 37.2% (Bonvecchio A, 2009). This demonstrated numerically the changes undergone by dietary patterns. The role of child-directed advertising, the constant bombardment of information on high-energy-value drinks, and the broad array of offers for this type of food has induced an important change in the childhood feeding pattern. Many interesting efforts have been made in applying marketing techniques to promote the consumption of fruits and vegetables and to revert in this manner the effects of the food-consumption behavior adopted over the last 40 years (Domínguez-Vázquez P, 2008).

2. Materials and methods

Considering the previously cited findings, the Health Department of the Mexico City-based Universidad Iberoamericana (UIA) took on the task of developing the Summer Course entitled "Playing to Gain Health", a model for the promotion of a healthy lifestyle for school-aged children, focused on the skills, attitudes, and knowledge concerning correct diet and the practice of physical activity in a playful, carefree, and non-violent atmosphere to promote the consumption of three servings of fruits and vegetables, water, and skin milk and practicing 30 min of moderate and 15 min of light physical activity and fruits during 3 weeks of morning sessions at schools of community centers during the summer vacation period. The strategy can be adapted for utilization in children's free time during the week or even on weekends in parks and schoolyards or open spaces in the community.

Eating habits that are acquired during childhood may persist into adulthood (Branen L, Fletcher J, 1999); thus, factors that influence food consumption should be identified in order to carry out more effective interventions that will promote a healthy diet throughout the entire lifespan (Pérez, 2004). Also, the physical-activity level tends to decline and sedentary behavior tends to increase prior to adolescence (Basterfield L, 2011); reinforcement of an active lifestyle is crucial at this age.

A number of behavioral theories are applied to eating habits research to describe the mechanisms by which attitudes and beliefs exert their influence on eating behavior (Jack I, 2010). It is expected that the efficiency and efficacy of individual and community interventions in the form of health programs, particularly food programs, would increase as our understanding of basic behavioral mechanisms through these theories also increases. The

Social Cognitive Theory (Bandura, 1977) proposes that an individual's behavioral and environmental conduct and personal characteristics interact in reciprocal relationship (reciprocal determination), explaining the subject's behavior. These characteristics are defined as the following: accessibility (the ease with which students were able to find ready-to-eat vegetables and fruits [VF]); expectancy (the value that the person places on a given outcome); self-efficacy (the person's confidence in engaging in a particular behavior and in overcoming barriers to that behavior); preference (what the child likes to eat), and knowledge (what the child knows about the function of VF in the body) (Baranowski T, 2002). Applying this theory to nutritional education has been successfully employed as the foundation in health education interventions in schools (Yngve A, 2005). Our model summer program and intervention were designed based on the social learning theory (Pérez-Lizaur AB, 2008) and constructivist pedagogy whereby summer-course participants construct their learning curve on the attitudes that they develop during the 3 weeks that the workshop lasts. The activities facilitate the knowledge and promote the skills and attitudes to comply with the program's objectives written in terms of didactic strategies that define the following: name of the activity; session number; objective of the activity; purpose or principle of thee strategy; theme, subtheme; duration; procedure; sponsorship; resources, and time.

"Playing to Gain Health" summer course has its pedagogical foundation on the constructivist teaching trend in which participants guide their learning process based on the activities that they develop during the workshop's 3-week duration. We developed a manual in which the activities are described that facilitate knowledge and that promote skills and attitudes to comply with the objectives of the program and that are described by means of didactic strategies that define:

- Name of the activity
- Session number
- Objective of the activity
- Purpose or principle of the activity
- Theme, subtheme
- Duration, procedure, sponsorship, resources, time.

The content of the Summer Course Manual was validated by a group of experts and the strategy has been evaluated on two occasions with respect to the eating habits and physical activity of the children.

The program is designed to be carried out during 3 weeks in a period of 4½ h daily, including breakfast and a snack for the children to have access to correct eating (especially tasting and consumption of vegetables, fruits, plain water, and skin milk). The games are focused on developing light- and moderate-intensity physical activity as well as some minutes of vigorously intense activity in a playful and non-violent environment.

In complementary fashion, we designed menus for the breakfasts and the snacks (refreshments) that were focused on compliance with the general guidelines established by the Ministry of Health and the Ministry of Public Education in Mexico for the sale or distribution of food and beverages in the school consumption establishments of basic-education centers (Secretaría de Educación Pública, 2010). With the purpose of providing access to a great variety of fruits and vegetables, we prepared and served raw and/or cooked vegetables and fruits, whether as an ingredient in a some typical dish (with zucchini squash "sopes", and purslane and cheese "tacos"), or a the main ingredient of some snack (frozen pineapple popsicle). In order to draw the children near to vegetables and fruits and to familiarize the children with these as part of the workshop's activities, the children prepared some recipes such as fruit kabobs, vegetarian robots, and diverse figures such as a ship with vegetables; similarly, they prepared a certain recipe such as a fruit and veggie rainbow (Figures 1-3).

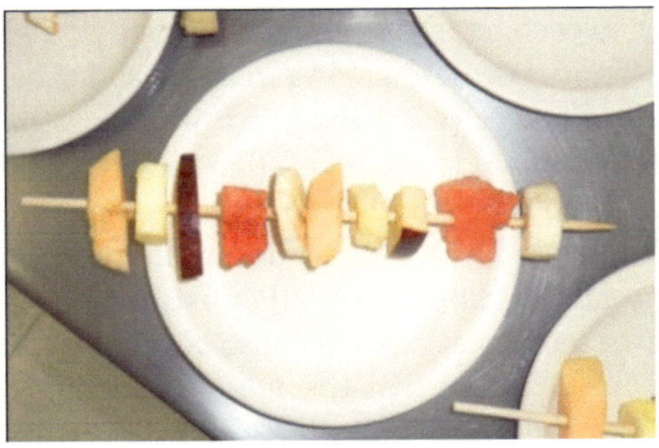

Fig. 1. Fruit kabob

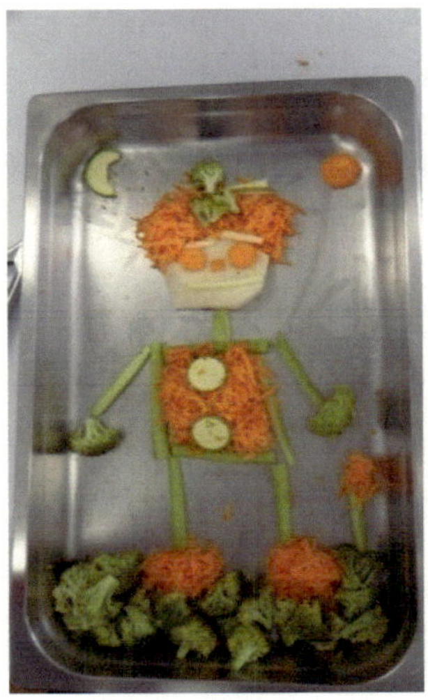

Fig. 2. Vegetarian robot

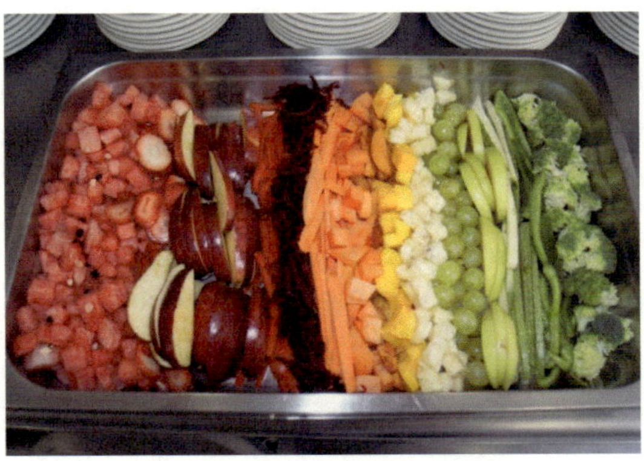

Fig. 3. Fruit and veggie rainbow

2.1 Subjects

The physical-activity education program was piloted in 45 boys and girls aged 6-13 years, belonging to a low socioeconomic level (classification D[1])(AMAI 200)(A.C., 2009), who regularly attend public schools in Mexico's Federal District. We received informed consent form the children's parents and the consent of the children themselves. For study participation, we requested a medical certificate as proof of the child's good health. We utilized convenience sampling, selecting all children who accepted the invitation to participate in the program. For recruitment, the invitation was issued by means of posters distributed in the neighborhood where the study was carried out. Interested parents attended an informative meeting in which we explained the program procedures and requested their written consent concerning the participation of their children. An additional population (n = 21) with characteristics equivalent to those of the summer-course attendee population was selected to make comparisons (age- and Body mass index [BMI]-paired) of the physical activity carried out in an environment designed for its promotion as a summer workshop, in contrast with the physical activity quantified in a common school environment. For selection of this population, we also had written informed consent from the children's parents.

For determination of the total vegetable and fruit consumption, we weighed the daily production of all fruits, vegetables, and prepared dishes, we weighed the leftovers of these dishes and the waste on the children's plates). We determined the percentage of leftovers/waste and the total percentage of fruits and vegetables consumed.

Water consumption was measured by the amount of large, plastic water containers consumed every day; this comprised free access and was offered at breakfast, during the practice of physical activity, and during snack time.

2.2 Instruments and procedures

The "Playing to Gain Health" program was carried out at the *Santa María Comedores* AC communal dining rooms and at public courts of the Colonia Tlapechico neighborhood in the Álvaro Obregón Delegation in Mexico's Federal District; these sites complied with the requirements of being a physical space with a kitchen, a dining room, and public space for outdoor activities and to conduct the activities planned.

A group of young people (cheerleaders (*animadores*) aged 18-22 years, at a 1:8 ratio of one youth per 8 children) trained in didactic strategies and coordinated by the program supervisor (see Figure 5) provided an emotionally and physically safe ambiance for development of the program. This tactic allowed for a dual function on providing activities for the youth population in contact with the children and the promotion of good health practices.

---

[1]Lower middle class (D+) – The head-of-household profile in these homes is one of individuals with a complete primary or secondary school academic level. The living spaces of this segment are, in the majority, owned by the family, while some persons rent their homes and some are social-.interest dwellings.

Lower Class (D) – This is the mid-section of the lower classes. The profile of the head of household in these homes is one of individuals with an average primary-school educative level (complete in the majority of cases). The dwellings of those belonging to this sector are owned or rented (it is easy to find typical tenement houses), which are in their majority social-interest or fixed/controlled-rent housing. Source: AMAI[16].

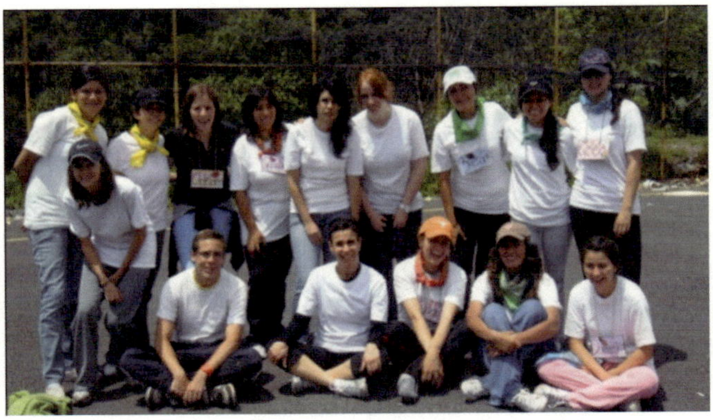

Fig. 4. Cheerleader Group 1.

The main strategy for complying with the objectives was the involvement of the children in a non-violent environment, in traditional games (children's songs and rounds, hoops, jump rope) and in sports such as soccer, basketball, volleyball, races, and rallies, which took place on the site's public sports courts and playing fields (Figures 5 and 6).

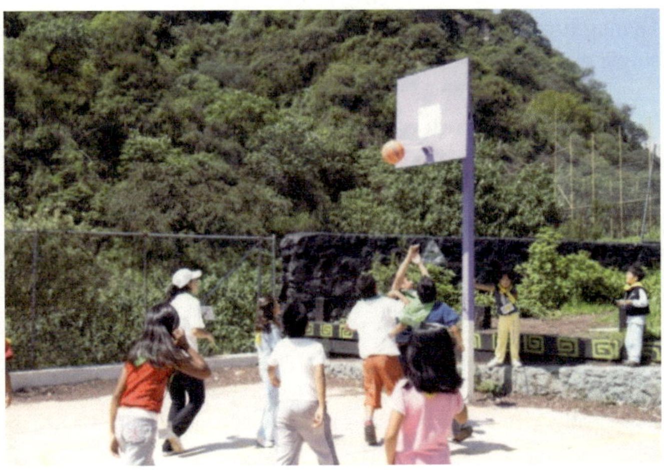

Fig. 5. Basketball.

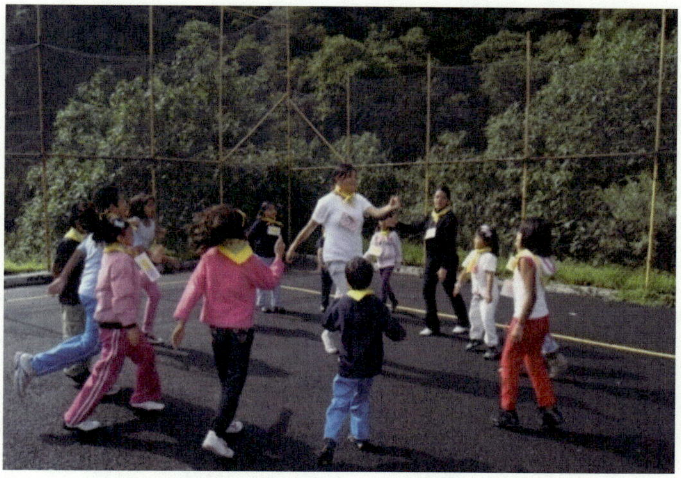

Fig. 6. Children's games and rounds.

Additionally, we included activities with basic healthy-eating Concepts, including knowledge of the Healthy Eating Dish, the practical concepts of the complete and varied diet, as well as the importance of the consumption of fruits, vegetables, and water (Figures 7 and 8).

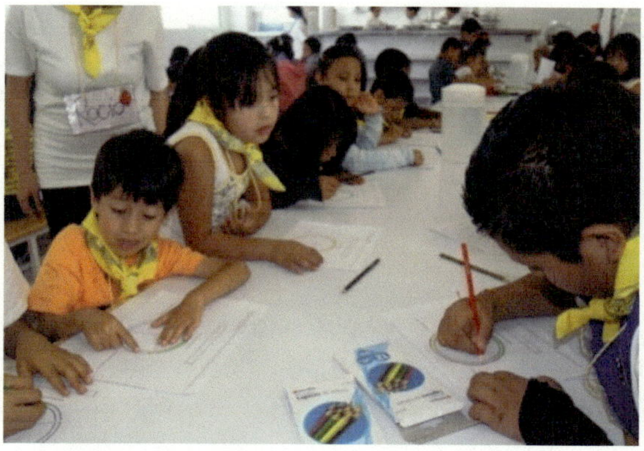

Fig. 7. Coloring "The Healthy Eating Dish".

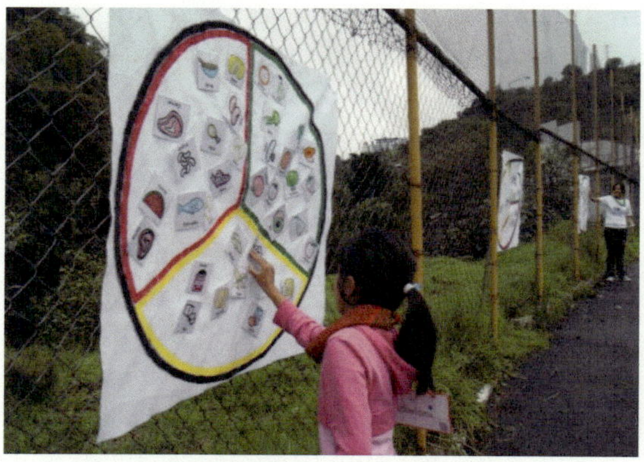

Fig. 8. Identifying foods on the "The Healthy Eating Dish".

The children ate their breakfast and snack in the workshops; the menus were designed based on Correct Diet characteristics (Salud, 2005) (Bandura, 1977) and following the general guidelines for the sale or distribution of foods and beverages in establishments catering to school consumption at basic-education centers (Ministry of Public Education, 2010). In Table 1, we are able to observe a nutrient-evaluation example of a breakfast and a snack. The requirement is that referred for children of Mexican population (Bourges et al., 2009), such as simple carbohydrates including lactose and sucrose (15 g); the remaining nutrients are covered on average at between 90 and 110% in all menus.

	Kcal	Simple carbo-hydrates	Protein	Lipids	Carbo-hydrates	Sodium	Calcium
Requirement	760.00	29.00	28.50	21.00	114.00	927.20	400.00
Water	0.00	0.00	0.00	0.00	0.00	7.20	0.00
Fruit kabob	120.82	24.05	1.39	0.54	31.26	4.94	0.00
Egg with corn tortilla	277.76	1.37	12.39	14.31	24.53	896.11	90
Milk	84.24	0.00	8.23	0.39	11.66	123.43	295.84
Watermelon with yogurt	229.79	13.02	6.20	7.46	38.09	36.51	54.32
	712.61	38.44	28.20	22.70	105.54	1,068.19	440.15
% of daily requirement	93.76	132.55	98.95	108.09	92.58	115.21	110.54

Table 1. Evaluation example of the nutrient composition of a menu

To evaluate the results of the program, we performed evaluations in week 1 and 3 (first and last weeks) of the workshop, including anthropometric variables (weight, height, BMI, waist circumference according to the technique proposed by Lohman) (Lohman TG, 1988), blood pressure, and physical activity measurement with accelerometers (ActiGraph GT3X). Anthropometric measurements of physical activity and blood pressure were carried out by nutritionists standardized for these measurements. Evaluations with accelerometers were performed in duplicate for each child, with measurement at the workshop's beginning and end. Measurements were considered valid if they had at least a 4-h duration. The main success indicator explored was the achievement of performing at least 30 min of moderate and 15 min of light physical activity. We performed a descriptive analysis of baseline (initial) and endline (final) conditions through calculation of central trend measurements and appropriate spread of variable type and distribution. Baseline-endline comparison of the workshop was conducted by means of analysis with the Wilcoxon test. In addition, we employed, by means of multiple regression analysis, the variables that could explain the physical activity carried out in the two measurements as well as the change between the first and second measurement. For comparison of physical activity performed by pilot-workshop participants, we paired them with a control group of 21 children (age- and BMI-matched) (Wilcoxon test).

3. Results

We studied 45 children, 60% (n = 27) were girls attending between 1st and 6th grade of primary school, with ages between 6 and 13 years. Comparison between baseline physical-activity measurements vs. those performed at endline show that there were no changes in anthropometric variables nor in blood pressure (Table 2).

	FIRST WEEK Med (min-max)	LAST WEEK Med (min-max)	Signifi-cance* (p =)
Weight (kg)	31.00 (18.00-54.00)	30.00 (18.00-48.00)	0.414
BMI	17.00 (14.00-25.00)	-17.00 (14.00-25.00)	0.317
Waist circumference (cm)	59.00 (48.00-76.00)	57.00 (49.00-76.00)	0.323
Systolic blood pressure	99.00 (77.00-142.00)	92.00 (77.00-133.00)	0.170
Diastolic blood pressure	62.00 (43.00-110.00)	59.50 (36.00-85.00)	0.26

*Wilcoxon test. Med = Media ; min = minimun ; max = maximun .

Table 2. Changes in anthropometric variables and blood pressure

With regard to observations on physical activity, there was a global increase in the physical activity engaged in by the children, which we evaluated with total counts registered by accelerometer (Wilcoxon test; p = 0.000). Specifically, changes in the intensity of the activity carried out showed a significant reduction in sedentary-type physical activity, while activities of light and moderate intensity increased (Figure 9).

Once the modifications were explored of the physical-activity amount and type carried out by the children, we evaluated the achievement of the main objectives of the study, which corresponded to engaging in at least 30 min of moderate- and 15 min of light-type physical activity. In terms of light physical activity, 95.5% (n = 43) of the participants had already covered the expected time in the baseline measurement and there was no modification under this heading in the final quantification, in contrast with moderate-type activity, which no child carried out for 30 min or more at the beginning of the program and which only 9.5% achieved at the end of the workshop. We identified, by means of multiple linear regression analysis (Stepwise), which of the variables collected (age, weight, height, BMI, waist circumference, and systolic and diastolic blood pressure) explained the physical-activity counts at the end of the workshop. We identified age as the sole predictor variable of the total counts registered for each child (p = 0.011).. On its part, change in physical activity at both dates (week 1 counts - week 3 counts) were not predicted in regression analysis by any of the variables analyzed (p = 0.983).

With respect to comparison of the physical activity engaged in by the workshop children vs. that carried out by the children during a school day, we observed that from week 1, the energy expenditure was significantly greater in the former (p <0.05), because these children initiated their games and activities from day 1 of the intervention (Table 3).

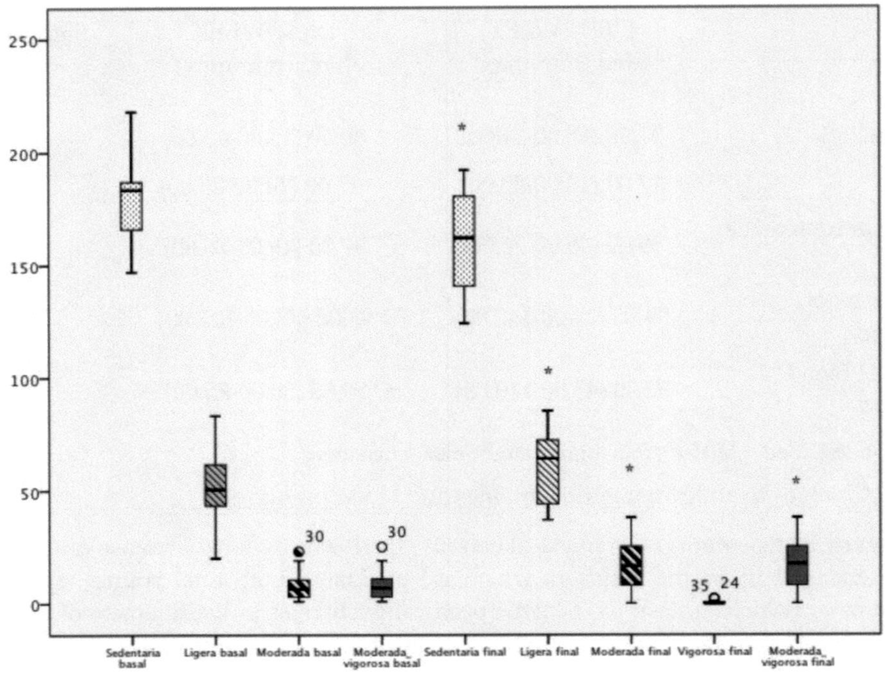

Baseline vs. endline activity comparison; Wilcoxon test; $p < 0.05$.
Sedentaria base = Baseline sedentary
Ligera base = Baseline light
Moderada base = Baseline moderate
Moderata, vigorosa base = Baseline moderate-to-vigorous
Sedentaria final = Endline sedentary
Ligera final = Endline light
Moderata final = Endline moderate
Vigorosa final = Endline vigorous
Moderata, vigorosa final = Endline moderate-to-vigorous

Fig. 9. Baseline and endline comparison of physical activity.

VARIABLE Minutes (mins)	SUMMER PROGRAM GROUP		GROUP IN SCHOOL	SIGNIFICANCE* (Intervention, baseline vs. control)	SIGNIFICANCE* (Intervention, (endline vs. control)
	Initial week Med (min-max)	Final week Med (min-max)	Med (min-max)		
Sedentary activity (mins)	183.50 (147.00-218.00)	162.00 (124.00-192.00)	213.00 (150.00-240.00)	0.000	0.000
Light activity (mins)	50.50 (20.00-83.00)	64.00 (37.00-85.00)	27.00 (0.00-77.00)	0.000	0.000
Moderate activity (mins)	5.00 (00-23.00)	16.50 (0.00-38.00)	1.00 (0.00-13.00)	0.007	0.000
Vigorous activity (mins)	0.00 (0.00-2.00)	0.00 (0.00-2.00)	0.00 (0.00-0.00)	0.102	0.038
Moderate + vigorous activity (mins)	7.00 (1.00-25.00)	17.50 (0.00-38.00)	1.00 (0.00-13.00)	0.004	0.000

*Wilcoxon test. Med = Media ; min = minimun ; max = maximun .

Table 3. Change of physical activity in workshop children vs. children in school

To determine vegetable and fruit consumption, we weighed the total production of each dish or food programmed, and the waste (what was no longer good and that remained in the casseroles in the kitchen) and we additionally weighed everything left on the children's plates (waste), separating vegetables and fruits from the remaining ingredients. Consumption of vegetables and fruits was determined by means of an average, which was 91.69%; it is noteworthy that the children accepted fruits better than vegetables and that in general, they consumed more raw than cooked fruits and vegetables. It is interesting to observe, in Table 4, the increase of fruit consumption from week 1 to week 3, and that during the morning, the children reached a consumption during of >60% of the World Health Organization (WHO) recommendation.

Consumption of vegetables and fruit (g/child)	Week 1	Week 3
Monday	90	363
Tuesday	313	221
Wednesday	248	218
Thursday	333	376
Friday	207	390

Table 4. Consumption of vegetables and fruits, total in grams (g) per child per day

Regarding water consumption, this was 52.66 l each day, which is equivalent to 0.612 l per child. It is important to remember that children had free access.

It is important to mention some of the barriers that presented themselves for the correct development of the workshop. Some members of the community did not respect the space in which the activities were developed and they met every day from 10 a.m. to smoke marijuana next to the soccer field, little by little impinging upon the space for the development of the programmed activities (Figure 10). This is a real example of what occurs in the few spaces designed for the practice of physical activity.

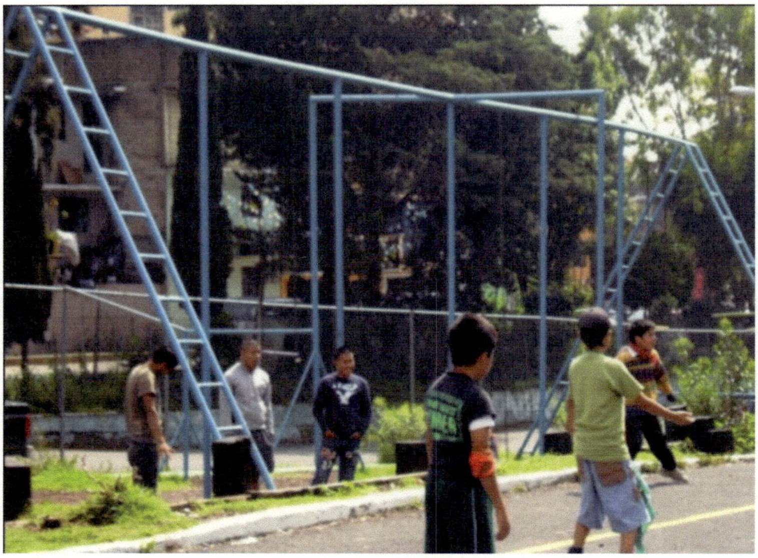

Fig. 10. Onlooking community members smoking marijuana.

On the other hand, eating behavior is a set of actions that establish the relationship of humans with food. Eating behaviors are acquired through direct experience with food, by imitating models, food availability, social status, affective symbolisms, and cultural traditions. It has been found that the most direct familial group, especially mothers, exerts an important influence on the way in which the child behaves in relation to eating; regrettably and although mothers and/or those charged with feeding children were invited to attend three, 2-4-h sessions at the installations where the workshop was offered, with the objective of their engaging in physical activity (dance, yoga) and diverse activities focused on food orientation, attendance of the mothers was very low (four mothers for 75 children); thus, lack of interest is considered a scarcely modifiable factor and impedes the prevention of childhood obesity and the change to a healthy individual and familial lifestyle.

During the workshop's 3-week duration, the children remain in direct contact with fruits and vegetables in diverse presentations, forming part of typical dishes, new, flavorful, and fun dishes. The children can touch textures and observe colors. At the same time, consumption of food in a non-violent, hygienic, and warm environment surely exerts a positive impact on the experience of the children with the foods prepared at the workshop. Availability of and accessibility to foods were factors that facilitated the consumption and acceptance of fruits and vegetables.

4. Discussion

Diverse evidence-based reports have cited the benefits of physical activity for school-aged children. These data deal with considerations of the impact on musculoskeletal and cardiovascular health as well as details on the conditions related with the metabolic syndrome, such as overweight, high blood pressure, and dyslipidemias (Jasen I, 2010; Hills AP, 2007; Lohman TG, 1988; Strong WB, 2005). In general terms, the majority of these benefits are visualized as long-term consequences and, in brief observations such as that which we report, they are hardly evaluable. In our study, the modifications in physical-activity type and amount achieved by the children during the summer workshop were unable to be associated statistically with changes in clinical and anthropometric markers such as blood pressure, weight, or waist circumference, which is very probably due to that the follow-up time was very short for verifying this. However, weight, waist circumference, and systolic and diastolic blood pressure exhibited changes of -3.2, -3.3, -7.07, and -4.03%, respectively, which could have positive clinical repercussions if these were conserved at the long term.

Other known benefits of physical activity can exert an impact on the everyday characteristics of perception in the child, such as those that affect self-perception, feelings associated with anxiety and depression, non-violence, as well as success in academic performance; thus, it is important to explore this in future implementations of the program (Strong WB, 2005).

International recommendations on physical activity tend to suggest that from the age of beginning school, children accumulate, on average, at least 60 min daily of moderate or more intense physical activity, although these recognize that certain benefits can be obtained from activities engaged in for 30 min daily (Jasen I, 2010; Services, 2008). In our study, we established as success parameter the achievement of 50% of this goal; despite that the children were involved for >4 h in an ambiance devoted predominantly to the promotion of physical activity, this was unable to be achieved in the majority of the children. It was expected that in the short term -3 weeks-, the children would achieve engaging in least 30 min of moderately intense and 15 min of slightly intense physical activity. Additionally, we sought to evaluate whether the workshop's activities achieved increasing physical activity performed under habitual conditions, taking as reference for this the physical activity engaged in within a school ambiance. These findings oblige us to reflect upon the difficulty of achieving physical-activity recommendations in daily surroundings, rendering it imperative to establish a very well-structured plan and with highly enthusiastic executors for its application in more daily ambits such as school. Examples of successes in Mexico have been reported; however, application at the long term appears to be a great challenge (Balas-Nakaxh M, 2010). Our comparative observations between children in a high-stimulus physical-activity environment and children in a daily school environment agree with other reports, evidencing the gravity of sedentariness in a large proportion of school-aged population in Mexico (Ciampa PJ, 2010).

Another serious problem confronting similar populations to that studied here is the lack of spaces adapted for the practice of physical activity, as well as the lack of friendly spaces or physically active communities of neighborhoods, which taken together impede children from carrying out some type of physical activity safely. In the Summer-vacation Workshop, although the spaces and all of the equipment were focused on the children's safety, the community did not offer an environment that adequately protected the children as team members.

Authors who are expert in fruit and vegetable consumption in children (Baranowski, 2002) conclude that in order to improve fruit and vegetable consumption, direct contact is important in diverse presentations, forming part of typical dishes, novel, tasty, and fun dishes that permit children to touch textures and to observe colors. At the same time, food consumption in a non-violent, hygienic, and emotionally warm environment surely exerts a positive impact on the experience of the children with the foods prepared in the workshop. Availability and accessibility were factors that facilitated consumption and acceptance of fruits and vegetables during the workshop, as witnessed by the increased consumption of these between weeks 1 and 3.

We consider that conducting the workshop in a playful ambiance promotes greater long-term adherence to better eating and physical-activity habits, because the children consumed adequate quantities of plain water, fruits, and vegetables and increased physical activity. The challenge for an intervention of this type is for the population in its milieu to maintain these habits and to adopt them as their own. The participation of parents and the community is basic for maintaining foods within the reach of the children and safe installations to encourage the practice of physical activity.

5. Declaration on conflict of interests

We declare that in the development of the present work, there was no conflict of interests for any of the authors.

6. Acknowledgments

The authors are grateful to the following persons who made execution of the program possible: LindaYafa Essesldi; Adriana Flores-López; Carla Sosa-Alvarado; Elena Paola Kegel-Sánchez; Jessika Bukrinsky; Tania Tostado; Pamela Morales; Rita Shlam; Vanessa Camacho, and Sandra Olvera, and likewise to *Comedores Santa María, A.C.* for facilitating their installations.

The present study was sponsored by the Universidad Iberoamericana (UIA), Mexico City, and the Fundación Mexicana para la Salud, A.C. (FUNSALUD).

7. References

American Heart Association. Policy Position Statement on the Treatment of Childhood Obesity in the Health Care Environment. American Heart Association. [Consulted January 18, 2011]. Available at: http://www.americanheart.org/downloadable/heart/1213386303597Treatment%20of%20Childhood%20Obesity%20in%20the%20Health%20Care%20Environment%20Position%20Statement%20with%20new%20logo.pdf

Asociación Mexicana de Agencias de Investigación de Mercado y Opinión Pública, A.C. Índice de niveles socioeconómicos. México: AMAE, 2009. [Consulted February 2011]. Available at: http://www.amai.org/niveles.php

Balas-Nakash M, Benítez-Arciniega A, Perichart-Perera O, Valdés-Ramos R, Vadillo-Ortega F. The effect of exercise on cardiovascular risk markers in Mexican school-aged children: comparison between two structured group routines. Salud Publica Mex 2010;52:398-405.

Bandura A. Self-efficacy: toward a unifying theory of behavioral change. Psychol Rev 1977;84:191-215.

Baranowski T, Perry C, Parcel G. How individuals, environments and health behavior interact. In: Glanz K, Rimer B, Lewis F, editors. Health Behavior and Health Education. Jossey-Bass, 2002.

Basterfield L, Adamson AJ, Frary JK, Parkinson KN, Pearce MS, Reilly JJ. Longitudinal study of physical activity and sedentary behavior in children. Pediatrics 2011;127:e24-e30.

Berenson GS, Srinivasan SR, Wattigney WA, Harsha DW. Obesity and cardiovascular risk in children. Ann N Y Acad Sci 1993;699:93-103.

Branen L, Fletcher J. (1999) Comparison of college students' current eating habits and recollections of their childhood food practices. J Nutr Educ 1999;31:304-310.

Briggs M. Position of the American Dietetic Association: Individual-, Family-, School-, and Community-Based Interventions for Pediatric Overweight. J Am Diet Assoc 2010;106(6):925-945.

Ciampa PJ, Kumar D, Barkin SL, Sanders LM, Yin HS, Perrin EM, et al. Interventions aimed at decreasing obesity in children younger than 2 years: a systematic review. Arch Pediatr Adolesc Med 2010;164(12):1098-1104.

de Onis M, Blössner M, Borghi E. Global prevalence and trends of overweight and obesity among preschool children. Am J Clin Nutr 2010;92(5):1257-1264.

Domínguez-Vázquez P, Olivares S. Influencia familiar sobre la conducta alimentaria y su relación con la obesidad infantil Arch Latinoam Nutr 2008;58(3):249-55.

Elizondo-Montemayor L, Serrano-González M, Ugalde-Casas PA, Cuello- García C, Borbolla-Escoboza JR. Metabolic syndrome risk factors among a sample of overweight and obese Mexican children. J Clin Hypertens (Greenwich) 2010;12(5):380-387.

Hills AP, King NA, Armstrong TP. The contribution of physical activity and sedentary behaviours to the growth and development of children and adolescents: implications for overweight and obesity. Sports Med 2007;37(6):533-545.

Jack I, Grim M, Gros T, Lynch S, McLin C. Theory in Health Promotion Programs. In: Fertman C, Allensworth D, editors. Health Promotion Programs. Soc Public Health Education; 2010.

Jansen I, Le Blanc AG. Systematic review of the health benefits of physical activity and fitness in school-aged children and youth. (Abstract). Int J Behav Nutr Phys Act 2010;7:40.

Jáuregui A, Villalpando S, Rangel-Baltazar E, Castro-Hernández J, Lara-Zamudio A., Méndez-Gómez-Humarán I. The physical activity level of Mexican children decreases upon entry to elementary school. Salud Publica Mex 2011;53:228-236.

Jennings-Aburto N, Nava F, Bonvecchio A, Safdie M, González- Casanova I, Gust T, et al. Physical activity during the school day in public primary schools in Mexico City. Salud Publica Mex 2009;51:141-147.

Lohman TG, Roche AF, Martorell R, editors. Anthropometric standardization reference manual. Abridged edition. Champaign, Illinois: Human KineticBooks; 1988.

O'Donovan G, Blazevich AJ, Boreham C, Cooper AR, Crank H, Ekelund U, Fox KR, Gately P, Giles-Corti B, Gill JM, Hamer M, McDermott I, Murphy M, Mutrie N, Reilly JJ, Saxton JM, Stamatakis E The ABC of Physical Activity for Health: a consensus statement from the British Association of Sport and Exercise Sciences. J Sports Sci 2010;28(6):573-591.

Olaiz-Fernández G, Rivera-Dommarco J, Shamah-Levy T, Rojas R, Villalpando-Hernández S, Hernández-Ávila M, et al. Encuesta nacional de salud y nutrición. 2° ed. Cuernavaca, Morelos, Mexico: INSP; 2006.

Papandreou D, Rousso I, Mavromichalis I. Update on non-alcoholic fatty liver disease in children. Clin Nutr 2007;26:409-415.

Pérez RC, Aranceta J, Brug H, Wind M. Estrategias educativas para la promoción del consumo de frutas y verduras en el medio escolar: proyecto pro children. ¿?? Arch Latinoam Nutr 2004;54:S14-S19.

Pérez-Lizaur AB, Kaufer M, Plazas M. Environmental and personal correlates of fruit and vegetable consumption in low income, urban Mexican children. J Hum Nutr Diet 2008;21: 63-71.

Pimenta AM, Beunza JJ, Sánchez-Villegas A, Bes Rastrollo M, Martínez-Gonzalez MA. Childhood underweight, weight gain during childhood to adolescence/young adulthood and incidence of adult metabolic syndrome in the SUN (Seguimiento Universidad de Navarra) Project. Public Health Nutr 2010;17:1-8.

Puyau MR, Adolph AL, Vohra FA, Butte NF. Validation and calibration of physical activity monitors in children. Obes Res 2002 Mar;10(3):150-157.

Ramírez-Silva I, Rivera J, Ponce X, Hernández M. Consumo de frutas y verduras en la población mexicana: datos de la Encuesta Nacional de Salud y Nutrición 2006. Salud Publica Mex 2009;51(4.

Secretaría de Salud (SSA). Norma Oficial Mexicana NOM-043-SSA2-2005, Servicios básicos de salud. Promoción y educación para la salud en materia alimentaria. Criterios para brindar orientación. http://bibliotecas.salud.gob.mx/gsdl/collect/nomssa/index/assoc/HASH0138/713924cd.dir/doc.pdf [Consulted August 15, 2011].

Secretaría de Educación Pública. Lineamientos para la venta o distribución de alimentos y bebidas en los establecimientos de educación básica. http://portal.salud.gob.mx/sites/salud/descargas/pdf/salud_alimentaria/programa_accion.pdf [Consulted August 15, 2011].

Strong WB, Malina RM, Blimkie CJ, Daniels SR, Dishman RK, Gutin B, Hergenroeder AC, Must A, Nixon PA, Pivarnik JM, Rowland T, Trost S, Trudeau F. Evidence based physical activity for school-age youth. J Pediatr 2005;146(6):732-737.

Summerbell CD, Waters E, Edmunds LD, Kelly S, Brown T, Campbell KJ. Interventions for preventing obesity in children. Cochrane Database Syst Rev 2005 Jul 20;(3):CD001871.

Tauman R, Gozal D. Obesity and obstructive sleep apnea in children. Paediatr Respir Rev 2006;7(4):247-259.

U.S. Department of Health and Human Services. 2008 Physical Activity Guidelines for Americans. Washington, D.C.: U.S. Department of Health and Human Services; 2008. [Consulted January 18, 2011]. Available at: http://www.health.gov/paguidelines/pdf/paguide.pdf

Yngve A, Wolf A, Poortvliet E, Elmadfa I, Brug J, Ehrenblad B, Franchini B, Haraldsdottir J, Krolner R, Maes L, Pérez-Rodrigo C, Sjostrom, M, Thorsdottir I, Klepp, KI. (2005) Fruit and vegetable intake in a sample of 11-year-old children in 9 European countries: The Pro Children Cross-sectional Survey. Ann Nutr Metab 2005;49:236-245.